T0234498

INTERNAL MEDICINE

The *Essential* Facts

INTERNAL MEDICINE
The *Essential* Facts

—————————SECOND EDITION—————————

Nicholas J Talley
MD PhD FRACP FAFPHM
FRCP(Edin) FACP FACG

Professor of Medicine
The University of Sydney
Nepean Hospital, Sydney

Brad Frankum
BMed FRACP

Staff Specialist in Immunology
Nepean Hospital, Sydney
Lecturer in Medical Education & Medicine
The University of Sydney

David Currow
BMed MPH FRACP

Senior Staff Specialist in Palliative Medicine
Nepean Hospital, Sydney
Lecturer in Medicine
The University of Sydney

Blackwell
Science

© 2000 MacLennan & Petty Pty Limited
PO Box 145, Rosebery NSW 1445, Australia

First published 1990
Reprinted 1992
Second edition 2000

Distributed in the United Kingdom, Europe,
the Middle East and Africa by
Blackwell Science Ltd
Osney Mead, Oxford OX2 0EL
Orders should be addressed to:
Marston Book Services Ltd
PO Box 269, Abingdon
Oxon OX14 4YN
Tel: 01235 465500
Fax: 01235 465555

Distributed in USA by:
Blackwell Science, Inc.
Commerce Place
350 Main Street
Malden, MA 02148
Tel: 800 215 1000
      781 388 8250
Fax: 781 388 8270

A catalogue record for this title is available from the
British Library and the Library of Congress

ISBN: 0 632 05613 4

Contents

Preface

I've got Bright's disease and he's got mine
S J Perelman (1904–1979)

They do certainly give very strange and new fangled names to diseases
Plato (427–347BC)

The first edition of *Internal Medicine* appeared in 1990, and soon proved a success with both senior medical students and post-graduates sitting their examinations in Europe, North America and Australasia. Senior clinicians have also found it useful to refresh their memory about a particular problem. The second edition has been completely revised and updated, but has retained all the elements so popular with students. Each chapter where relevant is now set out in a standard format, covering clinical clues, pathophysiology, diagnosis and therapeutics, which should allow the reader to easily follow and digest the text.

The book is designed to be a handy pocket-sized guide that can be carried conveniently and delved into frequently. Key facts are presented as skeleton lists and tables; they have been derived from a number of sources including eminent lectures, major textbooks and the medical literature, after careful review for relevance and clarity. The book emphasises essential areas that may be overlooked when one is reading major textbooks in medicine. However, it is not meant to replace major textbooks, or programs such as the Medical Knowledge Self Assessment Program (MKSAP) of the American College of Physicians, which are highly recommended revision tools.

We hope that this concise revision guide and *aide memoire* will assist all students of internal medicine.

Nicholas J Talley
Brad Frankum
David Currow
August, 1999

Acknowledgments

We would like to acknowledge the very generous help and assistance of staff from The University of Sydney and The University of Newcastle and associated hospitals. Those who have generously helped with the preparation of this book include Professor Philip Boyce, Dr James Branley, Dr Susan Coulshed, Associate Professor Bob Cummings, Dr John England, Dr Eddy Fischer, Dr Gayle Fischer, Dr Drew Fitzpatrick, Dr David Fulcher, Associate Professor David Gottlieb, Associate Professor Paul Harnett, Professor David Henry, Professor Les Irwig, Dr Andrew Keegan, Dr Susan Lawrence, Dr Cait Lonie, Dr Stephen MacNamara, Dr Nicholas Manolias, Dr Darryl MacKender, Dr Philip McManis, Professor Sirus Naraqi, Dr Simon O'Connor, Associate Professor Graeme Stewart, Dr David Sullivan, Dr Martin Weltmann, Dr Nicholas Wilcken, Professor Jim Wiley.

Abbreviations

A2	Aortic component of second heart sound
ABGs	Arterial blood gases
ACTH	Adrenocorticotrophic hormone
ADH	Antidiuretic hormone
ALS	Amyotrophic lateral sclerosis
ALT	Alanine aminotransferase
AML	Acute myeloid leukaemia
Anti-HBc	Anti-hepatitis B core antibody
Anti-HBs	Anti-hepatitis B surface antibody
APTT	Activated partial thromboplastin time
AR	Aortic regurgitation
AS	Aortic stenosis
ASD	Atrial septal defect
AST	Aspartate aminotransferase
AV	Atrioventricular
AVRT	Atrioventricular re-entrant tachycardia
AZT	Azidothymidine
BHL	Bilateral hilar lymphadenopathy
CABG	Coronary artery bypass graft
CAD	Coronary artery disease
CAL	Chronic airflow limitation
CLL	Chronic lymphocytic leukaemia
CML	Chronic myeloid leukaemia
CMV	Cytomegalovirus
CNS	Central nervous system
COAD	Chronic obstructive airways disease
COPD	Chronic obstructive pulmonary disease
CPAP	Continuous positive airways pressure
CREST	Calcinosis, Raynaud's, oesophageal dysmotility, sclerodactyly and telangiectasia
CRH	Corticotrophin releasing hormone
CSF	Cerebrospinal fluid
CT	Computerised tomography
CWP	Coal worker's pneumoconiosis
CXR	Chest X-ray
DIC	Disseminated intravascular coagulation
DIP	Distal interphalangeal joint
DLCO	Diffusion capacity for carbon monoxide

Abbreviations

EBV	Epstein-Barr virus
ECG	Electrocardiogram
EEG	Electroencephalogram
EPG	Electrophoretogram
ESR	Erythrocyte sedimentation rate
EST	Exercise stress test
FEV1	Forced expiratory volume in 1 second
FVC	Forced vital capacity
GBM	Glommerula basement membrane
GCSF	Granulocyte colony stimulating factor
GFR	Glommerula filtration rate
GH	Growth hormone
GI	Gastrointestinal
GMCSF	Granulocyte macrophage colony stimulating factor
GN	Glomerulonephritis
G-6-PG	Glucose-6-phosphate dehydrogenase
HCM	Hypertrophic cardiomyopathy
HAV	Hepatitis A virus
HBeAg	Hepatitis B e antigen
HBsAg	Hepatitis B surface antigen
HCV	Hepatitis C virus
HDL	High density lipoprotein
HDV	Hepatitis D virus
HEV	Hepatitis E virus
HIV	Human immunodeficiency virus
HLA	Human leucocyte antigen
HSV	Herpes simplex virus
IDL	Intermediate density lipoprotein
IEPG	Immunoelectrophoretogram
IL	Interleukin
INR	International normalised ratio
ITP	Immune thrombocytopenic purpura
IV	Intravenous
JVP	Jugular venous pressure
LDH	Lactate dehydrogenase
LDL	Low density lipoprotein
LFTs	Liver function tests
LHRH	Luteinising hormone releasing hormone
LMN	Lower motor neurone
LP	Lumbar puncture
LVF	Left ventricular failure
MB	Myocardial fraction of creatine kinase
MCHC	Mean corpuscular haemoglobin concentration
MCP	Metacarpophalangeal joint
MCTD	Mixed connective tissue disease

MGUS	Monoclonal gammopathy of uncertain significance
MI	Myocardial infarction
MRI	Magnetic resonance imaging
MS	Mitral stenosis, multiple sclerosis
MVP	Mitral valve prolapse
NAP	Neutrophil alkaline phosphatase
NHL	Non-Hodgkin's lymphoma
NSAIDs	Non-steroidal anti-inflammatory drugs
OCP	Oral contraceptive pill
P2	Pulmonary component of second heart sound
PAN	Polyarteritis nodosa
PDA	Patent ductus arteriosus
PEEP	Positive end-expiratory pressure
PIP	Proximal interphalangeal joint
PMF	Progressive massive fibrosis
PNH	Paroxysmal nocturnal haemoglobinuria
PPD	Purified protein derivative
PT	Prothrombin time
PTCA	Percutaneous transluminal coronary angioplasty
PTHrP	Parathyroid hormone related peptide
PVD	Peripheral vascular disease
RAST	Radio-allergosorbent test
RTA	Renal tubular acidosis
RVF	Right ventricular failure
S1 S2 S3 S4	First, second, third and fourth heart sounds
SAAG	Serum-ascites albumin gradient
SAP	Serum alkaline phosphatase
SIADH	Syndrome of inappropriate secretion of antidiuretic hormone
SLE	Systemic lupus erythematosus
TB	Tuberculosis
TBG	Thyroid binding globulin
TIA	Transient ischaemic attack
tPA	Tissue plasminogen activator
TSH	Thyroid stimulating hormone
TT	Thrombin time
TTP	Thrombotic thrombocytopenic purpura
UMN	Upper motor neurone
VC	Vital capacity
VLDL	Very low density lipoprotein
VSD	Ventricular septal defect
VZV	Varicella zoster virus

1
Epidemiology, Statistics and Evaluation of the Literature

To keep abreast of rapid developments in the management of disease, it is essential for clinicians to be able to appraise the literature and incorporate effective innovations into clinical practice. Some basic skills in epidemiology and statistics, and an understanding of recent international trends in the development of evidence-based medicine will be of assistance.

Clinicians should be applying these principles at three levels to reduce morbidity and mortality. These levels are:

Primary prevention: Preventing the onset of pathology (for example, by reducing the risk of an acute myocardial infarction by avoiding tobacco smoke).

Secondary prevention: Preventing the development of disease once pathology has occurred (for example, by managing hypertension to reduce the risk of an acute myocardial infarction).

Tertiary prevention: Preventing the sequelae of a disease once it has become manifest (for example, by preventing extension of an acute myocardial infarction by treatment with a fibrinolytic agent).

STUDY DESIGN

The range of study designs employed to determine treatment or program effects are presented in Table 1.1 with their strengths and weaknesses. The appropriate choice of study depends on the study objective.

DESCRIBING DATA AND RELATIONSHIPS

The following terms are often used to describe data and their distribution:

- **Mean:** the average of the observations $= \dfrac{\text{Sum of observations}}{\text{Number of observations}}$
- **Median:** value at which the number of observations above equals the number below.

Table 1.1 Study Designs

Study design	Strengths	Weaknesses
Randomised controlled trial (RCT). Participants are randomly assigned to either an intervention or non-intervention group. **This is the study design of choice for evaluating new clinical interventions.**	Reduces the effect of known and unknown confounders	Often expensive Difficult to follow all patients Need to analyse data on an intention-to-treat basis Ethical and feasibility difficulties can arise
Cohort study. A comparison of those with a certain exposure and those without. **This is the study design of choice for evaluating prognosis.**	Can sometimes answer questions which can't be answered by RCTs Can define causality Good for rare exposures Can measure incidence	Difficult to follow large populations over time Costly and time consuming
Case–control study. A comparison of those with a disease and those without.	Provides a mechanism to study rare conditions or those with a long latent period	Can only infer causality from this study design Cannot define incidence but only the odds ratio Prone to selection bias and recall bias
Cross-sectional study. Exposure or disease states defined in a population at a given time. **This is the study design of choice for evaluating diagnostic tests.**	Quick, inexpensive A good snapshot of current status Useful for looking at patient subgroups	Provides no information on causality
Correlational/ecological studies. Profile characteristics of whole populations.	Quick, inexpensive Can help generate hypotheses	Cannot define causality Represent average exposures
Case series or case reports, clinical experience or descriptive studies.	Able to generate hypotheses which can be more formally tested Can sometimes recognise important relationships	Not generalisable No ability to test for statistical association

- **Mode:** most frequently occurring value.
- **Frequency polygon:** the graphical representation of values with the variable value on the horizontal axis and the frequency on the vertical axis.
- **Normal (bell-shaped) distribution:** many biological variables are said to be normally distributed—this means that when they are graphed on a frequency polygon they form a bell-shaped curve which is symmetrical (Figure 1.1). Using this distribution, the distribution of the data can be described using the standard deviation.
- **Standard deviation (SD):** describes the distribution of the data around the mean. About two-thirds of the values are within one standard deviation (SD) of the mean, and 95% are within 2 standard deviations (Figure 1.1). The SD is the √Variance calculated by

$$\sqrt{\sum} \frac{(\text{Each observation} - \text{mean of all observations})^2}{\text{Number of observations} - 1}$$

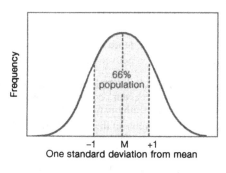

One standard deviation from mean

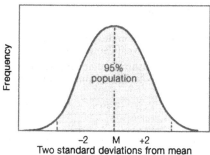

Two standard deviations from mean

Figure 1.1 *Normal distribution curve (frequency distribution of values from a homogeneous sample of a population).*

- **Standard error of the mean (SEM):** measures the variability of the sample mean as an estimate of the true mean of the population from which the sample was drawn. It is calculated by

$$\frac{SD}{\sqrt{\text{Number of observations}}}$$

Different types of measures are used to describe the relationships between the study factor and outcome in studies. These include incidence and prevalence rates, which can be standardised to certain populations and relative risks and odds ratios.

- **Incidence:** the proportion of a group initially free of a defined condition that develops the condition over a given time period.
- **Prevalence:** the proportion of a group possessing a defined condition at a given point in time.
- **Point estimate:** the result obtained from a sample at a given point in time.
- **Rate:** the number of cases occurring in a given population in a given time. It is calculated by the number of events occurring in a defined time period. The time period is usually one year.
- **Relative risk (RR):** this is a measure of how many times more likely persons exposed to a risk factor (e.g. smoking) get a disease (e.g. lung cancer) relative to those not exposed.

$$RR = \frac{\text{Incidence in exposed}}{\text{Incidence in non-exposed}}$$

  The stronger an association between exposure and disease, the higher the RR (or OR).
- **Relative risk reduction (RRR):** if a particular intervention works, there is reduction of the risk of an event occurring as a result of the intervention. This can be expressed mathematically as:

$$\frac{\begin{array}{c}\text{Number of events in the control arm}\\ -\text{ number of events in the intervention arm}\end{array}}{\text{Number of events in the control arm}} \times 100$$

- Unfortunately, this model fails to discriminate the size of the treatment effect. The magnitude of difference is captured as the **absolute risk reduction (ARR)** by:

$$\begin{array}{c}\text{Number of events in the control arm}\\ -\text{ number of events in the intervention arm}\end{array}$$

- **Odds ratio (OR):** in case-control studies, incidence cannot be computed. However, it is possible to obtain an estimate of the RR by calculating the odds ratio (OR):

	Cases	Non-cases
Exposed	A	B
Not exposed	C	D

$$OR = \frac{AD}{BC}$$

CHANCE

To minimise chance explaining the results, a range of statistical tests is used to determine the likelihood that any observed differences have occurred due to chance and not due to the study factor.

Differences between exposed and non-exposed groups can arise by chance alone. Statistical tests can be used to determine the probability that this has actually happened when a difference is found. The types of tests which are commonly used are:

- **Chi-square (χ^2):** compares counts of *discrete* variables.
- **Student's *t* test:** compares *two means*. The value *t* is the ratio of the difference in the means of two series compared to the uncertainty of the standard error of these means. The higher the value of *t*, the less the probability that the difference represents chance variation.
- **Analysis of variance (ANOVA):** compares ≥2 means.

The results of these are most commonly reported using probability *(P)* values and confidence intervals.

- A *P* **value** is a quantitative way of describing how likely an observed difference in a particular study could have occurred by chance. For example, $P < 0.05$ indicates that the likelihood of a difference being due to chance is less than 1 in 20. However, even very small *P* values do *not* indicate that the difference is clinically important (i.e. they do not indicate the magnitude). This may occur if a very large number of subjects is studied—the results may be highly significant but the magnitude too small to be clinically meaningful.
- **Confidence intervals** (CIs) are a range of values around the point estimate in a study in which the actual value will lie with a degree of certainty. Different levels of certainty can be used. For example, if the success rate of a certain treatment in a random sample of patients is 40% with a 95% confidence interval of 35%–45% then we can be 95% sure that the actual success rate in this group of patients lies between 35% and 45%.

TYPES OF ERRORS

There are two major types of errors which occur when using these types of tests:

- **Type I (α) error:** a significant result is found but in fact there is no true difference—e.g. on multiple comparison testing of 20 tests, by chance alone one will have a $P < 0.05$.
- **Type II (β) error:** no significant result is found but in fact there is a true difference. This occurs when the number of subjects studied is too small, so that the power of the study is too weak to detect a real difference.

Power of a study

The power of a study is a design concept for the investigators. It is necessary to establish that the study is big enough to answer the question. This is done by predicting the likely differences between the groups being studied that are clinically important, setting the alpha error (usually 0.05) and beta error (usually 0.20) and taking into account how the outcome will be expressed (e.g. continuous or nominal data). This in turn will predict the size of the study which needs to be done.

When reviewing a study it is also useful to consider the reliability (reproducibility—the extent to which repeated measurements are close to each other) and the validity (the degree to which measurement results correspond to the true result).

FACTORS AFFECTING THE QUALITY OF EVIDENCE

The quality of the evidence obtained from these studies is influenced by
- bias
- confounding

Bias is minimised by good study design. Confounding is best dealt with by good study design to ensure that information on confounders is collected (if possible), and data are analysed to take these factors into account.

BIAS

Bias is any deviation from the true value being examined. With bias, the difference between the true value and what is observed is not due to chance but due to a systematic problem. Bias affects the generalisabiltiy of the results of the study, and can cause an over or underestimation of the magnitude of the problem or effect. It is generally more of a problem when bias overestimates the effect, for example, of a new drug.

Selection bias is bias that occurs because of the way in which people are selected (by their own choice or that of the investigators) to go into various exposure groups in a study. Selection bias occurs when the study population is not defined adequately, and non-comparable criteria are used to identify participants in a study. This may result in an atypical group of patients being selected for a study—they may either have a higher level of disease or an atypical reaction to treatment. For example, if only hospitalised patients with depression are enrolled in a study they may have a different outcome to treatment compared with all patients with depression. A randomised controlled trial with no loss to follow-up and analysis by intention-to-treat can help to minimise selection bias.

Measurement or observation bias occurs because of invalid and/or unreliable measurement of study variables. Measurement bias may occur if non-comparable information is obtained in the two study groups. This may occur in the way the information is collected or interpreted (**interviewer bias**) or in the way study participants report the information (**recall bias**).

For example, interviewer bias may occur in a case-control study looking at the association between lung cancer and tobacco exposure if the interviewer knows the disease status of the individual and probes for the tobacco history in those with lung cancer more than in those without lung cancer.

Recall bias occurs when people with certain disease status or exposure remember their experiences differently from those not affected. For example, cases in a case-control study on the effect of asbestos exposure and the development of mesothelioma may over-report their exposure if they believe the exposure to have caused the cancer compared to those without the cancer.

In randomised controlled trials, measurement bias can be minimised by ensuring blind assessment of exposure and outcome variables.

Publication bias: journals tend to publish articles with a positive result. This can significantly skew the information available for making clinical decisions.

CONFOUNDING

Cohort and randomised controlled trials may analyse the relationship between an exposure and disease outcome. Confounding can occur if there is a third factor which is associated with the exposure and independently affects the disease outcome. For example, a study comparing a group of miners exposed to asbestos with a group of office workers with non-exposure may find the rate of mesothelioma in the miners is greater than in the office workers. However, if the miners are more likely to smoke than the office workers, the difference in the cancer rates may be largely due to this difference, and tobacco smoking is a confounder which would need to be considered before the true association between exposure and disease status could be determined.

A confounder must be associated with both the exposure and the disease outcome and must vary in the diseased and the non-diseased, or the exposed and the non-exposed, to have an effect on the study results.

Confounding is usually controlled for in studies, either through the study design or through data analysis. Study designs used to control confounding include restriction of the study population, and matching and randomisation of exposure. Analysis methods to control for confounding include stratification and multivariate analysis.

INTERPRETING TEST RESULTS

Every day the clinician is ordering and interpreting tests in light of a patient's history and clinical examination. Whenever a test is undertaken there are four possible results: the patient has the disease and the test is positive (true positive) or negative (false negative), or the patient doesn't have the disease and the test is negative (true negative) or positive (false positive). This relationship is often illustrated using a 2×2 table as follows:

DISEASE

		Truly present	Truly not present
TEST	**Positive**	TRUE POSITIVE a	FALSE POSITIVE b
	Negative	FALSE NEGATIVE c	TRUE NEGATIVE d

The test's sensitivity and specificity are used to describe how accurate the test is. The *sensitivity* is the true positive rate (i.e. the percentage of affected persons with a positive test) and the *specificity* is the true negative rate (i.e. the percentage of unaffected persons with a negative test). They are calculated as follows:

$$\text{Sensitivity} = \frac{a}{a+c} \qquad \text{Specificity} = \frac{d}{b+d}$$

These calculations are independent of the disease prevalence.

Taking into consideration the prevalence of disease in a population (the pre-test probability) will alter how useful tests can be. This can be determined by calculating the **positive predictive value (PPV)** of a test (the probability of disease in the case with a positive test) and the **negative predictive value (NPV)** (the probability of no disease in the case with a negative test result). These are calculated as follows:

$$\text{PPV} = \frac{a}{a+b} \qquad \text{NPV} = \frac{d}{c+d}$$

The predictive value of a test depends on the prevalence of the condition in the population. The disease prevalence can be calculated by $(a + c) / ((a + c) + (b + d))$.

This means a patient with a low pre-test probability of disease and a positive test result will have a lower probability of disease than a patient who has a high pre-test probability and a positive result. This is very useful when deciding which tests to order.

For example, take a test for which the normal range is based on the normal distribution using two standard deviations from the mean. If 100 tests are done, 5% will be false positives. However, if these tests are only done in patients who have a high pre-test probability, the PPV is improved and the number of false positives and their attendant costs are minimised.

SCREENING

A test's sensitivity and specificity are particularly important when evaluating a screening test. Screening is used to detect disease in affected individuals before it becomes symptomatic. For example, Papanicolou (Pap) smears and mammograms are used to detect cervical and breast cancer, respectively, to facilitate early treatment and reduce morbidity and mortality from these cancers. Before screening is introduced it must fulfil the following criteria:

- there must be a presymptomatic phase detectable by the screening test
- intervention at this time changes the natural history of the disease to reduce morbidity or mortality
- the screening test must be inexpensive, easy to administer and acceptable to patients
- the screening test will ideally be highly sensitive and specific (although this is not usually possible)
- the screening program is feasible and effective.

APPLICATION OF EVIDENCE-BASED MEDICINE

Ideally, all clinicians should be able to critically analyse the literature and introduce proven interventions into their practice. However, there is an ever increasing number of journals, and a limit to the time clinicians can put into critically appraising the literature and integrating the results. Much of what is published is important, but little of it should actually change clinical practice.

To assist busy clinicians to incorporate evidence-based medicine into their practice there are many international and national initiatives. The mainstay of these is the systematic review, which is a method of analysing the available information (both published and non-published if possible) and presenting it in a fashion which can be incorporated by the clinician.

RATING THE QUALITY OF THE EVIDENCE
OF INTERVENTION STUDIES
(such as a new drug being compared with the current 'gold-standard' drug)

Systematic reviews rate the quality of the evidence using a hierachy. Level 1 evidence (meta-analyses of well designed randomised controlled trials) carries more weight in most clinical decision making than Level 4 evidence (a single case report). An example of such a hierarchy is:

- *Level 1*: Systematic review of best quality evidence (e.g. meta-analysis of a group of well designed randomised controlled trials)
- *Level 2*: Properly designed randomised trial
- *Level 3*: *i* Controlled trial (non-randomised)
    - *ii* Cohort study or case-control study from more than one group or centre
    - *iii* Evidence obtained from multiple time series
- *Level 4*: Clinical experience in the form of a case series or expert opinion.

Overall, data are usually defined as being qualitative or quantitative. Generally, qualitative data are collected using focus groups or surveys using open-ended questions. These data are useful for generating hypotheses, or providing initial observations about the cause of disease or its impact which can be tested using more rigorous approaches.

SYSTEMATIC REVIEWS AND GUIDELINES

The Cochrane Collaboration is probably the most well known group which undertakes the production of systematic reviews on a range of topics using rigorous criteria and international consortia. They attempt to include both published and unpublished information and to maintain an ongoing process of updating the review to keep it current.

IMPORTANT QUESTIONS TO ASK WHEN EVALUATING A NEW INTERVENTION[1]

1. **Are the results of the study valid?**
   Are the treatment or effect in the true direction and magnitude of the expected effect? Are there biases which affect these results? Were the groups similar before the trial started?
2. **What were the results?**
   What is the size of the treatment effect and how precise is this effect?
3. **Were all the patients accounted for from the time of randomisation?**
4. **Were the investigators and the patients blinded to the arm they were assigned in the study?**
5. **Will the results help me in caring for my patients?**
   Are the results applicable to my particular patients?
   What is the net impact of treatment?

EVALUATING A NEW TEST IN THE LITERATURE

Often new tests are introduced without an adequate evaluation. Cross-sectional studies should be sought in your literature review when looking for studies defining the clinical usefulness of tests. The following is a useful checklist to use when analysing a study evaluating a new test.[2]

1. Was there an independent, 'blind' comparison with a 'gold standard' of diagnosis?
2. Was the setting for the study, as well as the filter through which study patients passed, adequately described?
3. Did the patient sample include an appropriate spectrum of mild and severe, treated and untreated disease, plus individuals with different but commonly confused disorders?
4. Were the tactics for carrying out the test described in sufficient detail to permit their exact replication?
5. Was the reproducibility of the test result (precision) and its interpretation (observer variation) determined?
6. Was the term 'normal' defined sensibly? (e.g. Gaussian, percentile, risk factor, culturally desirable, diagnostic, or therapeutic?)
7. If the test was advocated as part of a cluster or sequence of tests, was its contribution to the overall validity of the cluster or sequence determined?
8. Was the 'utility' of the test determined? (Were patients really better off for it?)

References

1. Guyatt GH, Sackett DL, Cook DJ. Users'guide to the medical literature. II. How to use an article about therapy or prevention. A. Are the results of the study valid? Evidence-Based Medicine Working Group. *JAMA* 1993; 270: 2598–2601.
2. Dans AL, Dans LF, Guyatt GH, Richardson S. Users' guide to the medical literature: XIV. How to decide on the applicability of clinical trial results to your patient. Evidence-Based Medicine Working Group. *JAMA* 1998; 279: 545–549.

2

Pharmacology

PRINCIPLES OF PHARMACOKINETICS AND PHARMACODYNAMICS

DRUG ABSORPTION

The extent of absorption depends on the drug formulation and the site or route of administration. The small bowel absorbs most orally administered drugs; the controlling rate is therefore primarily gastric emptying.

Drugs given orally with a high clearance (Cl) often undergo 'first pass' metabolism in the liver. In cirrhosis, the liver is bypassed, and systemic levels may increase tenfold.

DRUG DISTRIBUTION

This depends on the apparent volume of distribution (Vd).

$$Vd = \frac{Dose}{Plasma\ drug\ concentration}$$

Water soluble (polar) drugs that distribute through the aqueous compartment have relatively low volumes of distribution and high plasma concentrations. Drugs which are highly lipid soluble will have apparent large volumes of distribution and relatively low plasma concentrations.

DRUG ELIMINATION

This is described in terms of clearance (Cl).

First order pharmacokinetics: Clearance may be a first order process (a constant fraction is eliminated per unit time). For example, 20% of the drug may be eliminated every 2 hours. Elimination of the drug from the body under first order elimination is characterised by the half-life being constant throughout the elimination. A semi-logarithmic graph will therefore be linear. This accounts for almost all drugs.

Steady state for first order pharmacokinetics: This is achieved when the rate of intake of drug matches its elimination from the body. For drugs with first order pharmacokinetics, the accumulation of the drug can be predicted because it is also a linear process. Ninety percent of steady state levels will be reached between 3 and 4 half-lives.

Non-first order pharmacokinetics (dose-dependent or zero order process pharmacokinetics): Drugs which have non-first order pharmacokinetics have different rates of elimination at different drug levels in the body. A constant amount is eliminated per unit time. For example, 10 mg per hour is eliminated so that if there is drug toxicity, the time for clearance will increase with the higher blood level. Clearance tends to increase at lower levels of the drug. Frequently encountered drugs which have non-first order clearance include *phenytoin, theophylline, salicylates* and *ethanol.*

The major clinical importance of dose-dependent elimination is that small increases in the drug dose may lead to large increases in the amount of available drug.

Drug half-life: $T\frac{1}{2}$ (elimination half-life) is the time in hours necessary to reduce the drug concentration in serum to one half:

$$t\frac{1}{2} = \frac{0.693 \times Vd}{Cl}$$

The half-life of a drug can be prolonged by either low clearance and/or a high volume of distribution. If the half-life extension is due to increased volume of distribution, then there will be no accumulation of the drug. If there is low clearance causing the prolonged half-life, the drug will tend to accumulate.

Drug concentration (Cp)

$$Cp = \frac{\text{Dosing rate}}{Cl} \text{ (if the kinetics are first order)}$$

The target steady-state drug level in plasma chosen is usually the middle of the therapeutic range for drugs with narrow therapeutic windows (e.g. theophylline).

To choose a loading dose:

Loading dose = target level × Vd/bioavailability

A loading dose is only chosen if a condition needs treatment quickly and the time to acquire steady state is long.

To choose the maintenance dose:

Dose rate = target level × Cl T/bioavailability
(Cl T = total clearance).

DOSE RESPONSE CURVES (AGONIST AND ANTAGONIST)

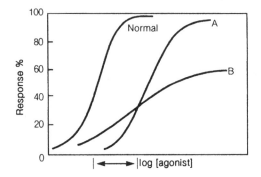

Figure 2.1 *Curve A: curve obtained when a known agonist is tested in the presence of a competitive antagonist, or an agonist with a potency less than that of a known agonist.*
Curve B: curve of a partial agonist, or a known agonist in the presence of a non-competitive antagonist.

DRUG HANDLING

EFFECTS OF AGEING

1. Drug distribution changes of importance in the elderly are:
    a) Half-life of *fat-soluble* drugs is *increased* (because of increased fat providing greater volumes of distribution).
    b) Concentration of *water-soluble* drugs is *increased* (because free water is decreased, providing smaller volumes of distribution).
    c) Level of active *protein-bound* drugs is *increased* (because albumin is decreased).
2. Drug metabolism and drug excretion decrease with ageing, which can reduce clearance leading to drug accumulation.
3. Changes in drug absorption are probably not clinically important.

EFFECTS OF RENAL DYSFUNCTION

For drugs that are eliminated by the kidney, decreased drug clearance will lead to accumulation of the drug. Renal clearance of a drug will mostly decline in a parallel fashion to the decline in glomerular filtration rate. The aim of adequate prescribing under these circumstances is that, by decreasing the dose or increasing the dose interval, normal drug levels can be maintained. Approximation of dose changes can be made by calculating the clearance with renal impairment and comparing this to normal clearance.

Note: A serum creatinine level within the laboratory's reported normal range may still reflect gross renal impairment with a markedly reduced creatinine clearance, especially in the elderly.

HEPATIC DYSFUNCTION

Hepatic impairment leads to much less predictable changes in drug clearance. It may either increase or decrease the amount of drug available, and careful monitoring of plasma levels or clinical response is needed. Responses are not predicted by liver function tests.

Drugs with high first pass clearance by the liver will accumulate if there is a significant decrease in hepatic blood flow, as is seen with right sided cardiac failure.

There are two major pathways for hepatic metabolism of drugs. The first of these is oxidation (performed by cytochrome P450) and the second is either glucuronidation or sulphation.

TOLERANCE TO DRUGS

Decreased efficacy (tolerance) is seen with the chronic administration of many drugs. Important classes include beta-agonists in the treatment of asthma and nitrates for angina. Physical tolerance to opioids occurs, but such tolerance is not the same as addiction. Addiction implies a psychological dependence and often manifests as drug seeking behaviour.

DRUG WITHDRAWAL

Withdrawal responses are seen when a chronically administered drug is ceased abruptly. Drugs with central nervous system (CNS) effects have the most common and often most vivid withdrawal syndromes. Most withdrawal syndromes are manifest by systemic sympathetic overactivity.

DRUG OVERDOSE AND POISONING

A history of the substance(s) used, the amount and time of ingestion and the intention of the drug use (suicidal or accidental) is important in the initial assessment. Initial management should be directed towards aggressive support of vital systems.

Complications can include rhabdomyolysis if there has been a long period between ingestion and discovery, especially with drugs which act on the CNS, and also the possibility of withdrawal from other drugs simultaneously.

The most common drugs used in overdoses (other than alcohol) are anti-depressants, analgesics (including paracetamol), illicit drugs and sedative-hypnotics.

Drugs which can cause stimulant syndromes (tachycardia, hypertension, hyper-reflexia, seizures, agitation and diaphoresis) in overdose include:

sympathomimetics e.g. amphetamines, cocaine
anticholinergics e.g. atropine, antihistamines
hallucinogens e.g. lysergic acid (LSD)

Drugs which cause depressant syndromes (lethargy, impaired consciousness and cardiorespiratory depression) include:

opioids, sedative-hypnotics, cholinergics and antidepressants

MANAGEMENT

1. A B C D: *airway* (clear if obstructed); *breathing* (intubate if there is respiratory arrest, or a comatosed patient, or there is an absent gag reflex); *circulation* (restore fluid volume if hypotensive); *determine* the level of consciousness and examine all major systems. Assess the electrolytes, urea and creatinine (and determine the anion* and osmolar gaps†), glucose, arterial blood gases, chest X-ray, and ECG. Measurement of drug levels can be helpful.
2. Give glucose and naloxone‡ if the patient is comatose (as these can rapidly reverse hypoglycaemia or opioid overdose).
3. Attempt to decrease the amount of drug in the gastrointestinal tract. Activated charcoal with or without cathartics is recommended. (Charcoal is not useful in iron or lithium overdoses.) The use of ipecac in conscious adults in order to induce vomiting is now controversial and outcomes are as good with charcoal/cathartics alone. Such measures should be used for up to 16 hours after an overdose. Never use ipecac in an unconscious patient or if there is a suspicion of ingestion of petroleum, distillates, or strong acid or alkali.
4. Specific antidote should be given if appropriate (Table 2.1). Always check serum paracetamol (acetaminophen) levels.
5. Alkalinise the urine in severe salicylate or phenobarbitol overdoses.
6. Haemodialysis is indicated early in methanol and ethylene glycol poisonings: it works because these drugs are water soluble and have a small volume of distribution.
7. Monitor level of consciousness and vital signs until normal.
8. ECG monitoring is indicated in tricyclic antidepressant, theophylline, propoxyphene, cocaine and amphetamine overdoses.
9. Psychiatric evaluation before discharge.

---

*High anion gaps are seen in methanol, ethylene glycol, paraldehyde or salicylate poisoning. They may also be seen with prolonged hypoxia or lactic acidosis.
† High osmolar gaps are seen in ethanol, methanol, ethylene glycol, acetone and isopropyl alcohol.
‡ It is important to remember that the half-life of some specific agonist drugs is much shorter than the drug which has been taken in overdose. In these patients repeated infusional therapy may be indicated.

Table 2.1   *Specific antidotes for overdoses and poisonings*

Poison	'Specific' antidote
Paracetamol (acetaminophen)	N-acetylcysteine
Salicylates	Urine alkalinisation, haemodialysis
Benzodiazepines	Flumazenil
Opioids	Naloxone
Barbiturates	Haemoperfusion
Atropine	Physostigmine
Organophosphates	Atropine and pralidoxime
Methanol, ethylene glycol	Ethanol, haemodialysis Methylpyrazole (inhibits alcohol dehydrogenase)
Digitalis	FAB fragment of specific IgG
Theophylline	Haemoperfusion
Cyanide	Amyl or sodium nitrite, sodium thiosulphate
Nitrite	Methylene blue
Carbon monoxide	Oxygen
Iron	Desferrioxamine
Lead	Calcium EDTA, d-penicillamine
Lithium	Haemodialysis
Arsenic	Dimercaprol
Mercury	Dimercaprol (acute exposure) N-acetyl-d-penicillamine (chronic)

Specific acute clinical syndromes

Anaphylaxis	Adrenaline, antihistamines
Oculogyric crises	Benzotropine
Neuroleptic malignant syndrome (seen in patients on neuroleptics with insidious onset over days. Central dopamine inhibition with fluctuating consciousness and autonomic instability)	Dantrolene, bromocriptine
Malignant hyperthermia (autosomal dominant post-synaptic muscle contraction secondary to inhalational anaesthetic agents such as halothane)	Dantrolene

3

Cardiology

IMPORTANT CLINICAL CLUES AND PATHOPHYSIOLOGY

FUNCTIONAL ASSESSMENT OF ANGINA

NEW YORK HEART ASSOCIATION CLASSIFICATION
OF PATIENTS WITH HEART DISEASE

Grade	Symptoms
I	Angina / dyspnoea on unusual activity
II	Angina / dyspnoea on ordinary activity
III	Angina / dyspnoea on less than ordinary activity
IV	Angina / dyspnoea at rest

Table 3.1 *Arterial pulse wave forms*

Type	Cause
Anacrotic	Aortic stenosis
Plateau	Aortic stenosis
Bisferiens	Aortic stenosis *and* regurgitation
Collapsing	Aortic regurgitation
	Hyperdynamic circulation
	Patent ductus arteriosus
	Peripheral arteriovenous fistula
	Arteriosclerotic aorta (elderly)
Small volume	Aortic stenosis
	Pericardial effusion
Alternans (alternating weak and strong beats)	Left ventricular failure
Jerky	Hypertrophic cardiomyopathy (HCM)
	Cardiac tamponade
Pulsus paradoxus*	Acute severe airways obstruction

Table 3.1 Continued

Type	Cause
Reversed pulsus paradoxus (pressure rises on inspiration)	Intermittent positive pressure respiration with left ventricular failure

*Pulsus paradoxus—decrease in volume of the arterial pulse of >10 mmHg during inspiration.
Kussmaul's sign—venous pressure either fails to fall with inspiration or rises with inspiration.

JUGULAR VENOUS PULSE (JVP)

CAUSES OF AN ELEVATED JVP

1. Right ventricular failure
2. Tricuspid regurgitation or stenosis
3. Pericardial effusion or constrictive pericarditis
4. Superior vena caval obstruction
5. Fluid overload
6. Hyperdynamic circulation

CAUSES OF ABNORMAL JVP WAVE FORMS (Figure 3.1)

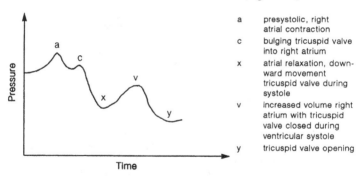

a	presystolic, right atrial contraction
c	bulging tricuspid valve into right atrium
x	atrial relaxation, downward movement tricuspid valve during systole
v	increased volume right atrium with tricuspid valve closed during ventricular systole
y	tricuspid valve opening

Figure 3.1 *Normal jugular venous pressure (JVP), showing a, c and v waves.*

DOMINANT 'a' WAVE

1. Tricuspid stenosis (also causes a slow y descent)
2. Pulmonary stenosis
3. Pulmonary hypertension

Internal Medicine

CANNON 'a' WAVES

1. Complete heart block
2. Nodal tachycardia with retrograde atrial conduction
3. Ventricular tachycardia with retrograde atrial conduction or atrioventricular (AV) dissociation

DOMINANT 'v' WAVES

1. Tricuspid regurgitation

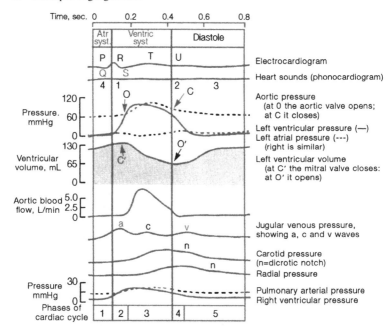

Figure 3.2 *Events of the cardiac cycle at a heart rate of 75 beats/minute. The phases of the cardiac cycle identified by the numbers at the bottom are as follows: 1 = atrial systole; 2 = isovolumetric ventricular contraction; 3 = ventricular ejection; 4 = isovolumetric ventricular relaxation; 5 = ventricular filling. Note that late in systole, aortic pressure actually exceeds left ventricular pressure. However, the momentum of the blood keeps it flowing out of the ventricle for a short period of time. The pressure relationships in the right ventricle and pulmonary artery are similar. Atr syst = atrial systole; Ventric syst = ventricular systole.*
Reproduced, with permission, from Ganong WF. Medical Physiology. 13th edition. Los Altos: Appleton & Lange, 1994.

ABNORMALITIES OF THE HEART SOUNDS

FIRST HEART SOUND (S1)

Loud
1. Mitral stenosis, tricuspid stenosis
2. Tachycardia, hyperdynamic circulation

Soft
1. Mitral regurgitation
2. First degree heart block, left bundle branch block
3. Severe, calcific mitral stenosis

SECOND HEART SOUND (S2)

AORTIC COMPONENT

Loud
1. Systemic hypertension

Soft
1. Calcific aortic stenosis
2. Aortic regurgitation (when the leaflets cannot coapt)

PULMONARY COMPONENT

Loud
1. Pulmonary hypertension

Soft
1. Pulmonary stenosis

SPLITTING OF S2

Increased normal splitting (wider on inspiration)
1. Right bundle branch block
2. Pulmonary stenosis
3. Mitral regurgitation
4. Ventricular septal defect

Fixed splitting (no respiratory variation)
1. Atrial septal defect

Reversed splitting
1. Left bundle branch block
2. Severe aortic stenosis

THIRD HEART SOUND (S3)

LEFT VENTRICULAR S3 (louder at apex and on expiration)

Causes
1. Physiological (<40 years of age, during pregnancy)
2. Left ventricular failure
3. Aortic regurgitation, mitral regurgitation

4. Ventricular septal defect, patent ductus arteriosus
5. Constrictive pericarditis

RIGHT VENTRICULAR S3 (louder at left sternal edge and on inspiration)

Causes
1. Right ventricular failure.
2. Constrictive pericarditis.

FOURTH HEART SOUND (S4)

LEFT VENTRICULAR S4

Causes
1. Aortic stenosis, acute mitral regurgitation
2. Systemic hypertension
3. Ischaemic heart disease

RIGHT VENTRICULAR S4

Causes
1. Pulmonary hypertension
2. Pulmonary stenosis

OTHER SYSTOLIC SOUNDS

1. Ejection click: may be aortic or pulmonary and be heard in normal hearts
2. Mid-systolic click: mitral valve prolapse

Table 3.2 Cardiac murmurs

Timing	Lesion
Pansystolic	Mitral regurgitation (MR), tricuspid regurgitation (TR)
	Ventricular septal defect
Midsystolic	Aortic stenosis (AS), pulmonary stenosis, HCM
	Pulmonary flow murmur of an atrial septal defect
Late systolic	Mitral valve prolapse (MVP)
	Papillary muscle dysfunction, e.g. ischaemia, HCM
Early diastolic	Aortic regurgitation (AR), pulmonary regurgitation
Mid-diastolic	Mitral stenosis (MS), tricuspid stenosis
	Atrial myxoma, Carey-Coombs murmur of acute rheumatic fever
	Austin Flint murmur of aortic regurgitation
Presystolic	Mitral stenosis, tricuspid stenosis, atrial myxoma
Continuous*	Patent ductus arteriosus
	Aortovenous connection
	Venous hum
	Rupture of sinus of Valsalva into right atrium or ventricle
	'Mammary souffle'

*AS and AR, or MS and MR may be confused with continuous murmurs.

OTHER DIASTOLIC SOUNDS

1. Opening snap: mitral stenosis

A *triple rhythm* IS DUE TO S3 OR S4
A *gallop rhythm* IS A TRIPLE RHYTHM OR QUADRUPLE RHYTHM

VALVULAR LESIONS

MITRAL STENOSIS (MS)

AETIOLOGY

Rheumatic heart disease (10–15 years earlier); rarely congenital

SYMPTOMS

1. Dyspnoea, orthopnoea, paroxysmal nocturnal dyspnoea (increased left atrial pressure)
2. Haemoptysis (ruptured bronchial veins)
3. Fatigue, ascites, oedema (pulmonary hypertension)

SIGNS

1. Pulse: small volume, atrial fibrillation (50%)
2. Blood pressure: low
3. Apex beat: tapping (palpable S1), right parasternal heave (pulmonary hypertension), diastolic thrill (very rare)
4. Heart sounds: loud S1 (mobile valve cusps in sinus rhythm), loud P2 (pulmonary hypertension), opening snap (sudden tensing of incompletely opened valves)
5. Murmur: low-pitched mid-diastolic rumbling presystolic murmur (absent in atrial fibrillation) accentuated by exercise
6. Evidence of distant emboli

CLINICAL SIGNS OF SEVERITY (valve area $<1\,cm^2$)

1. Small pulse pressure
2. Soft S1 (indicates immobile valve cusps)
3. Early opening snap (due to increased left atrial pressure)
4. Long diastolic murmur (persists as long as there is a gradient)
5. Diastolic thrill
6. Presence of pulmonary hypertension

COMPLICATIONS

1. Left atrial thrombi and systemic emboli (10–20%)
2. Bacterial endocarditis
3. Deep venous thrombosis and pulmonary emboli
4. Right heart failure

TIMING OF SURGICAL INTERVENTION

Consider operation if there is progressive dyspnoea, pulmonary oedema or haemoptysis that has failed medical therapy. Balloon valvuloplasty is indicated in patients with moderate to severe stenosis with pliable valves and no regurgitation through the valve.

1. Left atrial enlargement
2. Signs of pulmonary hypertension including dilated pulmonary artery and increased right ventricular size
3. Pulmonary venous congestion

MITRAL REGURGITATION (MR)

AETIOLOGY

Chronic
1. Abnormalities of mitral annulus: a) degenerative calcification
                                      b) dilatation secondary to left ventricular enlargement
2. Mitral valve prolapse
3. Rheumatic heart disease
4. Papillary muscle dysfunction (dilatation of the left ventricle or ring in left ventricular failure or ischaemia)
5. Connective tissue disease, Marfan's syndrome, congenital

Acute
1. Infective endocarditis (perforation of anterior leaflets)
2. Myocardial infarction (chordae rupture or papillary muscle dysfunction)

SYMPTOMS

Chronic
1. Dyspnoea (increased left atrial pressure and pulmonary venous congestion)
2. Fatigue (decreased cardiac output)

Acute
1. Pulmonary oedema

SIGNS

Chronic
1. Apex beat: displaced, diffuse, hyperdynamic
2. Heart sounds: S1 soft or absent, S2 widely split (early aortic component of S2), left ventricular S3
3. Murmur: pansystolic

Acute
1. Heart size is normal
2. Murmur (if present): apical ejection murmur (short because atrial pressure is increased). With anterior leaflet chordae rupture murmur radiates to axilla and back. With posterior leaflet rupture murmur radiates to base and carotids.

CLINICAL SIGNS OF SEVERITY OF CHRONIC MITRAL REGURGITATION

1. Small pulse volume
2. Enlarged left ventricle
3. S3 and an early diastolic rumble (important)
4. Soft S1 and early A2
5. Pulmonary hypertension

TIMING OF SURGICAL INTERVENTION

1. Chronic: consider operation if class III or IV dyspnoea, or if there is left ventricular dysfunction (especially falling ejection fraction).
2. Acute: operate in the presence of pulmonary oedema. Often acutely unwell as there is no compensation in either of the left heart chambers.

MITRAL VALVE PROLAPSE

AETIOLOGY

Most common cause of congenital heart disease, affecting 5% of the population and inherited as an autosomal dominant pattern in some families. Other causes include redundant mitral leaflets from myxomatous degeneration, associated with Marfan's syndrome. Higher rate of atrial septal defect also seen in these patients. It is more frequent in women.

SYMPTOMS

Usually none; atypical chest pain, palpitations, dizziness.
Left ventricular failure if there is significant mitral regurgitation.

SIGNS

Midsystolic click and late systolic murmur (click occurs later and murmur becomes softer as left ventricular size increases and mitral regurgitation worsens).

COMPLICATIONS (rare)

Arrhythmias, mitral regurgitation from ruptured chordae or progression of the prolapse, systemic embolisation, sudden death.

AORTIC STENOSIS (AS)

AETIOLOGY

1. Rheumatic (early adulthood)
2. Degenerative senile calcific aortic stenosis (most common cause in adults)
3. Calcified bicuspid valve: bicuspid valve (1% of the population) is the second most common congenital heart defect after mitral valve prolapse.

Internal Medicine

1. Exertional angina (50% have no coronary heart disease)
2. Exertional dyspnoea
3. Exertional syncope
4. Congestive cardiac failure

SIGNS

1. Pulse: plateau or anacrotic, narrow pulse pressure
2. Apex beat: hyperdynamic, sustained apical impulse, may be slightly displaced
3. Thrill: base of the heart (aortic area)
4. Heart sounds: narrowly split S2, soft or absent S2, S4
5. Murmur: harsh midsystolic ejection murmur maximal over aortic area radiating to carotids; ejection click with congenital AS

CLINICAL SIGNS OF SEVERITY (Severe: gradient >50 mmHg (6.67 kPa) or valve area <1.0 cm^2)

1. Plateau pulse
2. Aortic thrill
3. Long and late peaking systolic murmur
4. S4, and paradoxical splitting of S2 (delayed left ventricular ejection and aortic valve closure)
5. Left ventricular failure (very late sign)

DIFFERENTIATE AORTIC STENOSIS (AS) FROM:

1. Aortic sclerosis (usually elderly; no peripheral signs of AS)
2. Supravalvular aortic outflow obstruction (loud A2 and thrill in the sternal notch, associated with elfin facies, mental retardation and hypercalcaemia)
3. Subvalvular aortic outflow obstruction (AR commonly associated due to a jet lesion on the coronary cusp)
4. Chordae rupture of posterior mitral valve leaflet

ECG: left ventricular hypertrophy
CXR: valve calcification, post-stenotic aortic dilatation

TIMING OF SURGICAL INTERVENTION

1. Operate on symptomatic patients if possible.
2. Operate if there is critically severe AS and severe left ventricular hypertrophy even if asymptomatic.

AORTIC REGURGITATION (AR)

AETIOLOGY

May be valvular in origin or due to disease of the aortic root

Valvular
1. Chronic: rheumatic heart disease, congenital bicuspid valve
2. Acute: infective endocarditis

Aortic root
1. Chronic: Marfan's syndrome, aortitis (seronegative arthropathies, rheumatoid arthritis, temporal arteritis, tertiary syphilis), ageing
2. Acute—Marfan's syndrome, hypertension, dissecting aneurysm

SYMPTOMS

Late stages of disease
1. Palpitations, fatigue (hyperdynamic circulation)
2. Dyspnoea on exertion (not present early in disease as exertion decreases the length of diastole)
3. Exertional angina

Acute
Tachycardia, pulmonary oedema and hypotension

SIGNS

1. Pulse: collapsing
2. Carotid: prominent pulsations (Corrigan's sign)
3. Apex beat: displaced, hyperkinetic
4. Thrill: left sternal edge (on expiration)
5. Heart sounds: soft A2
6. Murmur: decrescendo high-pitched diastolic murmur maximal at the left sternal edge (valvular lesion) or right sternal border occasionally (root lesion); acute AR murmur may be soft because of increased left ventricular end-diastolic pressure

CLINICAL SIGNS OF SEVERITY

1. Collapsing pulse, wide pulse pressure
2. Displaced apex beat reflecting a dilated left ventricle (except in acute regurgitation)
3. Long diastolic murmur, Austin Flint murmur (like MS but no opening snap and the S1 is soft—regurgitant jet causes vibration of the mitral valves)
4. S3 (left ventricular), soft A2
5. Pulmonary oedema

ECG: left ventricular hypertrophy
CXR: cardiomegaly with aortic root dilatation, pulmonary venous congestion

TIMING OF SURGICAL INTERVENTION

1. Operate on all symptomatic patients (as this indicates late disease; survival <5 years) if possible
2. Operate if there is evidence of worsening left ventricular dysfunction (left ventricular end-diastolic diameter >65 mm or when size is rapidly increasing)

Table 3.3 Summary of clinical signs of severity of valve disease

Aortic stenosis	Aortic regurgitation
Plateau pulse	Collapsing pulse
Thrill	Wide pulse pressure
Length and lateness of murmur	Length of diastolic thrill, displaced apex beat
Paradoxical splitting of second heart sound	Soft A2
S4	S3
Pulmonary oedema	Austin Flint murmur
Mitral stenosis	**Mitral regurgitation**
Small pulse pressure	Small pulse volume
Right ventricular heave	Enlarged left ventricle
Diastolic thrill	Soft first heart sound
Early opening snap	Early aortic component
Length of diastolic murmur	S3
Pulmonary hypertension	Pulmonary hypertension

Table 3.4 Dynamic manoeuvres and systolic murmurs

Manoeuvre	HCM	Mitral valve prolapse	Aortic stenosis	Mitral regurgitation
Valsalva strain phase (decreased preload)	Louder	Longer	Softer	Softer
Squatting or leg raise (increased preload)	Softer	Shorter	Louder	Louder
Handgrip (increased afterload)	Softer	Shorter	Softer	Louder
Amyl nitrate (decreased afterload)	Louder	Longer	Louder	Softer
Post-premature ventricular contraction (increased contractility and decreased afterload)	Louder*	Longer	Louder	Same

*Peripheral pulse decreases because of increased outflow obstruction.

PROSTHETIC HEART VALVES

A bileaflet mechanical caged disk valve (St Jude) is currently recommended because of improved haemodynamic results.

Xenograft: indicated for patients with a short life expectancy (for example, over 70 years of age) and those who can't or won't take anticoagulant prophylaxis.

Homograft: has a longer life than other bioprosthetic valves.

CARDIAC FAILURE

The events of the cardiac cycle are shown in Figure 3.2.

Table 3.5 *Systolic and diastolic dysfunction*

Aspect	Systolic dysfunction	Diastolic dysfunction
Characteristics	Reduced ejection fraction Left ventricular dilatation Elevated filling pressures	Elevated end-diastolic ventricular pressures with normal or reduced diastolic volumes
	Impaired cardiac output/cardiac reserve	High diastolic pressures Often normal cardiac contractility
	Cardiac contractility and output reduced	Often normal cardiac output
Pathophysiology	A primary muscle problem Loss of muscle fibres Myocarditis Impaired myocyte function	Primarily infiltrative or hypertrophic fibrosis Hypertrophy: impaired left ventricular compliance Infiltration: amyloid, haemochromatosis, collagen diseases
Clinically difficult to distinguish	Accounts for 80% of cardiac failure	Accounts for 20% of cardiac failure with incidence more frequent in the elderly. A diagnosis of exclusion
Treatment	ACE inhibitors, diuretics, carvedilol, digoxin, amlodipine	Control hypertension, cautious use of diuretics

ANATOMY OF CORONARY ARTERIES (Figure 3.3)

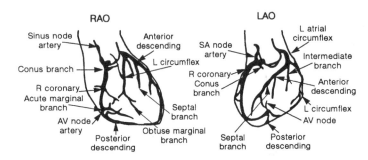

Figure 3.3 *Diagram of the coronary arterial tree as viewed in two projections commonly used in coronary arteriography, the right anterior oblique (RAO) and the left anterior oblique (LAO) projections. AV = atrioventricular; L = left; R = right; SA = sinoatrial.*

Reproduced, with permission, from Braunwald E, et al, editors. Harrison's Principles of Internal Medicine. 11th edition. New York: McGraw Hill, 1987.

LEFT MAIN

Supplies 45% to 60% of left ventricular muscle.

LEFT ANTERIOR DESCENDING

Supplies the apex, anterior 2/3 of the septum, the anterior wall, the right bundle and anterior division of the left bundle.

LEFT CIRCUMFLEX

Supplies the high lateral wall; it may supply the atrioventricular node and a variable amount of the inferior wall.

RIGHT CORONARY ARTERY

Supplies the right ventricle, posterior and diaphragmatic walls and usually the atrioventricular and sinus nodes.

DISEASE STATES

SYSTEMIC HYPERTENSION

CAUSES

Essential (95%)

Secondary (5%)
1. Renal disease
   a) Renovascular disease (renal artery atherosclerosis, fibromuscular disease, aneurysm, vasculitis)
   b) Chronic pyelonephritis, analgesic nephropathy, reflux nephropathy
   c) Glomerulonephritis, connective tissue diseases
   d) Polycystic disease, diabetic nephropathy
2. Endocrine disease: Cushing's syndrome, 17 and 11-beta hydroxylase defects, Conn's syndrome, phaeochromocytoma, acromegaly, hypothyroidism, hypercalcaemia
3. Drugs: contraceptive pill (oestrogens cause sodium retention, increased renin substrate and increased catecholamine receptor numbers), alcohol (mechanism unknown)
4. Coarctation of aorta
5. Other: polycythaemia rubra vera, toxaemia of pregnancy, hypercalcaemia, neurogenic (increased intracranial pressure, lead poisoning, acute porphyria), liquorice (mimics aldosterone)

CLINICAL CLUES SUGGESTING HYPERTENSION IS SECONDARY

1. Onset of hypertension before 20 or after 50 years of age
2. Very high blood pressure at diagnosis (>180/110) or evidence of end-organ damage
3. Radio-femoral delay (coarctation of aorta)
4. Abdominal bruit or retinopathy (renovascular hypertension)
5. Abdominal or flank mass, or a family history of renal disease (polycystic kidneys)
6. Truncal obesity, purple striae, central obesity, moon face (Cushing's syndrome)
7. Tachycardia, pallor, sweating, tremor, labile hypertension, hypertension in childhood (phaeochromocytoma, MEN IIa (page 241))
8. Neurofibromas (phaeochromocytoma, multiple endocrine neoplasia type II) (page 241)
9. Diastolic hypertension, muscle weakness, polyuria (Conn's syndrome)
10. Poor response to therapy
11. Proximal muscle weakness: hypokalaemia from Conn's syndrome

INITIAL SCREENING INVESTIGATIONS

1. Serum potassium (hypokalaemia may be due to diuretics, Conn's syndrome, potassium-losing nephropathy, renovascular disease, Cushing's syndrome, Liddle's syndrome)

2. Serum creatinine and urinalysis (renal disease)
3. Serum calcium (hypercalcaemia)
4. ECG (end-organ damage: left ventricular hypertrophy)
5. Coronary artery disease risk factors (glucose, lipids)
6. Complete blood count

Other tests depend on clinical evidence of disease.

PULMONARY HYPERTENSION

CAUSES

1. Primary (idiopathic)
2. Secondary (see page 296)
   a) Pulmonary emboli
   b) Lung disease: chronic obstructive pulmonary disease, obstructive sleep apnoea, interstitial lung disease
   c) Left-to-right cardiac shunt: atrial septal defect, ventricular septal defect, patent ductus arteriosus
   d) Restrictive lung disease, e.g. severe kyphoscoliosis
   e) Drug: e.g. contraceptive pill

SIGNS

1. Tachypnoea, peripheral cyanosis, small volume pulse
2. Prominent a wave in jugular venous pressure
3. Right ventricular heave, palpable P2
4. Loud P2, pulmonary systolic ejection murmur, occasionally pulmonary regurgitation
5. Signs of right ventricular failure (cor pulmonale), peripheral oedema

ISCHAEMIC HEART DISEASE

ANGINA MECHANISMS

1. Chronic atherosclerosis.
2. Thrombosis: occlusive.
   non-occlusive.
3. Coronary artery spasm (associated with other vascular phenomena such as migraine and Raynaud's syndrome). Often presents with ST elevation rather than depression.
4. Normal coronary arteries: associated with microvascular disease—abnormal exercise stress test.

UNSTABLE ANGINA

1. Recent onset of angina
2. Increased frequency of symptoms
3. Failure of pain to settle with rest or medication
4. Angina at rest
5. Angina in the immediate post-infarct period

NON-CARDIAC CAUSES OF ANGINA

1. Anaemia
2. Supraventricular tachycardia or any arrhythmias
3. Hyperthyroidism
4. Hypertension

MYOCARDIAL INFARCTION

CAUSES OF CHEST PAIN AFTER A MYOCARDIAL INFARCT

1. Extension of the infarct
2. Pericarditis
3. Pulmonary embolus
4. Aortic root dissection (rare)
5. Incipient myocardial rupture (often associated with nausea)

Table 3.6   *Cardiac enzymes for myocardial infarction (MI)*

Feature	Creatine kinase (MB)*	LDH isoenzymes LDH1 : LDH2**
Onset	6 to 12 hours	24 to 48 hours
Peak	24 hours	3 to 6 days
Duration	3 to 4 days	8 to 14 days
False positives	myocarditis, recent surgery, strenuous exercise	haemolysis, renal infarction

*≥Eightfold increase in creatine kinase associated with an increased mortality in the first years after infarction. Creatine kinase is also increased in muscle disease (e.g. muscular dystrophies) or with muscle injury (MM fraction predominantly), and in alcoholism and hypothyroidism.
**LDH1 : LDH2 >0.8 infarct likely, >1.0 infarct very likely.

An inferior MI often causes transient sinus bradycardia, junctional rhythms and heart block.

An anterior MI may cause right bundle branch block and left axis deviation; heart block suggests a very large infarct.

PROGNOSTIC FACTORS IN HOSPITAL PATIENTS FOLLOWING A MYOCARDIAL INFARCT

The best predictor of mortality after myocardial infarction is left ventricular function and the degree of underlying coronary artery disease.

FACTORS SUGGESTING A WORSE PROGNOSIS

1. Elderly
2. Anterior infarct

3. Hypertension prior to the infarct
4. Pulmonary oedema or pump failure
5. Unexplained sinus tachycardia or a new conduction system abnormality
6. Evidence of a large infarct (high creatine kinase, cardiomegaly on CXR, large defect on nuclear scanning, high wall motion score index on echocardiogram)
7. Extension of infarction
8. Mechanical complications: septal or papillary muscle rupture
9. Persistent ST elevation: aneurysm formation

The risk of complications for non-cardiac surgery in patients with a history of myocardial infarction is increased if:

1. Myocardial infarction within the last 6 months
2. S3 present
3. Coexistent aortic stenosis
4. Premature ventricular contractions on ECG

COMPLICATIONS OF MYOCARDIAL INFARCTION

1. Arrhythmias
2. Pump failure
3. Post-infarct angina and infarct extension
4. Left ventricular aneurysm (may cause ventricular tachycardia, cardiac failure, peripheral emboli, angina)
5. Free wall rupture
6. Mural thrombosis
7. Pericarditis and Dressler's syndrome
8. Ventricular septal rupture, rupture of a papillary muscle
9. Deep venous thrombosis, pulmonary embolism
10. Iatrogenic (drugs, pacing)

CAUSES OF A POST-MYOCARDIAL INFARCTION
SYSTOLIC MURMUR

1. Ventricular septal rupture.
   Usually in the first week after infarct; the murmur is at the left sternal edge (thrill in 50%) and a right ventricular heave is common. JVP may or may not be raised. Pulmonary artery catheter: O_2 saturation step-up between right atrium and right ventricle. Can usually be identified by colour Doppler.
2. Papillary muscle rupture.
   Murmur is at the apex usually without a thrill; pulmonary oedema is common. Echocardiogram may show a flail mitral leaflet. Colour Doppler may show mitral regurgitation. Pulmonary artery catheter: large v waves.
3. Papillary muscle dysfunction.
   Usually in the first week after infarct; with anterior leaflet dysfunction (usually anterior infarct) the murmur is at the apex and radiates to the axilla, while with posterior leaflet dysfunction (usually inferior

infarct) the murmur is at the apex or left sternal edge and radiates to the base.

Echocardiogram shows prolapse of the leaflet into the left atrium.

4. Functional mitral regurgitation secondary to left ventricular dilatation.
5. Pericardial friction rub. May be limited to systole.

FACTORS DECREASING POST-MYOCARDIAL INFARCT MORTALITY

1. Early thrombolysis
2. Beta-blockers and aspirin
3. Lipid control
4. Angiotensin converting enzyme inhibitors if ejection fraction is less than 40%
5. Exercise rehabilitation
6. Coronary artery by-pass grafting (CABG)

BENEFITS OF THROMBOLYTIC THERAPY

1. Decreases the size of the infarct and hence better maintains left ventricular function
2. Decreases the reported rate of congestive cardiac failure
3. Decreases the rate of pericarditis
4. Decreases the rate of ventricular arrhythmias
5. Increases short and long term survival

INDICATIONS FOR POST-MYOCARDIAL INFARCTION ANGIOGRAPHY

1. On-going ischaemia before hospital discharge
2. Prior myocardial infarction
3. Non-Q wave infarction on this presentation
4. Decreased left ventricular function
5. Ischaemia during pre-discharge exercise stress testing

RIGHT VENTRICULAR INFARCTION

A complication of transmural inferior infarction (30%)

Diagnosis

1. Clear lungs with an elevated jugular venous pressure
2. Hypotension may occur (due to underfilling of the left ventricle)
3. 2-D echocardiogram: dilated right ventricle with decreased wall motion
4. Haemodynamics: right atrial and right ventricular end-diastolic pressure $\geq$ pulmonary artery wedge (left ventricular end-diastolic pressure)

COMPLICATIONS

1. Pulmonary embolism from a mural thrombus
2. Tricuspid regurgitation from a ruptured papillary muscle
3. Cyanosis secondary to a left-to-right shunt through a stretched foramen ovale (rare)

THERAPY OF ACUTE MYOCARDIAL INFARCTION

Table 3.7 *Drugs of definite benefit after acute myocardial infarction*

Short term	Long term
aspirin	aspirin
thrombolytics	beta-blockers
intravenous beta-blockers	angiotensin converting enzyme inhibitors if ejection fraction is less than 40%
	lipid control

Table 3.8 *Unstable angina: treatments and investigations which are supported by level 1 evidence**

Thrombosis therapy
- Aspirin (indefinitely)
- Heparin for 2–5 days intravenously
- Low molecular weight heparin

Risk stratification
- Exercise testing
- Nuclear imaging or stress echocardiography

Interventions
- Coronary artery bypass surgery for left main coronary artery stenosis or three vessel disease with left ventricular dysfunction
- Incremental value of stenting with percutaneous transluminal coronary angioplasty
- Adjunctive use of platelet 11b/111a receptor antagonism with percutaneous transluminal coronary angioplasty

*See Chapter 1.

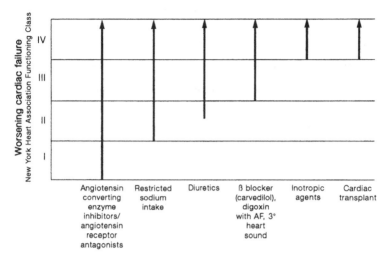

Figure 3.4 *Schema for treating cardiac failure.*

TREADMILL EXERCISE STRESS TEST (EST)

POSITIVE TEST FOR ISCHAEMIC HEART DISEASE

A 1 mm horizontal or downsloping ST segment depression beyond the baseline measured 80 msec after the J point.

Sensitivity: 70%; specificity: 80% (false positives 10% to 20%).

The test is most useful in patients with an intermediate risk level (a positive test in those with a low risk, e.g. women, younger patients, is likely to be a false positive.)

Patients with 32 mm ST segment depression at low workloads (<6 minutes on the Bruce protocol) or low heart rates (<85% of age-predicted maximum) generally have a poorer prognosis and more severe disease.

Contraindications	unstable angina
	unstable arrhythmias
	uncompensated heart failure
Difficulty interpreting EST	left bundle branch block
	digoxin
	pre-existing ST-T wave abnormalities

After myocardial infarction, a pre-discharge stress test that results in angina, ventricular arrhythmias or ST segment changes predicts a greatly increased mortality.

If the treadmill results are equivocal, a scintigraphic assessment for ischaemia (thallium-201 or radionuclide ventriculography) may be indicated.

PERCUTANEOUS TRANSLUMINAL CORONARY ANGIOPLASTY (PTCA)

CONSIDERATIONS

Acutely, PTCA may be useful with ongoing ischaemia in unstable angina pectoris or after a myocardial infarction.

Outcomes are improved for patients with haemodynamic compromise or anterior infarction following ischaemia.

Patients with one or two vessel disease may benefit from elective coronary angioplasty. Because 1% of patients undergoing angioplasty will have acute occlusion or need urgent surgery, left main coronary artery disease is an absolute contraindication unless protected by prior coronary bypass graft.

OUTCOMES

- 95% initial response
- 30–40% have symptoms or re-stenosis by 6 months
- 20–30% require repeat-PTCA
- Stenting appears to lower the acute occlusion rate to >1%, and the re-stenosis rate to 20–30%

Patients with an occluded artery may be suitable for PTCA. Consider this when there has been a sudden increase in the frequency and severity of exertional angina without infarction, or angina at rest. Success rates for symptoms of less than 3 months' duration are 80%, but fall to 20% if symptoms present for more than 3 months. These vessels have an increased risk of restenosis and reocclusion.

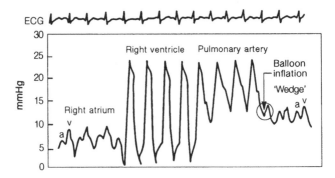

Figure 3.5 *Tracing of pressures in passage of a pulmonary artery catheter from the internal jugular vein to the pulmonary artery. Pressure wave forms are normal.*

Table 3.9 *Haemodynamic measurements after myocardial infarction*

Cardiac index normal: 3.4 L/min m², range 2.4–3.8	Pulmonary artery wedge pressure normal: 10 mmHg (1.3 kPa), range 6–15 mmHg (0.8–2 kPa)	Therapy to consider
>2.5	10 to 18 (1.3 to 2.4)	Nil
>2.5	>18 (2.4)	Frusemide
<2.5	<10 (1.3)	Fluids
<2.5	>18 (2.4)	Dobutamine or nitroprusside

CARDIAC FAILURE

LEFT VENTRICULAR FAILURE (LVF)

CAUSES

1. Volume overload
   a) Aortic regurgitation, mitral regurgitation
   b) Patent ductus arteriosus
2. Pressure overload
   a) Systemic hypertension
   b) Aortic stenosis
3. Myocardial disease
   a) Ischaemic heart disease
   b) Cardiomyopathy
      i) Dilated cardiomyopathy: idiopathic, alcohol, myocarditis, chronic uncontrolled tachycardia, familial, peripartum, neuromuscular disease (e.g. dystrophia myotonica), connective tissue disease (e.g. scleroderma), diabetes mellitus, haemochromatosis, sarcoidosis, drugs (e.g. doxorubicin), radiation
      ii) Restrictive cardiomyopathy: idiopathic, eosinophilic endomyocardial disease, endomyocardial fibrosis, infiltrations (e.g. amyloid), granulomas (e.g. sarcoid)
      iii) Hypertrophic cardiomyopathy

SYMPTOMS

1. Exertional dyspnoea
2. Orthopnoea
3. Paroxysmal nocturnal dyspnoea, pulmonary oedema

SIGNS

1. Tachycardia (occasionally pulsus alternans), displaced apex (volume or pressure overload impulse)
2. Gallop rhythm, mitral regurgitation (stretched atrioventricular ring)
3. Medium late or pan-inspiratory crackles in the lung bases

N.B. Always rule out ventricular septal defect, pericardial disease, ventricular aneurysm, hypertrophic cardiomyopathy and hypothyroidism if there is pulmonary oedema and a normal heart size.

FACTORS PRECIPITATING LEFT VENTRICULAR FAILURE (LVF)

1. Arrhythmias
2. Anaemia
3. Infection, fever
4. Myocardial infarction
5. Pregnancy
6. Thyrotoxicosis
7. Prolonged hypotension e.g. sepsis
8. Pulmonary emboli
9. Acute exacerbation of chronic airflow limitation
10. Discontinuation of therapy
11. Excessive physical exertion, high salt intake

RIGHT VENTRICULAR FAILURE (RVF)

CAUSES

1   Volume overload
   a) Atrial septal defect
   b) Tricuspid regurgitation
2   Pressure overload
   a) Pulmonary stenosis
   b) Pulmonary hypertension
3   Myocardial disease
   a) Secondary to left ventricular failure
   b) Right ventricular myocardial infarction

SYMPTOMS

1. Oedema, ascites
2. Anorexia, nausea

SIGNS

1. Elevated jugular venous pressure
2. Tricuspid regurgitation (stretched atrioventricular ring)
3. Large tender liver, oedema, ascites, pleural effusion

CARDIOMYOPATHY

Broadly divided into hypertrophic, restrictive and dilated.

HYPERTROPHIC CARDIOMYOPATHY (HCM)

AETIOLOGY

Idiopathic; autosomal dominant with multiple genes affecting the myosin heavy chain, variable expressivity.

SYMPTOMS

1. Dyspnoea (increased left ventricular end-diastolic pressure due to abnormal diastolic compliance)
2. Angina
3. Syncope, sudden death (secondary to ventricular fibrillation or sudden increase in outflow obstruction)
4. Pulmonary oedema with paroxysmal onset of atrial fibrillation (frequent presentation)

SIGNS

1. Pulse: sharp rising and jerky (rapid ejection followed by outflow obstruction)
2. JVP: prominent 'a' wave (forceful atrial contraction against a non-compliant right ventricle)
3. Apex beat: double or triple impulse (presystolic ventricular expansion following atrial contraction)
4. Murmur: pansystolic (apex, from mitral regurgitation in 50%), late systolic (left sternal edge) affected by dynamic manoeuvres; S4
5. Decreased carotid pulse after a premature ventricular contraction (increased contractility causes increased outflow obstruction)

COMPLICATIONS

1. Atrial fibrillation and other arrhythmias (may lead to rapid cardiac decompensation)
2. Systemic embolism
3. Infective endocarditis
4. Dilated cardiomyopathy

THERAPY

1. Beta-blockers reduce gradients and relieve symptoms
2. Calcium channel blockers reduce outflow obstruction and improve abnormal diastolic properties
3. Surgery (myectomy) is reserved for severe disease uncontrolled by medical therapy
4. *Avoid* glyceryl trinitrate, diuretics, afterload-reducing drugs, digitalis

CARDIAC TRANSPLANTATION

INDICATIONS

- Left ventricular ejection fraction <15–20% especially if seen with serious ventricular arrhythmias where life expectancy is limited despite optimal medical and/or surgical treatment.
- Medically compliant patient with adequate support (social and psychological)

CONTRAINDICATIONS

- Extensive end organ damage, especially from diabetes or collagen vascular disease
- Severe chronic lung disease
- Active infectious processes
- Active or recent malignancy
- Peripheral or cerebrovascular disease
- Active peptic ulceration
- Substance or alcohol misuse

MATCHING

Size of heart, ABO blood typing, negative lymphocyte cross match, cytomegalovirus compatability.

In the operation, the right and left atrium are left intact. There is therefore a double p wave postoperatively, as there are two sinoatrial nodes still in place.

COMPLICATIONS

- Immediate right heart failure
- Rejection (hyperacute, acute and chronic)
- Infection (acutely bacterial, long-term opportunistic infections)
- Long term: accelerated atherosclerosis

HEART-LUNG TRANSPLANTATION

INDICATIONS

- Eisenmenger's syndrome
- Primary pulmonary hypertension

CONTRAINDICATIONS as above

CLASSIFICATION OF CONGENITAL HEART DISEASE

ACYANOTIC

WITH LEFT-TO-RIGHT SHUNT

1. **Ventricular septal defect (VSD):** commonest congenital heart lesion after bicuspid aortic valve
   Small ($<0.5\,cm^2$)
   - may close spontaneously up to 10 years of age
   - left parasternal thrill
   - holosystolic murmur
   Large
   - increased pulmonary blood flow leading to pulmonary hypertension
   - needs surgical closure before pulmonary hypertension becomes established

2. **Atrial septal defect (ASD)**
   Secundum 90%
   - parasternal lift
   - midsystolic murmur, fixed split S2, loud P2
   - CXR: right ventricular dilatation, increased pulmonary vascular markings
   - ECG: right axis deviation, incomplete right bundle branch block
   - surgery indicated if pulmonary:systemic shunt >2:1

   Primum 10%
   - often associated with Down syndrome
   - associated with mitral and tricuspid regurgitation
   - ECG: changes can include first degree block, left axis deviation, incomplete right bundle branch block
3. **Patent ductus arteriosus (PDA)**
   - small: asymptomatic
   - large: continuous murmur, late systolic accentuation loudest in the left infraclavicular region

WITH NO SHUNT

1. Bicuspid aortic valve
2. Coarctation of aorta (associations: bicuspid aortic valve, berry aneurysms, polycystic kidneys)
3. Dextrocardia
4. Pulmonary stenosis, tricuspid stenosis

CYANOTIC (mnemonic ET)

- E—Eisenmenger's syndrome (reversal of a left-to-right shunt following the development of pulmonary hypertension). Polycythaemia common and needs to be treated to maintain haematocrit at <65%.
- Ebstein's Anomaly: the septal, posterior leaflets of the tricuspid valve are attached to the right ventricular wall below the tricuspid annulus. A right-to-left shunt may develop through a patent foramen ovale.
- T—Tetralogy of Fallot (combination of VSD, over-riding aorta, right ventricular outflow obstruction (subpulmonic stenosis) and right ventricular hypertrophy). As right ventricular hypertrophy worsens, right-to-left shunt and cyanosis worsen.
- Other, e.g. truncus arteriosus, transposition of the great vessels, tricuspid atresia, total anomalous pulmonary venous drainage.

ASSOCIATIONS WITH CONGENITAL HEART DISEASE

1. Down syndrome (trisomy 21): endocardial cushion defect, ASD, VSD, tetralogy of Fallot
2. Turner's syndrome (XO): coarctation of aorta, bicuspid aortic valve (with webbed neck, broad chest, lymphoedema)
3. Congenital rubella: patent ductus arteriosus, pulmonary artery stenosis
4. Holt Oram syndrome: atrial septal defect or endocardial cushion defect (with skeletal upper limb defect, hypoplasia of clavicles)

5. Noonan's syndrome: pulmonary stenosis (with cardiomyopathy, webbed neck, pectus excavatum, cryptorchidism)

ARRHYTHMIAS

SUPRAVENTRICULAR TACHYARRHYTHMIAS

ATRIAL FIBRILLATION

Causes
1. Ischaemic heart disease
2. Rheumatic heart disease, particularly mitral stenosis
3. Thyrotoxicosis
4. Other: hypertension, pulmonary embolus, chronic constrictive pericarditis, cardiomyopathy, atrial septal defect, atrial myxoma, mitral valve prolapse, idiopathic lone fibrillator

N.B. If there are grouped beats, digitalis toxicity may be present.

If there is a long-short interval before a wide complex tachycardia, the rhythm is likely to be atrial fibrillation with aberrancy (*not* ventricular tachycardia): this is termed the Ashmann phenomenon.

Anticoagulation is recommended in patients with chronic atrial fibrillation (including before and after cardioversion). Warfarin is recommended to keep the International Standardised Ratio (INR) between 2 and 2.5 (1.5–2.0 in patients over 60 years or those with left atrial enlargement, mitral valve disease, hypertension or left ventricular dysfunction).

Therapy
Acutely, beta-blockers or calcium channel blockers are likely to reduce the ventricular rate more rapidly than digoxin. Intravenous amiodarone can be used in haemodynamically compromised patients. Oral flecainide may be effective and is safe for patients without other heart disease.

When precipitating causes are optimally treated and atrial fibrillation persists, elective cardioversion (with anticoagulant cover) is the treatment of choice. Once chronic atrial fibrillation is established irreversibly, the main therapeutic aim is to control the ventricular rate.

ATRIAL FLUTTER

Associated with abnormal hearts (ischaemic heart disease, alcoholic cardiomyopathy, lung disease). It is best seen in leads II, III and AVF.

Carotid sinus pressure decreases ventricular rate.

Treatment
- Direct current cardioversion
- Rapid atrial pacing
- Drugs: class 1 antiarrhythmics, amiodarone or sotalol

With recurrent atrial flutter, options would include:

- Chronic administration of drugs
- Atrial pacing pacemaker

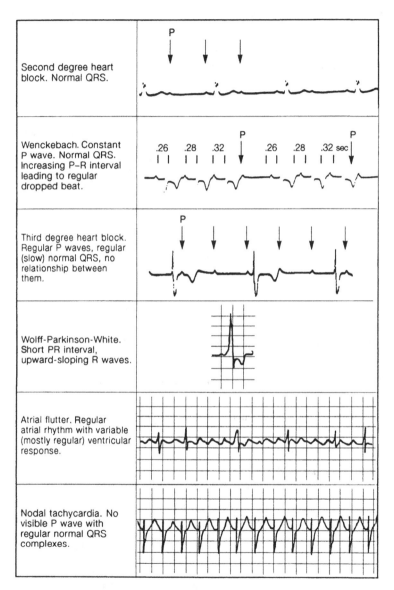

Second degree heart block. Normal QRS.	P
Wenckebach. Constant P wave. Normal QRS. Increasing P–R interval leading to regular dropped beat.	P P .26 .28 .32 .26 .28 .32 sec
Third degree heart block. Regular P waves, regular (slow) normal QRS, no relationship between them.	P
Wolff-Parkinson-White. Short PR interval, upward-sloping R waves.	
Atrial flutter. Regular atrial rhythm with variable (mostly regular) ventricular response.	
Nodal tachycardia. No visible P wave with regular normal QRS complexes.	

Figure 3.6 Arrhythmias.

- Radiofrequency ablation of isthmus between crista terminalis and tricuspid valve

OTHER SUPRAVENTRICULAR TACHYARRHYTHMIAS

Atrio-ventricular junction re-entrant tachycardia (AVJRT)
(Most common cause)
1. Concealed: a unidirectional bypass tract
2. Wolff-Parkinson-White (Figure 3.6)
   This is a re-entrant tachycardia circuit with forward conduction through the atrio-ventricular node with the circuit completed by an accessory pathway back into the atrium from the ventricle (bundle of Kent). Electrocardiographic clues include: Short P-R interval

   Delta wave in the QRS complex

   Broad complex atrial fibrillation

   Definitive treatment and cure are best achieved by radiofrequency ablation of the accessory pathway.

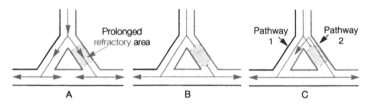

Figure 3.7 *Principle of re-entry arrhythmias: 2 pathways with differing refractory properties.*

Paroxysmal atrial tachycardia with heart block: consider digoxin toxicity.

Multifocal atrial tachycardia
This diagnosis can only be made with the presence of at least 3 distinct P wave morphologies.

BRADYARRHYTHMIAS

Atrioventricular block
First degree:	Lengthened P-R interval
Second degree	
Mobitz Type I*	Increasing P-R interval until a beat is dropped (Wenckebach). This is usually associated with A-V nodal disease.
Mobitz Type II*	Sudden dropped QRS with no preceding change in PR interval. Reflects infranodal disease. High chance of progression to complete heart block.
Third degree	Complete atrioventricular dissociation

*In 2:1 block, it is impossible to distinguish Type I from Type II.

COMPLETE HEART BLOCK

CAUSES

- Congenital (female propensity)
- Damaged myocardium (male propensity)
- Ischaemic heart disease, infective endocarditis, infiltrative cardiomyopathies, aortic or mitral valve disease
- Idiopathic (degenerative)

CLINICALLY

Varying intensity of the 'a' wave in the jugular venous pressure, varying intensity of the first heart sound, varying strength of the pulse.

ECG: atrioventricular dissociation.

A pacemaker is the treatment of choice for complete heart block especially if there is evidence of a broad complex QRS complex indicating a low ventricular pacemaker.

SICK SINUS SYNDROME

SYMPTOMS

- Lightheadedness, dizziness
- Syncope
- Most have ischaemic heart disease or long-standing hypertension
- Slow response to asystole from other spontaneous pacemakers accounts for most symptoms
- There is an increased risk of atrioventricular node disease (symptomatic episodes known as Stokes-Adams attacks) in these patients

Sick sinus syndrome can manifest as both bradyarrhythmias and tachyarrhythmias of atrial origin.

bradyarrhythmias: sinus bradycardia, sinus pauses, sinus block
tachyarrhythmias: atrial fibrillation, atrial flutter

VENTRICULAR ARRHYTHMIAS

VENTRICULAR TACHYCARDIA

Non-sustained asymptomatic runs of ventricular tachycardia are predictive of increased risk of sudden death in patients with impaired ventricular function.

Almost all sustained episodes of ventricular tachycardia occur in hearts with damaged myocardium (ischaemic heart disease, other cardiomyopathies). Risk of sudden death depends on the degree of cardiac compromise.

ECG: wide (>120 ms) QRS complex with atrioventricular dissociation.

Potential treatment
- Pharmacological: amiodarone, sotalol
- Altering the myocardial source of the arrhythmia: radiofrequency ablation, surgery

Internal Medicine

- Pacing procedures: over-drive pacing with pacing wire (acutely) or implantable cardiodefibrillator (ICD)

VENTRICULAR FIBRILLATION

1. Primary (no myocardial infarction associated): there is an 80% chance of recurrence and electrophysiological studies are indicated.
2. Secondary (associated with myocardial infarction within the first 48 hours): this does not need further evaluation.

WIDE COMPLEX TACHYCARDIA: DISTINGUISHING VENTRICULAR TACHYCARDIA (VT) AND SUPRAVENTRICULAR TACHYCARDIA (SVT) WITH ABERRATION

Clinically, adenosine can be used to help make this distinction, especially if the following criteria (Table 3.10) do not yield an answer. Adenosine is a short

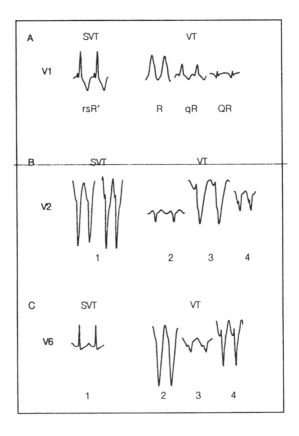

Table 3.10 *Features distinguishing VT and SVT with aberration*

Feature	Ventricular tachycardia (VT)	Supraventricular tachycardia (SVT) with aberration
QRS	Often >0.14 secs	Usually 0.12–0.14 seconds
AV dissociation	+	−
Left axis deviation	+	−
Fusion beats	+	−
Deep S in V6	+	−
QRS morphology in lead V1		
Right bundle branch block	Monomorphic R wave Biphasic qR or QR	Right 'rabbit ear' taller than left 'rabbit ear' (rsR)
Left bundle branch block	r wave >30 ms qS interval >60 ms Notched downstroke of S wave	− −

Exceptions to these rules for SVT with aberration: Wolff-Parkinson-White syndrome

◄────────────────────────────────

Figure 3.8 **A. Tracings of ECG lead V1 typical of SVT and VT with a right bundle branch block configuration.** *During SVT, V1 typically displays an rSR' wave. During VT, multiple configurations of V1 may be seen, including a monophasic R wave, a qR (amplitude of Q wave less than the R wave amplitude), or QR (amplitude of Q wave equal to amplitude of R wave).*
B. Tracings of ECG lead V1 typical of SVT and VT with a left bundle branch block configuration. *During SVT lead V1 typically displays no r wave or a very narrow initial r wave, with a rapid downstroke to the S wave (illustrative tracings in '1'). During VT lead V1 typically displays a wide initial r wave having a duration >30 msec (illustrative tracing in '2'), or long duration from the onset of the r wave to the nadir of the S wave, >60 msec (illustrative tracing in '3'), or notching on the downstroke of the S wave (illustrative tracing in '4').*
C. Tracings of ECG lead V6 typical of SVT and VT with a right bundle branch block configuration. *During SVT lead V6 typically displays an initial R wave amplitude greater than the S wave (illustrative tracing in '1'). In contrast, during VT lead V6 typically displays no r wave (illustrative tracings in '2' and '3'), or an r wave amplitude less than the S wave (illustrative tracing in '4'). Notching on the downstroke of the S wave (illustrative tracing in '3') is also much more typical of VT than SVT.*
Reproduced from MKSAP IX, with permission.

Table 3.11 Differential diagnosis of common arrhythmias

Arrhythmia	Rate	Rhythm	QRS shape	Atrial activity	P-QRS relation	Carotid sinus massage
Sinus tachycardia	100 to 200	Regular	Normal	P wave normal	Yes	Slows
Supraventricular tachycardia	160 to 190	Regular	Normal	Absent	Often masked	No change or reverts
Atrial flutter	140 to 160 (typically 150)	Regular (may be irregular with shifts from 2:1 to 3:1)	Normal	Flutter waves	Often masked	Increases block
Atrial fibrillation	160 to 190	Irregularly irregular	Normal	Absent	Not applicable	No response
Ventricular tachycardia	100 to 230	Regular	Abnormal*	P waves march through QRS	No	No response

*Abnormal with an intraventricular conduction disturbance.

acting intravenous antiarrhythmic agent for possible VT (immediate onset of action, 10 second half-life). Verapamil should *not* be used (unless Wolff-Parkinson-White syndrome has been already definitely excluded).

Table 3.12 Anti-arrhythmic drugs

Class	Examples	Pharmacology
IA	Quinidine, disopyramide, procainamide	Sodium channel blockade reduces phase O depolarisation (V max); increases action potential duration
IB	Lignocaine, phenytoin, mexilitine	Moderate phase O depression at faster rate
		No change or decreases action potential duration
IC	Flecainide, encainide	Marked phase O depression at normal rate
		Minimal effect on action potential duration
II	Propranolol, metoprolol	β-receptor blockade
		Lengthens atrioventricular node refractory period and conduction velocity
III	Sotalol, amiodarone	Prolongs action potential duration in atrium, ventricle and Purkinje fibres
IV	Verapamil	Calcium channel blockade decreases conduction velocity, and increases AV node refractoriness
—	Adenosine	Decreased atrial activity, no effect on ventricles

AV: atrioventricular.

Table 3.13 Chronic therapeutic options for arrhythmias

Arrhythmia	Therapy
Premature atrial contractions	Usually none needed. β-blocker, verapamil
Paroxysmal atrial fibrillation or flutter	To control rate—digoxin, β-blocker, verapamil
	To prevent paroxysms—sotalol, flecainide, amiodarone (if severe and uncontrolled)
Supraventricular tachycardia	Verapamil, digoxin, β-blocker, flecainide
Wolff-Parkinson-White and recurrent atrial fibrillation or supraventricular tachycardia	Acutely—adenosine
	Recurrent—sotalol, flecainide, amiodarone
	Avoid digitalis, verapamil, and β-blockers (all may shorten the refractory period of the accessory pathway)

Table 3.13 Continued

Arrhythmia	Therapy
Premature ventricular ectopics	Rarely indicated
Ventricular tachycardia	Amiodarone, sotalol

Adenosine, amiodarone, β-adrenergic blockers, calcium channel blockers, and digoxin slow atrioventricular node conduction.

Type IA, IC and III slow conduction in myocardium and prolong the QT interval predisposing to Torsades de pointes.

REMEMBER THESE IMPORTANT INTERACTIONS

1. Verapamil and quinidine increase digoxin levels (by decreasing renal clearance)
2. Propranolol (and cardiac failure) increase lignocaine levels (as clearance is decreased)

REMEMBER THESE IMPORTANT SIDE EFFECTS

1. Digitalis: nausea, green-red visual disturbances, arrhythmias (brady-arrhythmias; with toxicity paroxysmal atrial tachycardia, ventricular fibrillation)
2. Quinidine: thrombocytopenia, sudden death (?related to ventricular tachycardia and prolonged QT interval)
3. Lignocaine: drowsiness, dysarthria (may be confused with stroke), seizures

RHEUMATIC FEVER

Table 3.14 Diagnostic criteria (modified Jones' criteria)

Major manifestations	Minor manifestations
Carditis	Fever
Migratory polyarthritis	Arthralgia
Sydenham's chorea	Elevated ESR or C-reactive protein
Erythema marginatum	Prolonged P-R interval on ECG
Subcutaneous nodules	

Diagnosis: 2 major criteria *or* 1 major and 2 minor criteria *plus* evidence of preceding streptococcal infection (positive throat culture and/or positive antigen detection test, and/or elevated or increasing streptococcal antibody test).

SECONDARY PROPHYLAXIS

Highest risk of recurrence under 40 years of age, and in the first 5 years following rheumatic fever.

- Penicillin G 1.2 million units intramuscularly monthly *or*
- Penicillin V 125–250 mg bd orally
- Sulfadiazine or erythromycin may be substituted in patients unable to take penicillin

INFECTIVE ENDOCARDITIS

PROPHYLAXIS

High-dose, short-term antibiotic therapy is required (although proof of efficacy is lacking).

Patients with known or suspected valvular heart disease, congenital heart disease (except for uncomplicated atrial septal defect), asymmetrical septal hypertrophy, prosthetic valve replacement or a past history of infective endocarditis need prophylaxis. The role of prophylaxis in mitral valve prolapse is less well defined but is indicated when mitral regurgitation is present.

1. Dental procedures causing bleeding, oral surgery or procedures to the upper respiratory tract (*Streptococcus viridans*)
2. Procedures to the gastrointestinal or urinary tracts including urinary catheterisation, and certain endoscopic procedures e.g. oesophageal dilatation (*Enterococcus; Streptococcus bovis*)

ANTIBIOTIC REGIMES FOR PROPHYLAXIS IN ADULTS (AMERICAN HEART ASSOCIATION)

- *Streptococcus viridans* likely: amoxycillin 3 g orally 1 hour before procedure, then 1.5 g 6 hours later (if risk is high [e.g. prosthetic valve or prior endocarditis] initially give ampicillin and gentamicin as below). If allergic to penicillin, give erythromycin 1 g orally 2 hours before the procedure then 500 mg 6 hours later; or clindamycin 300 mg orally 1 hour before the procedure, and 150 mg six hours later.
- *Enterococcus** likely: ampicillin 2 g and gentamicin (1.5 mg/kg) IM or IV (to a maximum of 80 mg) 30 minutes before the procedure, then amoxycillin 1.5 g orally 6 hours later. In cases of penicillin allergy, vancomycin/gentamicin is an alternative.
  *20% of enterococci are now resistant to aminoglycosides; cephalosporins are *not* of value.

AORTIC DISSECTION

A tear in the intima leads to blood surging into the aortic media separating the intima and adventitia. This may be acute (presentation within 2 weeks) or chronic (presentation after 2 weeks).

CLASSIFICATION

Type I   begins in the ascending aorta and extends proximally and distally.
Type II limited to the ascending aorta and aortic arch (commonly associated with Marfan's syndrome).
Type III begins distal to the left subclavian artery and extends more distally (clinical clue: pain limited to back); this has the best prognosis.

PRESENTATIONS

1. Chest pain (typically very severe, radiating to the back, maximum in intensity at the time of onset) and hypertension—always think about the possibility of dissection.
2. Stroke, syncope (associated with tamponade), left ventricular failure (acute aortic regurgitation).
3. Atypical presentations include mesenteric ischaemia, ischaemic limb, paraplegia from spinal cord ischaemia, uncontrollable hypertension due to renin release from ischaemia of the kidney.

SIGNS

1. Decreased or absent pulses (proximal > distal dissections)—may wax and wane.
2. Hypertension (distal > proximal) unless rupture occurs (proximal > distal).
3. Acute aortic regurgitation (cardiac failure may mask peripheral signs).
4. Acute cardiac tamponade may occur (pulsus paradoxus; raised JVP, Kussmaul's sign, prominent x but absent y descent; impalpable apex with reduced heart sounds; tachycardia and hypotension).

INVESTIGATIONS

1. Trans-oesophageal echocardiography
2. Contrast CT scan of the thorax

MANAGEMENT

1. Early short-term therapy: sodium nitroprusside and beta-blockade to reduce blood pressure to a safe level.
2. Definitive therapy
   a) Acute proximal dissections: surgery.
   b) Acute distal dissections: medical therapy unless there is extension or rupture, hypertension is uncontrollable, or in Marfan's syndrome.
3. Long-term management: antihypertensive therapy, e.g. beta-blocker, calcium channel blocker (avoid hydralazine and minoxidil, which produce a hyperdynamic circulation).

SHOCK

A state in which there is generalised, serious reduction in tissue perfusion that leads to cellular dysfunction if prolonged.

CAUSES

1. Hypovolaemia
   a) External fluid losses, e.g. blood, gut (vomiting, diarrhoea), renal (diabetes, diuretics etc), skin burns, excess sweat not replaced
   b) Sequestration of fluids, e.g. ascites, haemothorax, haemoperitoneum, intestinal obstruction
2. Cardiogenic
   a) Pump failure, e.g. myocardial infarction, acute aortic regurgitation
   b) Arrhythmia
   c) Cardiac tamponade
   d) Dissecting aortic aneurysm
   e) Massive pulmonary embolus
3. Sepsis
4. Anaphylaxis
5. Addison's disease
6. Neuropathic
   a) Drugs, e.g. anaesthesia, ganglion blockers
   b) Spinal cord injury
   c) Orthostatic hypotension

ACUTE PERICARDITIS

CAUSES

- Idiopathic
- Viral
- Post infarct (Dressler's syndrome)
- Drugs: hydralazine, procainamide
- Systemic illnesses: chronic renal failure, rheumatoid arthritis, rheumatic fever, scleroderma, systemic lupus erythematosus
- Malignancy
- Trauma
- Irradiation
- Bloodstained pericardial fluid: uraemia, malignancy, tuberculosis

SYMPTOMS

- Chest pain
- Sometimes fever

SIGNS

- Pericardial rub (may be absent)
- Sinus tachycardia
- Fever

CHRONIC CONSTRICTIVE PERICARDITIS

CAUSES

1. Tuberculosis; pyogenic infection, e.g. secondary to pneumonia; histoplasmosis
2. Neoplastic disease, e.g. lung, breast; mediastinal irradiation.
3. Cardiac operation or trauma.
4. Connective tissue disease, e.g. rheumatoid arthritis; systemic lupus erythematosus
5. Acute viral infection
6. Uraemia treated by dialysis

SIGNS

Predominantly right ventricular failure
1. Cachexia, pulsus paradoxus, hypotension
2. Raised jugular venous pressure (Kussmaul's sign is rare; prominent x and y descents)
3. Impalpable apex beat, distant heart sounds, early S3, early pericardial knock
4. Hepatosplenomegaly, ascites, oedema

INVESTIGATIONS

1. ECG: low voltage QRS, diffuse T-wave flattening or inversion
2. Chest X-ray: pericardial calcification (in 50% with long-standing disease)
3. Echocardiography: pericardial thickening, abnormal septal motion
4. CT scan: increased pericardial thickness; calcification
5. Cardiac catheterisation: shows the 'square root sign' and equalisation of end-diastolic pressures

PERICARDIAL TAMPONADE

Clinical manifestations of tamponade become apparent when ventricular filling is impaired during diastole and cardiac output drops.

The common causes of tamponade are malignant pericardial effusions, viral pericarditis, uraemia and trauma (surgery, percutaneous cardiac procedures and violent trauma). The volume of fluid in the pericardial sac is not predictive of tamponade as it is the rate at which it accumulates which is more significant.

Acutely, it presents with falling arterial pressure, rising venous pressures and muffling of heart sounds. Chronically, it may present as cardiac failure.

Other clinical factors which may point to this are: paradoxical pulse (greater than 10mmHg decline in systolic pressure during inspiration), enlarged cardiac silhouette, decreased amplitude on ECG and electrical alternans.

Table 3.15 *Differentiating chronic constrictive pericarditis from acute cardiac tamponade*

Feature	Constrictive pericarditis	Tamponade
Pulsus paradoxus	absent	present
Kussmaul's sign	present	absent
ECG: electrical alternans	absent	may be present
Thickened pericardium	often present	absent
Pericardial effusion	absent	present

HYPERLIPOPROTEINAEMIAS

LDL* (in mmol/L or mg/dL) can be calculated as follows:

$$\text{LDL (mmol/L or mg/dL)} = \text{total cholesterol} - \frac{[\text{HDL} + \text{total triglycerides (mmol/L or mg/dL)}]}{5}$$

The most important predictor of coronary artery disease risk from hypercholesterolaemia is most likely the LDL: HDL ratio rather than an absolute number for either.

Best evidence of the effect of lowering cholesterol is seen in secondary prevention models where, with established CAD, lowering cholesterol decreases mortality rates.

DIET THERAPY FOR HYPERCHOLESTEROLAEMIA

INDICATIONS

When the LDL cholesterol is >3.4 mmol/L (160 mg/dL), or >3.3 mmol/L (130 mg/dL) and two or more risk factors are present (male sex, family history of premature coronary artery disease, hypertension, diabetes, vascular disease, extreme obesity, smoking, low HDL levels).

The aim of dietary intervention is to reduce total caloric intake, total fat intake and saturated fat intake.

Cholesterol levels above 6.2 mmol/L (240 mg/dL) will increase coronary mortality.

DRUGS FOR HYPERLIPIDAEMIA

Drug therapy for hypercholesterolaemia is indicated for those who on diet therapy have LDL levels >3.5 mmol/L (190 mg/dL), or >3.4 mmol/L (160 mg/dL) with two or more risk factors.

Secondary prevention with medication is indicated in patients with known coronary artery disease in whom the the total cholesterol level exceeds 5.5 mmol/L (211 mg/dL).

---

*N.B. Triglyceride levels >7.8 mmol/L (300 mm/dL) result in spuriously low LDL values using this formula.

Table 3.16 *Hyperlipoproteinaemias*

Type	Lipoprotein elevated	Electrophoretic mobility	Mechanism	Secondary causes	Clinical features	Associations
I	Chylomicrons	Origin	Deficiency of extrahepatic lipoprotein lipase or Apo CII	Rarely SLE	Eruptive xanthomata, lipaemia retinalis	Pancreatitis
IIa	LDL	β	Receptor defect	Cushing's; hypothyroidism	Xanthelasma; corneal arcus; tendon xanthomata	CAD, PVD
IIb	LDL & VLDL	β & pre-β		Cholestasis; nephrotic syndrome		
III	IDL	Broad β	Oversynthesis and/or abnormal apoprotein E	Renal and liver disease	Palmar crease and tuboeruptive xanthomata; xanthelasma	CAD, PVD
IV	VLDL	Pre β	Oversynthesis and/or undercatabolism of VLDL	Diabetes mellitus, alcoholism, chronic renal failure	Usually no xanthomata	
V	VLDL & chylomicrons	Origin and pre β	Saturation lipoprotein lipase by VLDL	As for IV	As for I	As for I

LDL = low density lipoprotein, VLDL = very low density lipoprotein, IDL = intermediate density lipoprotein; CAD = coronary artery disease, PVD = peripheral vascular disease; SLE = systemic lupus erythematosus.

Table 3.17 *Drugs for hyperlipidaemia*

Class of drug	Drug examples	Indication/ranking for use	Side effects
HMG-CoA reductase inhibitors ('statins')	Fluvastatin Pravastatin Simvastatin	Hypercholesterolaemia (1)	Elevated transaminases, myositis, abdominal pain, insomnia
Resin	Cholestyramine Colestipol	Hypercholesterolaemia (2)	Constipation, flatulence, nausea, reduced absorption of drugs
Gemfibrozil		Hypercholesterolaemia (3) Hypertriglyceridaemia (1)	Nausea, myositis, impotence, abnormal liver function tests
Niacin (nicotinic acid)		Hypercholesterolaemia (4) Hypertriglyceridaemia (3)	Flushing, pruritus, dry skin, nausea, abnormal liver function tests, hyperglycaemia, hyperuricaemia
Fish oil	Over the counter	Hypertriglyceridaemia (2)	

PHARMACOLOGY/THERAPY

Table 3.18 *Therapy for cardiac failure*

Drug	Pre-load reduction	After-load reduction
Nitrates	+	−
Angiotensin converting enzyme inhibitors	+	+
Nitroprusside	+	+
Beta-blockers	−	+
Hydralazine	−	+
Loop diuretic	+	−

Digoxin is most useful in the subgroup with atrial fibrillation but also improves symptoms for patients in sinus rhythm.

Table 3.19 Haemodynamic effects of nitrates and beta-blockers

Feature	Nitrates	Beta-blocker
Systolic blood pressure	Decreased	Decreased
Heart rate	Increased	Decreased
Left ventricular size	Decreased	Increased
Contractility	Increased	Decreased
Cardiac output	—	Decreased
Coronary arteries	Dilatation	May potentiate spasm

ANGIOTENSIN CONVERTING ENZYME INHIBITORS (ACE INHIBITORS)

These are currently the drugs of choice (±diuretics) in congestive cardiac failure and left ventricular dysfunction, as they may prolong life.

SIDE EFFECTS OF ACE INHIBITORS

(T_{50} 2 hours; excreted by the kidneys)
1. Hypotension (often a first-dose phenomenon in volume-depleted patients)
2. Taste disturbance (captopril)
3. Skin rash (10%): may be severe (captopril)
4. Proteinuria
5. Neutropenia (especially in patients with impaired kidney function and connective tissue diseases)
6. Worsening renal function with severe bilateral renal artery stenosis
7. Hyperkalaemia in patients with renal insufficiency or hyporeninaemic hypoaldosteronism
8. Cough
9. Angioneurotic oedema

Side effects are related to the sulphydryl group of the drug.

THERAPEUTIC APPROACH TO HYPERTENSION

Aim to normalise blood pressure (<140/90 mmHg) with the fewest number of drugs.

INITIAL THERAPY

Consider one of the drug classes in Table 3.20.

CONTRAINDICATIONS TO BETA-BLOCKERS

• Asthma
• Peripheral vascular disease

Drug class	Drug	Mode of action	Side effects	Contraindications
Diuretics	Thiazide	↓ Na⁺ absorption	↑ cholesterol, ↑ LDL, impaired glucose tolerance, ↑ uric acid	Gout, interstitial nephropathy, syndrome of inappropriate antidiuretic hormone (SIADH) secretion
β-blockers	β₁ selective metoprolol, atenolol	CNS β blockade Cardiac β blockade Renin β blockade	Asthma, negative inotrope, bradycardia, fatigue, depression, impotence, ↓HDL, ↑ triglycerides	Heart block, cardiac failure, asthma, peripheral vascular disease
Dihydropyridine calcium channel blockers (L-type)	Nifedipine Felodipine Amlodipine	Affect calcium channels in myocardium, myocardial conducting system and neurohormonal systems	Peripheral oedema ↑ sympathetic activity, headache, flushing	
Angiotensin converting enzyme inhibitors	'-pril'	Block conversion of angiotensin I to angiotensin II	Cough, hyperkalaemia	Bilateral renal artery stenosis
Angiotensin II receptor blockers	'-sartan'	Block angiotensin II type I receptor in adrenal cortex inhibiting aldosterone release	Hyperkalaemia	Bilateral renal artery stenosis
Centrally acting agents	Alpha methyldopa	CNS alpha₂ agonist	Fatigue, nightmares, Coombs' +ve haemolytic anaemia, hepatitis	
	Clonidine	Alpha₂ agonist	Withdrawal rebound	
Peripheral arteriolar vasodilator	Hydralazine	Direct vasodilator	SLE, tachycardia, fluid retention, headache	Aortic aneurysm, cerebral haemorrhage, ischaemic heart disease

CNS = central nervous system, SLE = systemic lupus erythematosus.

Internal Medicine

- Insulin-dependent diabetes mellitus (relative contraindication)
- Depression
- Cardiac conduction problems

Table 3.21 *Calcium channel blockers*

Characteristic	Verapamil	Nifedipine (sustained release), Amlodipine	Diltiazem
Negatively ionotropic	+ + +	+	+ +
Depresses AV node conduction	+ + + +	−	+ + +
Peripheral vasodilation	+ + +	+ + + +	+ +
Half-life	3 to 7 hours	2 to 5 hours	3 to 5 hours
Active metabolites	Yes	No	Yes
Metabolism	Hepatic (85% first pass)	Hepatic	Hepatic (50% first pass)

*Side effects: flushing, tachycardia, palpitations, headaches; may precipitate cardiac failure, severe sinus bradycardia or increase heart block if combined with beta-blockers.
May be most useful in patients with 'low renin' hypertension (elderly).

THROMBOLYTIC THERAPY

Maximum benefit derived from treating with thrombolytic therapy in the first hour after the onset of symptoms

INDICATIONS

- Ischaemic chest pain for more than 30 minutes
    and
- ST elevation of more than 1 mm in 2 contiguous leads or new left bundle branch block
    and
- Less than 12 hours since onset

ABSOLUTE CONTRAINDICATIONS:

- Active internal bleeding
- Central nervous system pathology (intracranial neoplasm, previous intracranial bleed, cerebrovascular accident in last 6 months)
- Head trauma in the last 6 months

RELATIVE CONTRAINDICATIONS:

- Age (the risk of thrombolysis-induced intracranial bleeds increases with age)

- Recent bleeding or high risk of bleeding (surgery, gastrointestinal bleed, postpartum, trauma)
- Pregnancy
- Blood pressure greater than 200/110 mmHg

SPECIFIC DRUGS

Agents activate plasminogen to plasmin which in turn breaks down fibrin and fibrinogen.

STREPTOKINASE

- Less specific for fibrin—often breaks down fibrinogen causing fibrin degradation products with antiplatelet and anticoagulant effects
- Anaphylaxis rate 0.1%. Dose cannot be repeated between 5 days and 1 year after administration
- Same patency rates at 6 hours as tPA

TISSUE PLASMINOGEN ACTIVATOR (tPA)

- Selectively binds to fibrin clot. Rapid thrombolysis
- Very short half-life (approx 5 minutes)
- Higher rate of acute intracerebral bleed especially if high-dose heparin started with high-dose tPA
- Better 30 day mortality rate than streptokinase
- Give to patients with < 4 hours of symptoms
  <75 years of age
  anterior infarcts

ELECTROCARDIOGRAPHY

To interpret the ECG, determine:
1. Rate (count the number of large squares between two QRS complexes and divide by 300)
2. Rhythm
3. Mean frontal QRS axis
   a) The normal axis is 0 to +90 degrees
   b) Use the following general rule to *estimate* the axis:
      QRS is *negative* in lead II with significant *left axis deviation*
      QRS is *negative* in lead I with significant *right axis deviation*
   c) Use the following approach to *calculate* the axis: (Figure 3.9)
      The axis is closest to the standard lead (I, II, III) with the *largest* net deflection (the axis is *positive* with an upward deflection and *negative* with a downward deflection).
      If the net deflection in any two leads is equally large, the axis is midway between them.
      Then look at the standard lead with the *smallest* deflection: if this is slightly positive or negative, add or subtract 15 degrees to the axis calculation.

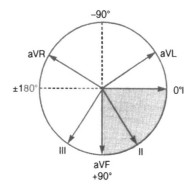

Figure 3.9 *Calculation of the mean frontal axis.*

4. Look at each lead for:
    a) P waves (normal, absent, distorted, inverted, multiple)
    b) P-R interval (normal, prolonged, short, variable)
    c) QRS complex (abnormal Q wave, widened QRS, low or high voltage QRS, abnormal shape)
    d) Q-T interval (normal, prolonged, short)
       Measure this from the beginning of the QRS to the end of the T wave:

Rate	*Normal Q-T interval* (approximately)
60	0.43
75	0.39
100	0.34

    e) S-T segment (normal, depressed, elevated)
    f) T-wave (normal, tall and peaked, flattened, inverted)
    g) U wave (absent or normal, inverted, prominent)

ECG PATTERNS

MYOCARDIAL INFARCTION

Anterior	
Superior	I, aVL
Anteroseptal	I, AVL, V1–3: Q waves, ST elevation, T wave inversion.
Anterolateral	I, AVL, V4–6: Q waves, ST elevation, T wave inversion.
Inferior	II, III, AVF: Q waves, ST elevation, T wave inversion.
Posterior	V1–2: Tall broad R wave, ST depression, tall upright T wave (usually associated with inferior or lateral infarct).
Right ventricular	V1: ST elevation (usually associated with inferior infarct).

DIFFERENTIAL DIAGNOSIS OF R WAVE > S WAVE IN V1

1. Posterior infarction
2. Right ventricular hypertrophy

3. Right bundle branch block
4. Wolff-Parkinson-White syndrome

ATRIAL ENLARGEMENT CRITERIA

Left atrium
P mitrale (notched, slurred P in I, II) (early)
P wave duration ≥0.12 secs
Biphasic P wave in VI (late)

Right atrium
P pulmonale (tall, peaked 2.5 mm amplitude in inferior leads)

VENTRTICULAR HYPERTROPHY CRITERIA

Left ventricle
R wave in V5 or V6 and S wave in V1 > 35 mm
S wave in V1, V2 or V ≥ 30 mm
R or S wave in limb lead ≥20 mm
Strain pattern (depressed ST and inverted T wave in lateral leads)
Left axis ≥30 degrees

Right ventricle
Tall R wave over right praecordium

Deep S wave over left praecordium
Strain pattern over right praecordium
Right axis deviation

BUNDLE BRANCH BLOCK CRITERIA

Left bundle branch block (LBBB)
QRS duration ≥0.12 secs
R waves notched, slurred or broad in lateral leads (I, AVL, V5–6)
QS or rS pattern over anterior praecordium
Secondary ST-T wave changes

Right bundle branch block (RBBB)
QRS duration ≥0.12 secs
R1 wave large in V1
S wave deep in V6
Q waves normal

Secondary T wave in V1

Left anterior hemiblock
Left axis deviation >–45 degrees
QRS duration 0.10 secs
rS pattern in inferior leads
qR pattern in I and AVL

Left posterior hemiblock
Right axis deviation >+90 degrees
QRS duration 0.10–0.12 secs
qR pattern in inferior leads
rS pattern in I and AVL
Exclude other causes of right axis deviation

Transient non-specific changes may occur including

Acutely
1. SI, QIII, TIII (an S wave in lead I, a Q wave in lead III and an inverted T wave in lead III: often associated with anterior ST depression—'right ventricular strain')

Internal Medicine

Chronically with pulmonary hypertension
1. P pulmonale
2. Right axis deviation and clockwise rotation
3. Right bundle branch block
4. T wave inversion in the praecordial leads
5. Atrial arrhythmias

POTASSIUM AND THE ECG

Hyperkalaemia
Tall T waves (symmetrical)
Prolonged PR interval
Widened QRS
Flattened or absent P waves
Arrhythmias—bradycardia, sinus
  arrest, nodal rhythm, ventricular
  tachycardia or fibrillation, asystole

Hypokalaemia
Flattened T waves
Depressed ST segment; prolonged QT
Tall U waves
Arrhythmias—atrial or
  ventricular tachycardia,
  ventricular fibrillation

CALCIUM AND THE ECG

Hypercalcaemia
QT shortens

Hypocalcaemia
QT lengthens

DIFFERENTIAL DIAGNOSIS OF A PROLONGED QT INTERVAL

1. Drugs, e.g. quinidine, disopyramide, procainamide, tricyclic antidepressants, antihistamines, amiodarone, sotalol
2. Electrolyte changes, e.g. hypokalaemia, hypocalcaemia, hypomagnesaemia
3. Hypothermia
4. Familial, e.g. Lange-Nielsen syndrome (autosomal recessive associated with nerve deafness); Romano-Ward syndrome (autosomal dominant)
5. Idiopathic

Table 3.22 *M-mode echocardiograms*

Disease	Characteristic findings
Hypertrophic cardiomyopathy (HCM)	Systolic anterior motion (SAM) and midsystolic closure of aortic valve
	Asymmetrical septal hypertrophy (ASH)
Mitral stenosis	Delayed mitral closure with decreased E-F slope
	Heavy echoes from thickened or calcified mitral leaflets
	Anterior motion of posterior mitral leaflet in diastole
Aortic regurgitation (chronic)	Flutter of the anterior mitral leaflet in diastole
Aortic regurgitation (acute)	Premature closure of mitral valve

66

Table 3.22 *Continued*

Disease	Characteristic findings
Mitral valve prolapse	Posterior displacement of posterior or both mitral leaflets in systole
Left atrial myxoma	Dense echoes behind anterior mitral leaflet
Pericardial effusion	Echo-free space anterior and posterior to the heart

Doppler echocardiography: important for calculating the pressure gradient across valves, and for assessing intracardiac shunts and fistulae.

Transoesophageal echocardiography: better ability to define vegetations and abscesses, aortic dissection and left atrial pathology (thrombi, masses).

PACEMAKERS

Pacemakers have three designated letters which denote the sensing and pacing activities of the machine.

The first letter designates the chamber(s) paced: atrium (a), ventricle (v) or dual (d).

The second letter denotes the chamber(s) sensed: (a), (v) or (d).

The third letter denotes how the pacemaker responds to sensing: triggered (t), inhibited (i) or dual (d). Triggered means that the pacemaker can fire during a QRS complex and inhibited has this switched off.

The letter 'R' after these three letters means that the unit has a rate-responsive ventricular pacing capability, making it responsive to normal physiological stimuli such as exercise.

RADIOFREQUENCY ABLATION

Radiofrequency ablation is the use of radiowaves to destroy electrical conduction pathways in the heart. It is performed as a percutaneous procedure.

INDICATIONS

- Re-entrant atrioventricular tachycardia and atrioventricular junction re-entrant tachycardias
- Bundle branch re-entrant ventricular tachycardia
- Re-entry / atrial tachycardias
- Monomorphic ventricular tachycardias which are stable haemodynamically

ELECTROPHYSIOLOGICAL TESTING (EPS)

These studies directly measure electrical activity in various areas of both chambers of the heart and the conducting pathways including the atrioventricular node by multipolar leads. EPS is useful for localising problems in the conducting system. Most catheters are able to sense and pace, and may be introduced through the venous or arterial system.

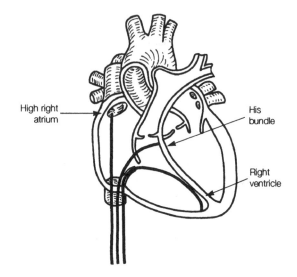

High right atrium

His bundle

Right ventricle

Figure 3.10 *Standardised lead placement for EPS.*

Programmed stimulation paces the heart with frequent low amplitude impulses. These impulses can reproduce and terminate most tachyarrhythmias.

INDICATIONS

1. DIAGNOSTIC

- Undiagnosed supraventricular tachycardias
- Undiagnosed wide complex tachycardias
- Unexplained syncope (in the presence of previous heart disease) where tachyarrhythmias are suspected
- Patients for whom implantable defibrillators are being considered

2. ASSESSING THERAPEUTIC RESPONSE

- A guide to sites for radiofrequency ablation
- A guide to efficacy of pacing devices implanted for tachyarrhythmias

4

Respiratory Medicine

IMPORTANT CLINICAL CLUES

GRADING DYSPNOEA

GRADE DEGREE

0	None
1	Slight: on walking up a hill have to stop for breath
2	Moderate: on walking on the level
3	Severe: on walking 100 metres
4	Very severe: on dressing or undressing

CLUBBING

COMMON CAUSES

CARDIAC

1. Cyanotic congenital heart disease
2. Infective endocarditis

RESPIRATORY

1. Lung carcinoma* (usually not small cell carcinoma)
2. Chronic pulmonary suppuration:
   a) Bronchiectasis
   b) Lung abscess
   c) Empyema
   d) Cystic fibrosis
3. Lung fibrosis (note—sarcoidosis is a very rare cause of clubbing)

UNCOMMON CAUSES

RESPIRATORY

1. Tuberculosis
2. Benign fibrous pleural mesothelioma* (not malignant mesothelioma)

---

*Hypertrophic pulmonary osteoarthropathy particularly associated.

Internal Medicine

GASTROINTESTINAL

1. Cirrhosis, especially biliary
2. Inflammatory bowel disease
3. Coeliac disease

ENDOCRINE

1. Thyrotoxicosis

RARE

1. Familial
2. Neurogenic diaphragmatic tumours
3. Unilateral: bronchial arteriovenous aneurysm; axillary artery aneurysm

HAEMOPTYSIS

CAUSES

RESPIRATORY

1. Lung carcinoma
2. Chronic bronchitis
3. Pulmonary infarction
4. Bronchiectasis
5. Lung abscess
6. Pneumonia
7. Tuberculosis
8. Foreign body
9. Post-traumatic
10. Vasculitic syndromes e.g. Goodpasture's syndrome
11. Idiopathic pulmonary haemosiderosis
12. Rupture of a mucosal vessel after vigorous coughing
13. Parasitic lung infection e.g. fluke

CARDIOVASCULAR

1. Mitral stenosis
2. Acute left ventricular failure
3. Mouth bleeding e.g. dental or gum disease

BLEEDING DIATHESIS

SPURIOUS

1. Nasal bleeding
2. Haematemesis

CAUSES OF MASSIVE HAEMOPTYSIS

1. Lung cancer
2. Bronchiectasis
3. Tuberculosis
4. Fungus ball
5. Lung abscess

In massive haemoptysis (200 to 600 mL in 24 hours), the cause of death is usually asphyxiation, not hypovolaemia.

HYPERVENTILATION

Tachypnoea in the absence of clinical signs of lung disease and with a normal chest X ray can be due to:
1. Psychiatric disease (panic disorder, anxiety disorder)
2. Multiple pulmonary emboli
3. Early pulmonary oedema
4. Interstitial lung disease
5. Metabolic acidosis
6. Salicylates
7. Hyperthyroidism
8. Fever or pain
9. Respiratory muscle weakness
10. Lymphangitis carcinomatosis
11. Brain disease e.g. stroke, encephalitis

CHRONIC COUGH

CAUSES

1. Postnasal drip (allergic rhinitis, chronic sinusitis)
2. Asthma
3. Gastroesophageal reflux
4. Chronic bronchitis
5. Congestive heart failure
6. Bronchiectasis
7. Interstitial lung disease
8. Drugs e.g. angiotensin converting enzyme inhibitors

COIN LESIONS

CAUSES

1. Primary lung cancer
3. Metastatic tumour
3. Granuloma
4. Hamartoma
5. Fungus ball
6. Lung abscess

FACTORS FAVOURING A SOLITARY LESION
BEING MALIGNANT

- Smoker
- Increasing age of patient
- Previous lung malignancy
- Lesion >3 cm in diameter
- Lesion not present on old X-rays
- Non-calcification of the lesion
- Irregular border of lesion on X-ray or CT scan

PATHOPHYSIOLOGY

ARTERIAL BLOOD GAS ANALYSIS

ACID-BASE DISTURBANCES

RESPIRATORY ACIDOSIS

- Acute respiratory acidosis can be detected by a lowered pH, elevated $PaCO_2$, and a rise in HCO_3^- by 1 mmol/L for every 10 mmHg increase in $PaCO_2$.
- In chronic respiratory acidosis, HCO_3^- increases by around 3.5 mmol/L for every 10 mmHg increase in $PaCO_2$.
- If the HCO_3^- is **lower** than the calculated value, there is a concurrent metabolic acidosis.
- If the HCO_3^- is **higher** than the calculated value, there is a concurrent metabolic alkalosis.

RESPIRATORY ALKALOSIS

- In acute respiratory alkalosis, there is an elevated pH, reduced $PaCO_2$, and a decrease in HCO_3^- by 2 mmol/L for every 10 mmHg decrease in $PaCO_2$.
- In chronic respiratory alkalosis, HCO_3^- should decrease 5 mmol/L for every 10 mmHg decrease in $PaCO_2$.
- If the HCO_3^- is **lower** than calculated, there is a concurrent metabolic acidosis.
- If the HCO_3^- is **higher** than calculated, there is a concurrent metabolic alkalosis.

THE AA GRADIENT

- The alveolar (PAO_2)—arterial (PaO_2) gradient is normally between 8 and 20 mmHg.

- The Aa gradient is calculated in the following way:

$$150 - \left[PaO_2 + (1.25 \times PaCO_2)\right] \text{ mmHg at sea level}$$
$$\text{breathing room air at rest}$$

- A small increase in the gradient may be due to hypoventilation, but a large increase indicates ventilation-perfusion mismatch.

DETECTING PULMONARY SHUNTING

- If the PaO_2 on 100% oxygen is known, left-to-right pulmonary shunting can be calculated in the following way:

$$\% \text{ shunt} = (620 - PaO_2 \text{ observed on } 100\% \text{ } O_2) \times 5$$

- Normally, the shunt does not exceed 7%. A 20–30% shunt is usually due to significant lung disease, and a >30% shunt is life-threatening.

HYPOXAEMIA

Causes
- Hypoventilation
- Ventilation-perfusion mismatch
- Shunt
- Impaired diffusion
- Low inspired environmental O_2, or excessive desaturation of venous blood (e.g. carboxyhaemoglobin).

HYPERCAPNIA

Causes
- Hypoventilation
- Increased perfusion over ventilation, i.e. increased physiological dead space
- Increased inspired CO_2

Table 4.1 A clinical classification of causes of respiratory failure

Hypoxaemia without CO_2 retention, clear CXR	Hypoxaemia without CO_2 retention, infiltrate on CXR	Hypoxaemia, CO_2 retention, clear CXR
Pulmonary emboli	Cardiac failure	Chronic airflow limitation
Acute airway obstruction	Interstitial disease	Severe asthma
Intracardiac shunt	Pneumonia	
	Adult respiratory distress syndrome	

CXR = chest X-ray.

OXYGEN–HAEMOGLOBIN DISSOCIATION CURVE

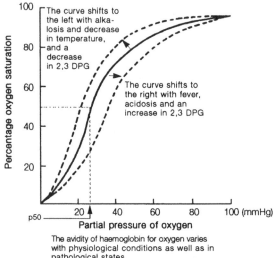

The avidity of haemoglobin for oxygen varies
with physiological conditions as well as in
pathological states.

Figure 4.1 Oxygen-haemoglobin dissociation curve.

The p_{50} is the PaO_2 at which oxygen is 50% saturated, and is normally 26 mmHg.

Causes of an **increased** affinity for O_2 (curve shifts to the left):

1. Increased pH
2. Decreased $PaCO_2$
3. Carboxyhaemoglobin and abnormal haemoglobin, e.g. fetal
4. Methaemoglobin
5. Decreased 2,3-DPG (2,3 diphosphoglycerate)

Causes of a **decreased** affinity for O_2 (curve shifts to the right):

1. Decreased pH
2. Increased $PaCO_2$
3. Abnormal haemoglobin, e.g. Kansas
4. Anaemia
5. Increased 2,3,DPG

PULMONARY FUNCTION TESTS

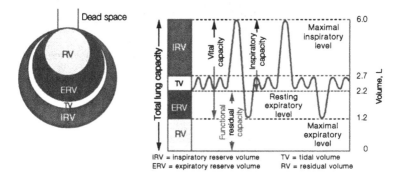

Figure 4.2 *Lung volumes and some measurements related to the mechanics of breathing.*
Adapted from Comroe JH Jr., et al. The Lung: Clinical Physiology and Pulmonary Function Tests. 2nd ed. Year Book, 1962.

INTERPRETATION OF PULMONARY FUNCTION TESTS

1. ASSESS VOLUMES

Normally vital capacity (VC) = forced vital capacity (FVC). VC is not affected by collapse of the airways, unlike FVC which is low with airway collapse.

Increases in total lung capacity (TLC), functional residual capacity (FRC), and residual volume (RV) indicate hyperinflation and gas trapping, while decreases indicate loss of lung volume or restrictive lung disease.

2. ASSESS FLOWS

Forced expiratory volume in 1 second (FEV1) is decreased in both obstructive airways disease and restrictive lung disease, but a reduced ratio of FEV1 to FVC occurs in obstruction, whereas the ratio is preserved or increased in restrictive disease.

Maximal voluntary ventilation is low in severe CAL and in neuromuscular disease, but is normal in restrictive lung disease.

3. ASSESS DIFFUSING CAPACITY (DLCO)

DLCO is the diffusing capacity for carbon monoxide. It depends on the alveolar surface area as well as pulmonary capillary volume and the haemoglobin level.

DLCO is low in emphysema, pulmonary oedema, restrictive lung disease, recurrent pulmonary emboli and anaemia.

DLCO is increased in polycythaemia, diffuse lung haemorrhage (e.g. Goodpasture's syndrome), and with an increased pulmonary capillary bed.

Table 4.2 *Characteristic pulmonary function changes in lung disease and in the elderly*

Pulmonary function test	Chronic airflow limitation	Restrictive lung disease	Elderly
FEV1/ FVC ratio	Decreased	Increased or normal	Normal
Vital capacity (VC)	Decreased or normal	Decreased	Decreased
Residual volume (RV)	Increased	Decreased	Increased
Maximum mid-expiratory flow rate (MMFR)	Decreased	Decreased or normal	Decreased
Total lung capacity (TLC)	Increased or normal	Decreased	Unchanged
DLCO	Decreased or normal	Decreased or normal	Decreased

FEV1 = Forced expiratory volume in 1 second.
FVC = Forced vital capacity.
DLCO = Diffusing capacity for carbon monoxide.

SPIROMETRY AND FLOW VOLUME LOOPS

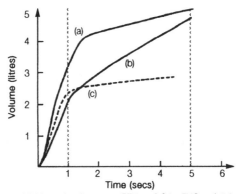

Curve (a) Normal spirometry. FEV_1 = 4.2 L, FVC = 4.8 L
(b) Obstructive defect. FEV_1 = 2.2 L, FVC = 4.5 L
(c) Restrictive defect. FEV_1 = 2.4 L, FVC = 2.8 L

Figure 4.3a *Example of spirometry.*

Flow volume loops are a sensitive way of detecting large airways obstruction, and help identify the site of obstruction. Maximum expiratory and inspiratory flows are plotted against lung volume during maximally forced inspiration and expiration.

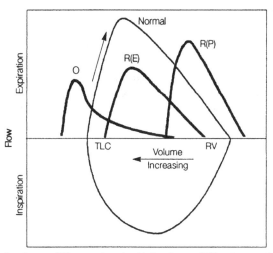

O, obstructive disease; R(P), parenchymal restrictive disease; (R(E), extraparenchymal restrictive disease with limitation in inspiration and expiration. Forced expiration is plotted in all conditions; forced inspiration is shown only for the normal curve. TLC, total lung capacity; RV, residual volume. By convention, lung volume increases to the left on the abscissa. The arrow alongside the normal curve indicates the direction of expiration from TLC to RV.

Figure 4.3b *Flow volume curves in different conditions.*
From Fauci AS, et al (editors). Harrison's Principles of Internal Medicine, 14th ed. New York: McGraw-Hill, 1998. Reproduced with permission.

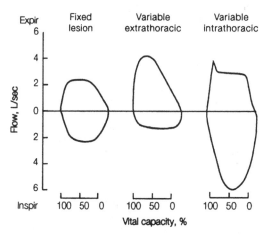

Figure 4.3c *Characteristic flow volume loops produced by major airway obstructive lesions. Expir = expiration. Inspir = inspiration*

Table 4.3 *Flow volume loops*

Pattern	Expiratory peak	Inspiratory peak
Fixed obstruction	Plateau	Plateau
Variable intrathoracic obstruction	Plateau	Preserved
Variable extrathoracic obstruction	Preserved	Plateau

DISEASE STATES

OBSTRUCTIVE LUNG DISEASE

ASTHMA

DEFINITION

Asthma is a common condition characterised by eosinophilic airway inflammation, bronchial hyper-reactivity and a reversible obstructive ventilatory defect.

DIFFERENTIAL DIAGNOSIS

1. Upper airways obstruction (inspiratory stridor usually present rather than expiratory wheeze)
2. Foreign body aspiration, tumour or bronchial stenosis (resulting in localised wheeze, often monophasic in character)
3. Bronchospasm due to chronic airflow limitation, carcinoid syndrome, recurrent pulmonary emboli, cardiogenic pulmonary oedema, systemic vasculitis, or eosinophilic pulmonary syndromes
4. Bronchospasm induced by drugs (e.g. beta-blockers, aspirin, any nebulised drug)

PATHOPHYSIOLOGY OF ALLERGIC ASTHMA

- Airway response to an inhaled allergen frequently involves an early bronchoconstrictive response which peaks within 30 minutes and resolves in 1–2 hours, followed by a late phase response from 3 to 9 hours later.
- Early asthmatic responses reflect the concentration of specific IgE, and the extent of non-specific bronchial hyper-responsiveness.
- Early responses are mediated through degranulation of mast cells and release of preformed and newly formed inflammatory mediators.
- Late phase responses are characterised by the influx of inflammatory cells.
- Late phase responses are IgE independent, with the metabolism of mast cell membrane phospholipids such as leukotrienes, platelet activating factor, and prostaglandins being chemotactic for inflammatory cells.

- Inflammatory cells, especially eosinophils, neutrophils, and T helper cells, then release further inflammatory mediators.
- Occupational exposures can induce asthma (see below).

SIGNS OF SEVERE ASTHMA

1. Exhaustion, apprehension
2. Use of accessory muscles of respiration
3. Inability to speak because of dyspnoea
4. Drowsiness—hypercapnia is a preterminal state
5. Cyanosis—preterminal
6. Tachycardia >130 beats/minute
7. Pulsus paradoxus >20 mmHg
8. Reduced breath sounds or a silent chest
9. Pneumothorax or pneumomediastinum
10. FEV1 <50% predicted
11. Respiratory failure on arterial blood gases (ABGs) ($PaO_2 < 50$ or $PaCO_2 > 50$ mmHg)

The above abnormalities indicate the need for hospital admission and urgent treatment.

TREATMENT OF ACUTE SEVERE ASTHMA

- High-flow oxygen via non-rebreather mask
- Continuous SaO_2 monitoring
- Continuous inhaled beta-agonist via nebuliser (or intravenously if patient's ventilatory effort is failing)
- Regular intravenous hydrocortisone (100 mg every 6 hours)
- Intravenous aminophylline may benefit some patients (but beware of toxicity)
- Ventilatory support if worsening respiratory failure, with mask continuous positive airway pressure (CPAP) or intubation

ALLERGIC BRONCHOPULMONARY ASPERGILLOSIS

This is a rare condition which may complicate asthma, in which a hypersensitivity reaction to the colonising organism *Aspergillus fumigatus* results in cough, dyspnoea and, frequently, worsening asthma control.

DIAGNOSTIC CRITERIA

1. Asthma
2. Pulmonary infiltrates
3. Peripheral eosinophilia
4. Immediate wheal-and-flare response to *Aspergillus fumigatus*
5. Serum precipitins to *A. fumigatus*
6. Serum IgE elevated
7. Proximal bronchiectasis

BRONCHIECTASIS

DEFINITION

Pathological dilatation of the bronchi

CAUSES

Congenital
1. Immotile cilia syndrome (0.5%). There are 2 major types of defect in this syndrome:
   a) *Dynein* arm loss—associated with sinusitis, bronchiectasis, infertility in males, and situs inversus (Kartagener's syndrome)
   b) *Radial spoke deficiency*—associated with sinusitis, nasal polyps, otitis, mastoiditis, recurrent bronchitis, and infertility in both sexes
2. Cystic fibrosis
3. Immunodeficiency (IgA deficiency, common variable immunodeficiency)

Acquired
1. Childhood infection e.g. pneumonia, pertussis, measles
2. Localised disease e.g. bronchial adenoma, tuberculosis, foreign body
3. Allergic bronchopulmonary aspergillosis (causing proximal bronchiectasis)

COMPLICATIONS

Lung
1. Pneumonia, pleurisy
2. Empyema
3. Lung abscess

Extrapulmonary
1. Cor pulmonale
2. Cerebral abscess
3. Amyloidosis

BRONCHIOLITIS

DEFINITION

Inflammation of the small airways. Bronchiolitis may be constrictive, or bronchiolitis obliterans with organising pneumonia (BOOP).

Constrictive bronchiolitis (obliterative bronchiolitis)
Results from concentric narrowing of small airways due to intramural fibrotic tissue causing scarring of bronchiolar walls and surrounding tissue.

Bronchiolitis obliterans with organising pneumonia (cryptogenic organising pneumonia)
Results from plugging of airways by granulation tissue, often with extension of the inflammation into the alveolar spaces and surrounding parenchyma. This commonly results in a restrictive pattern of abnormal lung function tests.

CAUSES

(of both forms of bronchiolitis)

1. Cigarette smoking
2. Post-infectious, e.g. adenovirus, influenza, mycoplasma
3. Connective tissue disease
4. Toxin inhalation (nitrogen oxides, chlorine, ammonia)
5. Chronic rejection after lung transplantation
6. Chronic graft-versus-host disease

CYSTIC FIBROSIS

This is an autosomal recessive disorder caused by muttiple mutations of a single gene on the long arm of chromosome 7, with its major effects on the lungs and pancreatic exocrine function.

DIAGNOSTIC CRITERIA (3 or more of the following):

1. Sweat chloride >80 mEq/L (80 mmol/L)
2. Positive clinical features—chronic sinusitis, nasal polyps, haemoptysis, atelectasis
3. Exocrine pancreatic insufficiency
4. Positive family history
5. Abnormal mucous gland biopsy

PATHOPHYSIOLOGY

- Recurrent pulmonary infection, predominantly with *Pseudomonas aeruginosa* and *Staphylococcus aureus*
- Inspissated secretions
- Bronchiectasis
- Malabsorption
- Progressive respiratory failure and cor pulmonale
- Median survival approximately 30 years

CHRONIC AIRFLOW LIMITATION—CAL (COAD, COPD)

DEFINITION

This is a spectrum of disease ranging from predominant emphysema to predominant chronic bronchitis.

Emphysema is defined pathologically as an abnormal enlargement in the size of the air spaces distal to the terminal bronchioles.

Chronic bronchitis is defined clinically as persistent cough or sputum for more than 3 months a year for 2 consecutive years.

CAUSES

1. Cigarette smoking
2. Alpha-1-antitrypsin deficiency (emphysema)
3. Occupational exposure e.g. coal, haematite (centrilobular emphysema), bauxite (bullous emphysema), cadmium (generalised emphysema)

Emphysema: Destruction of alveolar walls by enzymes released from inflammatory cells results in loss of airway tethering, with airway obstruction, and loss of alveolar-capillary units, which is reflected by a decrease in the DLCO (diffusing capacity for carbon monoxide).

Chronic bronchitis: airway obstruction results from mucous gland enlargement and smooth muscle hypertrophy, with consequent bronchial wall thickening and luminal narrowing. Recurrent bacterial infection may also be an important factor.

DIFFERENTIAL DIAGNOSIS

1. Adult onset asthma: may be non-smoker, atopic, family history of atopic disease, attacks may be episodic. Lung function may be near normal between exacerbations.
2. Bronchiectasis: daily large volume sputum production, clubbing, onset often in childhood, haemoptysis common.

COMPLICATIONS

- Chronic respiratory failure
- Cor pulmonale
- Spontaneous pneumothorax
- Recurrent lower respiratory tract infection

DIFFUSE PARENCHYMAL LUNG DISEASE

Diffuse parenchymal lung disease comprises interstitial and alveolar disorders.

A. PREDOMINANT INTERSTITIAL DISORDERS

SARCOIDOSIS

This is a systemic non-caseating granulomatous disease of unknown aetiology, typically with a predominant pulmonary component.

CLINICAL FEATURES

1. Bilateral hilar lymphadenopathy (BHL) (80%)—almost always asymptomatic.
2. Lung disease stages:
   0. No lung involvement
   1. BHL only (DLCO may be decreased)
   2. BHL and pulmonary infiltrate
   3. Fibrosing infiltrate (usually midzone) without lymphadenopathy
   4. End-stage pulmonary fibrosis
3. Skin—erythema nodosum (with BHL), lupus pernio, pink nodules in scars
4. Lymphadenopathy (generalised 7%)
5. Eyes—acute uveitis, uveoparotid fever (uveitis, parotid swelling, 7th cranial nerve palsy)

6. Nervous system—cranial nerve palsy, neuropathy, myopathy
7. Liver granulomas
8. Skeletal—bone cysts, arthritis
9. Heart—heart block, cardiomyopathy
10. Hypercalcaemia

DIAGNOSIS

Requires histological confirmation, usually via lung biopsy. Transbronchial biopsy will give a result in the majority of cases, but at times thorascopic or open lung biopsy, or biopsy of other involved tissue, is needed. Serum angiotensin converting enzyme levels may be elevated in sarcoidosis, but also in primary biliary cirrhosis, leprosy, atypical mycobacterial infection, miliary tuberculosis, silicosis, acute histoplasmosis and hyperparathyroidism. CXR reveals BHL and parenchymal infiltrates. Pulmonary function tests generally demonstrate a restrictive pattern and reduced DLCO.

IDIOPATHIC PULMONARY FIBROSIS

This is a disease of unknown aetiology with inflammation and fibrosis of alveolar walls. Without treatment there is often an inexorable deterioration to chronic respiratory failure.

DIAGNOSIS

Typical CXR appearance of diffuse interstitial opacities (and 'honeycombing' in more advanced stages of disease) and pulmonary function tests showing reduced DLCO, arterial hypoxaemia, and a restrictive ventilatory impairment suggest the diagnosis, but a lung biopsy is necessary in most cases for definitive diagnosis.

CONNECTIVE TISSUE DISEASES

Interstitial pneumonitis is a feature of a number of the multisystem autoimmune disorders. Systemic lupus erythematosus (SLE), rheumatoid arthritis, scleroderma, Sjögren's syndrome and polymyositis can all be associated with various forms of lung disease including interstitial pneumonitis and pulmonary fibrosis.

DRUG-INDUCED INTERSTITIAL LUNG DISEASE

A large number of drugs have been found to produce parenchymal lung disease. Below are some examples.

CATEGORY OF DRUG	EXAMPLE
Chemotherapeutic agents	methotrexate, busulphan
Antibiotics	nitrofurantoin
Anti-arrhythmics	amiodarone, procainamide
Disease-modifying anti-rheumatics	gold salts, D-penicillamine
Recreational	'crack' cocaine

PNEUMOCONIOSES

(See under Occupational Lung Disease)

CAUSES OF PULMONARY FIBROSIS

UPPER LOBE (mnemonic SCATO)

S—silicosis, sarcoidosis
C—coal miner's pneumoconiosis
A—ankylosing spondylitis, allergic bronchopulmonary aspergillosis, allergic alveolitis
T—tuberculosis
O—other: drugs, radiation, berylliosis, eosinophilic granuloma, necrobiotic nodular form of rheumatoid arthritis

LOWER LOBE (mnemonic RASHO)

R—rheumatoid arthritis
A—asbestosis
S—scleroderma
H—Hamman-Rich syndrome, other types of idiopathic pulmonary fibrosis
O—other: drugs (busulphan, bleomycin, nitrofurantoin, hydralazine, methotrexate, amiodarone, methysergide, sulfasalazine, gold, d-penicillamine, drugs which induce SLE, intravenous talc, aspirated oil, oxygen), radiation

CHEST X-RAY PATTERNS OF VALUE IN DIFFERENTIAL DIAGNOSIS IN INTERSTITIAL LUNG DISEASE

1. Adenopathy (hilar, mediastinal)—sarcoid, lymphoma, lymphangial carcinoma, berylliosis
2. Pleural disease associated—connective tissue disease (not dermatomyositis), asbestosis, lymphoma, carcinoma, radiation, nitrofurantoin, cardiac failure
3. Spontaneous pneumothorax—eosinophilic granuloma, lymphangioleiomyomatosis
4. Lytic rib—eosinophilic granuloma, carcinoma
5. Subcutaneous calcinosis—scleroderma, dermatomyositis

B. PREDOMINANT ALVEOLAR DISORDERS

DIFFUSE ALVEOLAR HAEMORRHAGE

CAUSES

1. Vasculitides (especially Goodpasture's syndrome)
2. Toxic injury e.g. chemical inhalation
3. Coagulopathy
4. Increased pulmonary venous hydrostatic pressure e.g. mitral stenosis
5. Idiopathic pulmonary haemosiderosis

GRANULOMATOUS VASCULITIDES

Of these, Wegener's granulomatosis and sarcoidosis are the most important. Sarcoidosis usually causes a predominant interstitial disease, but can lead to diffuse alveolar damage. Wegener's is a systemic granulomatous vasculitis with prominent upper and lower respiratory tract involvement.

CLINICAL FEATURES OF WEGENER'S GRANULOMATOSIS

- Fevers, night sweats, lethargy, malaise, weight loss
- Haemopurulent nasal discharge, nasal blockage, sinus pain
- Cough, haemoptysis, dyspnoea
- Arthralgia, arthritis
- Haematuria, hypertension

DIAGNOSIS

Over 90% of patients have positive anti-neutrophil cytoplasmic antibodies (ANCA) in the cytoplasmic pattern (c-ANCA), and anti-proteinase 3 antibodies. A combination of the typical clinical features and positive c-ANCA is sufficient to establish the diagnosis in many cases. In less clear-cut circumstances, upper airway, lung or renal biopsy will be required.

EOSINOPHILIC PULMONARY DISORDERS

ACUTE EOSINOPHILIC PNEUMONIA

This is a rare disease of unknown aetiology.

Clinical features
- Fever
- Acute hypoxaemic respiratory failure
- Diffuse pulmonary (alveolar) infiltrates on CXR
- >25% eosinophils in bronchoalveolar lavage (BAL) fluid

CHRONIC EOSINOPHILIC PNEUMONIA

Another rare disease with unknown aetiology.

Clinical features
- Constitutional symptoms—fevers, night sweats, malaise, weight loss
- Asthma, often pre-dating the disease, in the majority of cases
- Dyspnoea
- Bilateral peripheral pulmonary infiltrates
- Raised acute phase reactants
- Peripheral blood eosinophilia
- >25% eosinophils in BAL fluid

PULMONARY INFILTRATE WITH EOSINOPHILIA

CAUSES (mnemonic **PLATE**)

Prolonged pulmonary eosinophilia may be due to:
1. Drugs e.g. sulfonamides, sulfasalazine, salicylates, acute nitrofurantoin use, penicillin, isoniazid, para-aminosalicylic acid (PAS), methotrexate, procarbazine, carbamazepine, imipramine

2. Parasites e.g. ascaris
3. Idiopathic

Loeffler's syndrome: benign acute eosinophilic infiltration with few clinical manifestations
Allergic bronchopulmonary aspergillosis
Tropical e.g. microfilaria
Eosinophilic pneumonia
Other: vasculitis e.g. polyarteritis nodosa, Churg-Strauss syndrome

CLINICAL CLUES TO AETIOLOGY OF DIFFUSE PULMONARY DISEASE

1. Raynaud's phenomenon—scleroderma, pulmonary hypertension
2. Symptom onset 4–6 hours after exposure—hypersensitivity pneumonitis
3. Less dyspnoea than expected from CXR appearance—sarcoidosis, silicosis, Langerhan's cell granulomatosis (histiocytosis X)
4. Erythema nodosum—sarcoidosis, histoplasmosis
5. Dysphagia—scleroderma, dermatomyositis, metastatic cancer
6. Haemoptysis—pulmonary emboli, heart failure, bronchiectasis, Goodpasture's syndrome, idiopathic pulmonary haemosiderosis
8. Haematuria—Wegener's, Goodpasture's, SLE, polyarteritis nodosa (PAN), scleroderma.

OCCUPATIONAL LUNG DISEASE

1. PNEUMOCONIOSIS

This is lung disease due to inhalation of inorganic dust.

a) **Asbestosis**—mainly found in asbestos miners, but also in workers in the building industry, especially demolition or ships lagging workers. Asbestosis is a form of diffuse interstitial fibrosis. Asbestos exposure can also result in pleural plaque formation, and is an important risk factor for carcinoma of the lung, and mesothelioma.
b) **Silicosis**—mainly found in mining and quarrying industries. Nodular pulmonary fibrosis may progress to progressive massive fibrosis (PMF). Calcification of hilar nodes (eggshell pattern) occurs in 20%.
c) **Coal worker's pneumoconiosis (CWP)**—seen in >10% of all miners. A form of pulmonary fibrosis, there is frequently an associated obstructive lung disease due to concurrent cigarette smoking. A small percentage also develop PMF.
d) **Berylliosis**—results from exposure in the electronics, computer and ceramics industries. Beryllium can rarely cause an acute pneumonitis, and more frequently a chronic granulomatous interstitial pneumonitis. A risk factor for carcinoma of the lung.

2. ASTHMA

Occupational asthma can occur in:

a) **Biological detergent** workers (*Bacillus subtilis*)
b) **Grain and flour** workers
c) **Electronic industry** workers (colophory in solder flux)
d) **Animal** workers (urinary proteins)

e) **Paint sprayers and polyurethane** workers (isocyanates)
f) **Epoxy resins and platinum salt** workers

3. EXTRINSIC ALLERGIC ALVEOLITIS

This is a Type III hypersensitivity reaction to inhaled organic dusts or animal proteins which can manifest in acute and chronic forms.

a) **Acute**—4 to 6 hours after exposure a sensitised subject develops dyspnoea, cough, and fever without wheeze. CXR reveals nodular or reticulonodular infiltrates with apical sparing.
b) **Chronic**—repeated attacks result in lung fibrosis.

Examples

* Farmer's Lung—thermophilic bacteria from mouldy hay
* Pigeon fancier's lung—animal protein from bird droppings

Diagnosis
A consistent clinical picture in association with serum precipitins to an appropriate antigen.

4. PULMONARY OEDEMA

Due to irritant gas exposure e.g. chlorine

PULMONARY INFECTIONS

A. BACTERIAL

ORGANISMS COMMONLY IMPLICATED IN COMMUNITY-ACQUIRED PNEUMONIA

* *Streptococcus pneumoniae*
* *Mycoplasma* species
* *Legionella* species
* *Haemophilus influenzae*
* *Moraxella catarrhalis*
* *Staphylococcus aureus*

RISK FACTORS FOR NOSOCOMIAL PNEUMONIA

* Increasing age
* Underlying chronic lung disease
* Altered neurological state
* Intubation
* Immobilisation

ORGANISMS COMMONLY IMPLICATED IN NOSOCOMIAL PNEUMONIA

* Gram-negative bacilli
* *Staphylococcus aureus*
* Anaerobic bacteria
* *Streptococcus pneumoniae*

Table 4.4 Pneumonia: underlying diseases and common associated pathogens

Disease	Common pathogens to consider
Obstructing lung cancer	Pneumococcus, oral anaerobes
Chronic airflow limitation (CAL)	Pneumococcus, *H. influenzae*
Cystic fibrosis	*Pseudomonas aeruginosa, S. aureus*
Influenza virus	Pneumococcus, *S. aureus*, influenza A and B
Alcoholism	Klebsiella, oral anaerobes
Alvéolar proteinosis	Nocardia
Hypogammaglobulinaemia	Encapsulated bacteria (pneumococcus, *H. influenzae*)
Neutropenia	Gram-negative bacilli, *A. fumigatus*

Table 4.5 Atypical pneumonias

Type	Manifestations	Diagnosis	Therapy
Mycoplasma	Dry cough, headache, fever, bullous myringitis, patchy pneumonitis with few chest signs in young adults, haemolysis, Guillain-Barré, hepatitis, rash, Raynaud's	CXR; cold agglutinins; specific complement fixation test; culture	Erythromycin Tetracycline Roxithromycin
Legionnaire's disease	Dry cough, pleuritic chest pain, bilateral coarse crackles with patchy pneumonitis, hyponatraemia, hypophosphataemia, abnormal LFTs, fever	CXR; serology (single titre >1 : 256 suggestive, 4-fold rise at 2–6 weeks); fluorescent antibody sputum test	Erythromycin Rifampicin (if immunocompromised) Tetracycline Roxithromycin
Q fever	Dry cough, pleuritic chest pain, headache, fever, myalgia, granulomatous hepatitis Livestock workers	Lower lobe consolidation on CXR; complement fixation test in those with hepatitis/endocarditis	Tetracycline
Psittacosis	Dry cough, pleuritic chest pain, headache, fever, patchy pneumonitis Bird handlers	CXR; complement fixation test	Tetracycline

LFTs = liver function tests.

88

CAUSES OF RECURRENT PNEUMONIA

(2 or more episodes in 6 months)
1. Bronchial obstruction by a lung cancer
2. Bronchiectasis
3. Recurrent pulmonary infarction
4. Recurrent aspiration of gastric contents
5. Hypogammaglobulinaemia (congenital or acquired)
6. Pulmonary eosinophilia
7. HIV infection

CAUSES OF A SLOWLY RESOLVING PNEUMONIA

1. Bronchial obstruction by a cancer or foreign body
2. Complications of pneumonia—abscess, empyema
3. Inappropriate therapy
4. Decreased host resistance
5. Pharyngeal pouch with spilling

B. VIRAL

VIRUSES WHICH MAY CAUSE PNEUMONIA IN ADULTS

- Influenza A or B
- Adenovirus
- Respiratory syncytial virus
- Parainfluenza

C. FUNGI

FUNGI WHICH MAY CAUSE LUNG INFECTION

- *Histoplasma capsulatum*
- *Aspergillus fumigatus*
- *Cryptococcus neoformans*
- *Blastomyces dermatiditis*
- *Coccidioides immitis*
- *Nocardia* species
- *Actinomyces*

CHEST X-RAY FINDINGS IN FUNGAL LUNG INFECTION

CXR findings	Associated fungal infection
Lung calcification	Histoplasmosis (spleen often also calcified)
Hilar lymphadenopathy	Histoplasmosis, blastomycosis, coccidiodomycosis
Cavitary disease	Nocardiosis, blastomycosis (thick-walled) Coccidiodomycosis (thin-walled)
Round opacity, with halo of translucency	Aspergilloma
Pleural effusion	Actinomycosis, nocardiosis, coccidiodomycosis

FUNGAL INFECTIONS OF THE LUNG AND EXTRAPULMONARY DISEASE

Anatomical sites	Possible fungal infection
Lung and skin	Blastomycosis (erythema nodosum)

89

	Coccidiodomycosis (erythema nodosum, morbilliform rash)
	Nocardiosis (subcutaneous abscess)
	Cryptococcosis (tiny papules, progress to ulcers)
Lung, nose, palate	Mucormycosis, aspergillosis
Lung, bone	Actinomycosis, blastomycosis, coccidiodomycosis
Lung, gut	Candida, histoplasmosis, aspergillus, actinomycosis
Lung, urinary tract	Blastomycosis (males)

MORPHOLOGICAL CLUES TO DIAGNOSIS OF FUNGAL INFECTION

Morphology	**Fungus**
45 degree angled branching	Aspergillus
90 degree angled branching & non-septate hyphae	Nocardia
Thick cell wall	Cryptococcus
Broad neck budding	Blastomycosis
Acid-fast fungus	Nocardia

D. MYCOBACTERIA

TUBERCULOSIS

(infection with *Mycobacterium tuberculosis*)
1. Primary infection—subject never previously exposed.
   Primary complex consists of Ghon focus in mid or lower lung zone and hilar lymphadenopathy
2. Secondary—usually reactivation of dormant infection.
   Lesions develop in the upper lobe or apex of the lower lobe with minimal lymphadenopathy
3. Extrapulmonary involvement occurs in up to 20% of patients.

DIAGNOSIS

1. Mantoux (PPD)—≥ 5 mm induration signifies previous or current infection, or BCG immunisation. False negatives may occur in miliary TB, immunosuppressed patients (e.g. HIV infection, malnutrition, concurrent use of corticosteroids), elderly individuals, sarcoidosis, coexisting infection (e.g. lepromatous leprosy), or due to technical error.
2. Chest X-ray abnormalities.
3. Microbiology—acid-fast staining on sputum, bronchoalveolar lavage fluid, or gastric washings.

MANAGEMENT

1. Chemoprophylaxis with daily isoniazid for 12 months is indicated if:
   - conversion to positive Mantoux test (10 mm or more <35 years, 15 mm or more >35 years) within last 2 years
   - HIV positive with Mantoux reaction 5 mm or more
   - recent contact with infectious patient, Mantoux 10 mm or more
   - chronic illness or immunosuppressed, Mantoux 10 mm or more

- high-incidence group, Mantoux 10 mm or more, <35 years of age (from endemic area, nursing home or institution)
2. Standard therapy
   - Isoniazid plus rifampicin for 9 months
     OR
   - Isoniazid plus rifampicin for 6 months with pyrazinamide for first 2 months
3. Therapy for drug-resistant cases
   - Suspect resistance in HIV-positive patients, injecting drug users, institutionalised individuals, and immigrants from endemic areas
   - Add in a fourth drug such as ethambutol or streptomycin

Table 4.6 *Drugs for tuberculosis*

Drug	Side effects	Comments
Isoniazid	Hepatitis (<1%; fast acetylators; increased >35 years)	Supplemental vitamin B_6 (pyridoxine) reduces the risk of peripheral neuropathy
	Peripheral neuropathy (especially slow acetylators)	
	Flu-like illness, fever	
	Skin rash, purpura, arthritis, lupus phenomenon	
Rifampicin	Hepatitis	Increases metabolism of OCP*, steroids, warfarin, digoxin, and oral hypoglycaemic agents
	Fever	
	Thrombocytopenia, haemolytic anaemia (rare)	
	Light chain proteinuria	
	Orange discoloration of urine	
Ethambutol	Retrobulbar optic neuritis (reversible)	Screen for side effects with red-green colour discrimination and visual acuity testing
	Skin rash	

*OCP = oral contraceptive pill.

NON-TUBERCULOUS MYCOBACTERIAL INFECTION

Organisms
- *Mycobacterium avium*
- *Mycobacterium kansasii*

Clinical manifestations in non-immunosuppressed patients
- Chronic, slowly progressive pneumonitis
- Usually elderly patients with chronic airflow limitation

ENVIRONMENTAL FACTORS IN PULMONARY INFECTION

ENVIRONMENTAL EXPOSURE HISTORY INFECTIONS TO CONSIDER

Water cooling units	Legionella
Military camps	Mycoplasma
Birds	Psittacosis, histoplasmosis, aspergillus
Dogs, cats, rats, pigs, cattle	Leptospirosis
Goats, pigs, cattle	Q fever
Abattoirs, vets	Brucellosis
Soil	Blastomycosis
Decaying wood, caves, chickens	Histoplasmosis
Florists, gardeners, plants, straw	Sporotrichosis

PLEURAL DISEASE

PLEURAL EFFUSION

EXUDATE

Features
- protein >3 g/100 mL (30 g/L)
- pleural/serum protein >0.5
- lactate dehydrogenase (LDH) >200 IU/L
- pleural/serum lactate dehydrogenase (IU/L) >0.6

Causes
- Pneumonia
- Neoplasm—lung carcinoma, metastatic carcinoma, mesothelioma
- Tuberculosis
- Pulmonary infarction
- Subphrenic abscess
- Pancreatitis
- Connective tissue disease (SLE, rheumatoid arthritis)
- Drugs—nitrofurantoin (acute)
          methysergide (chronic)
          chemotherapy
- Radiation
- Trauma

TRANSUDATE

Features
- Protein <3 g/100 mL
- Pleural/serum protein <0.5
- LDH <200 IU/L
- pleural/serum LDH <0.6

Causes
- Cardiac failure
- Nephrotic syndrome

- Liver failure
- Meigs' syndrome (ovarian fibroma and effusion)
- Hypothyroidism

PLEURAL FLUID CHANGES IN DIFFERENT DISEASE STATES

Pleural fluid analysis	Disease associated
pH <7.2	empyema (except *Proteus* where pH >7.8) TB, neoplasm, rheumatoid arthritis, oesophageal rupture
Glucose <3.3 mmol/L (<60 mg/dL)	infection, neoplasm, rheumatoid arthritis, mesothelioma
Red blood cells >5000/uL	pulmonary embolism, neoplasm, trauma, asbestosis, pancreatitis
Amylase >200 units/100 mL	pancreatitis, ruptured abdominal viscera, oesophageal rupture (salivary amylase)
Complement decreased	SLE, rheumatoid arthritis
Chylous (triglycerides >1.26 mmol/L [110 mg/dL])	tumour, thoracic duct trauma, TB, tuberous sclerosis
Cholesterol effusion	rheumatoid arthritis, nephrotic syndrome, old TB

PNEUMOTHORAX

CAUSES

1. Spontaneous
   a) Subpleural bullae (apical) that rupture usually young adults
   b) Emphysema
   c) Rare causes
      asthma
      eosinophilic granuloma
      lymphangioleiomyomatosis
      lung abscess
      carcinoma
      end-stage fibrosis
      Langerhan's cell granulomatosis
      Marfan's syndrome
      Pneumocystis carinii pneumonia
2. Traumatic
   a) Rib fracture
   b) Penetrating injury
   c) Pleural aspiration
   d) High positive end-expiratory pressure (PEEP) or mechanical ventilation
   e) Oesophageal rupture

1. >30% pneumothorax
2. Tension pneumothorax
3. Respiratory compromise, e.g. hypoxaemia

LUNG CANCER

CLASSIFICATION

1. Squamous cell carcinoma—30%
2. Small cell carcinoma—25%
   a) oat cell
   b) intermediate cell
3. Adenocarcinoma—30%
   c) acinar, papillary, solid with mucus
   d) bronchoalveolar (solitary peripheral lesion, or diffuse disease which may be confused with pneumonia)
4. Large cell carcinoma—15%
   e) giant cell
   f) clear cell

CLINICAL PRESENTATION

- cough
- haemoptysis
- chest pain
- dyspnoea
- incidental finding on a chest X-ray

RISK FACTORS

1. Smoking (80–90% of all cases)
2. Increasing age
3. Asbestos exposure (both carcinoma and mesothelioma). Smoking is synergistic
4. Radiation exposure—especially in uranium workers. Smoking is synergistic
5. Other occupational exposure (aromatic hydrocarbons, arsenic, vinyl chloride, chromium, nickel, haematite, chromate, methyl ether)
6. Previous lung cancer resected—5% per year risk of a second primary
7. Pulmonary fibrosis

COMPLICATIONS

LOCAL EXTENSION

1. Pleural effusion
2. Rib fractures
3. Nerve involvement:
   — Pancoast's syndrome (apical tumour causing T1 nerve root lesion and Horner's syndrome)

— Left recurrent laryngeal nerve palsy, usually due to a left hilar tumour
— Diaphragmatic paralysis due to phrenic nerve palsy
4. Superior vena caval obstruction
5. Pericardial disease
6. Oesophageal obstruction
7. Tracheal obstruction
8. Lymphangitis

DISTANT METASTASES

Most commonly to cervical nodes, brain, liver, bone and adrenal glands.

Table 4.7 Lung cancer

Feature	Small cell lung cancer (≤25% of lung cancers)	Non-small cell lung cancer (adenocarcinoma, squamous cell carcinoma, large cell undifferentiated)
Origin	Neuroendocrine	Bronchial mucosa
Chest X-ray	Tends to involve the hilum.	Central or peripheral lesion.
Clinically	Rapid progression of symptoms, fast growing, not associated with clubbing.	Slower growing, clubbing more common, often subtle onset of symptoms.
Staging	Limited extent—limited to one hemithorax including ipsilateral supraclavicular fossa. Extensive—all other patterns of spread.	Stage I*—localised to one lobe of the lung. Stage II—involvement of ipsilateral bronchial or hilar lymph nodes. Stage III—involvement of pleura ± mediastinal or supraclavicular lymph nodes. Stage IV—distant disease.
Treatment	Limited disease—very responsive to chemotherapy and radiotherapy. Combined treatment significantly prolongs life and 5–10% of patients are long-term survivors. Extensive disease— combination chemotherapy doubles life-expectancy to approximately 9 months.	Stage I, II—surgery or radiotherapy if surgery contraindicated. Long-term survival of 15%. Stage III—management is controversial but may involve chemotherapy, radiotherapy and surgery. Stage IV—palliative management.

Table 4.7 *Continued*

Feature	Small cell lung cancer (≤25% of lung cancers)	Non-small cell lung cancer (adenocarcinoma, squamous cell carcinoma, large cell undifferentiated)
Metastatic spread	Bone, liver, adrenals. 50% of patients will have evidence of central nervous system involvement.	Bone, liver, brain, adrenals.

*For formal staging a Tumour/Node/Metastases (TNM) classification is used, but this provides a useful clinical framework.

METASTATIC CARCINOMA TO THE LUNG: CHEST X-RAY PATTERNS

Nodular pattern	**Infiltrative pattern**
Renal cell carcinoma	Adenocarcinomas e.g. prostate, stomach, pancreas
Testicular	Lymphoma
Transitional cell bladder	Follicular cell thyroid
Colon	
Breast	
Melanoma	

MEDIASTINAL MASSES ON CHEST X-RAY

Anterior (the 5 'T's)	**Middle**	**Posterior**
Thyroid	Bronchogenic cyst	Aortic aneurysm
Thymoma	Pleuropericardial cyst	Paravertebral abscess
Teratoma		Neurogenic tumour
Terrible lymphoma or carcinoma		e.g. neurofibroma
Tortuous vessels		Hiatus hernia

PULMONARY VASCULAR DISEASE

PULMONARY HYPERTENSION

DEFINITION

Pulmonary hypertension exists when mean pulmonary artery pressure is greater than 20 mmHg.

CAUSES

1. Primary pulmonary hypertension
2. Secondary pulmonary hypertension

a) recurrent pulmonary embolism
b) parenchymal disease (e.g. emphysema)
c) reactive hypoxic vasoconstriction (e.g. sleep apnoea)
d) mechanical compression (e.g. kyphoscoliosis)
e) overperfusion (e.g. left-to-right shunt)
f) cardiac disease (e.g. mitral stenosis)
g) pulmonary veno-occlusive disease

PULMONARY EMBOLISM

- 10% of deep venous thromboses result in pulmonary embolism
- 10% of pulmonary emboli are fatal
- The majority of pulmonary emboli remain undiagnosed

SLEEP-DISORDERED BREATHING

SLEEP APNOEA

TYPES

1. Obstructive
2. Central
3. Mixed

RISK FACTORS FOR OBSTRUCTIVE SLEEP APNOEA

- Obesity
- Male sex
- Increasing age
- Upper airway anatomical abnormalities
- Use of sedative medications including alcohol
- Hypothyroidism

CLINICAL FEATURES OF OBSTRUCTIVE SLEEP APNOEA

- Loud snoring
- Apnoeic spells
- Daytime hypersomnolence
- Morning headache
- Pulmonary hypertension
- Cardiac arrhythmias
- Stroke

DIAGNOSIS

- Overnight sleep study, demonstrating repetitive apnoeas (cessation of airflow >10 seconds) and oxygen desaturation

TREATMENT OF OBSTRUCTIVE SLEEP APNOEA

- Weight loss
- Nasal CPAP

PHARMACOLOGY

BRONCHODILATORS

BETA-ADRENOCEPTOR AGONISTS

Examples
- Salbutamol, terbutaline (short-acting)
- Salmeterol, eformoterol (long-acting)

Actions
- Relax bronchial smooth muscle
- Inhibit mediator release from mast cells
- May increase mucus clearance through effect on cilia

Uses
- Asthma
- Chronic airflow limitation if some reversibility present

Side effects
- Tremor
- Hypokalaemia
- Tachycardia

METHYLXANTHINES

Examples
- Theophylline, aminophylline

Actions
- Inhibit phosphodiesterase, increase intracellular cyclic AMP
- Relax bronchial smooth muscle
- Possibly inhibit inflammatory cell activation

Uses
- Second line therapy in asthma, but low therapeutic index
- Clearance increased by tobacco, marijuana and phenobarbitone
- Clearance decreased by hepatic failure, cimetidine, phenytoin, the oral contraceptive pill, propranolol, erythromycin and cardiac failure

Side effects
- Nausea, diarrhoea
- Arrhythmias
- Tremor
- Seizures

ANTICHOLINERGICS

Example
- Ipratropium bromide

Actions
- Relax bronchial smooth muscle by inhibiting vagal tone

Uses
- Asthma
- Chronic airflow limitation

Side effects
- Nil significant

ANTI-INFLAMMATORY AGENTS

SODIUM CROMOGLYCATE AND NEDOCROMIL SODIUM

Actions
- Reduce bronchial hyper-responsiveness and both immediate and late phases of the asthmatic reaction through unknown mechanisms

Uses
- Asthma
- Exercise-induced asthma

Side effects
- Nil significant

INHALED CORTICOSTEROIDS (BUDESONIDE, FLUTICASONE, BECLOMETHASONE)

Actions
- Reduce airway inflammation, predominantly through inhibition of the generation of leukotrienes and prostaglandins, thereby limiting chemotaxis of inflammatory cells, especially eosinophils. With regular use, they inhibit both the early and late phases of the allergic response in the lungs.

Uses
- Regular inhaled steroids should be used in any patient with symptoms of chronic asthma.
- Courses of inhaled steroids should be used in asthmatics who have intermittent symptoms for all but mild exacerbations.

Side effects
- Oropharyngeal candidiasis
- Dysphonia
- Adrenal suppression and systemic steroid side effects are unusual, even with high chronic doses

5

Gastroenterology

OESOPHAGUS

CLINICAL CLUES

1. Differentiate odynophagia (painful swallowing) from difficulty swallowing and pharyngeal dysphagia.
2. Pharyngeal dysphagia presents with difficulty initiating swallowing (e.g. motor neurone disease) or nasal regurgitation and choking on ingestion (e.g. bulbar or pseudobulbar palsy).
3. Oesophageal dysphagia—ask
   a) What type of food produces dysphagia (*solids only*—consider structural problems e.g. strictures, carcinoma; *solids and liquids*—consider motor problems e.g. achalasia, diffuse oesophageal spasm)?
   b) What is the symptom course (*intermittent*—suggests a lower oesophageal ring or oesophageal spasm; *progressive*—suggests stricture, carcinoma, achalasia)?
   c) Is heartburn present (if yes: consider reflux with stricture formation, scleroderma or reflux with Barrett's oesophagus and cancer)?

PATHOPHYSIOLOGY

Gastro-oesophageal reflux disease usually presents with heartburn. Atypical presentations include adult-onset asthma, chronic cough, non-cardiac chest pain, dental caries and nausea.

The major mechanism implicated is transient lower oesophageal sphincter relaxation.

FACTORS INFLUENCING LOWER OESOPHAGEAL SPHINCTER PRESSURE

Pressure is increased by:
1. Gastrin (pharmacological but not physiological doses)
2. Dopaminergic receptor blockers, e.g. metoclopramide
3. Antacids (not alginic acid)
4. Cholinergic drugs

Pressure is decreased by:
1. Cholecystokinin, progesterone
2. Fatty meal, chocolate
3. Nicotine, alcohol
4. Theophylline
5. Anticholinergic drugs, calcium channel blockers, nitrates

DISEASE STATES

ODYNOPHAGIA (PAIN ON SWALLOWING)

CAUSES

Infections
- Herpes simplex
- Cytomegalovirus
- Candidiasis

Chemical or inflammatory
- Gastro-oesophageal reflux
- Drug-induced—slow-release potassium chloride, alendronate, tetracyclines, quinidine
- Radiation
- Graft *vs* host disease
- Crohn's disease
- Dermatological diseases (pemphigus, pemphigoid)
- Swallowing corrosive chemicals (alkalis)

OESOPHAGEAL DYSPHAGIA

CAUSES

Structural disorders
- Stricture (peptic, caustic, pill-induced, radiation-induced)
- Tumour
- Rings and webs
- Extrinsic compression (e.g. enlarged left atrium, aberrant right subclavian artery)

Oesophageal motor disorders
- Achalasia
    - Incomplete lower oesophageal sphincter relaxation
    - Aperistalsis in the oesophageal body
    - Elevated basal lower oesophageal sphincter (LOS) pressure, >25 mmHg (3.3 kPa)
- Diffuse oesophageal spasm
  Simultaneous ('spastic') non-peristaltic contractions that are repetitive (>2 peaks) and of increased duration (>5.5 seconds) with normal peristalsis intermittently

- Scleroderma
  Low to absent lower oesophageal sphincter pressure, weak to absent peristalsis in distal oesophagus and normal upper oesophageal sphincter and peristalsis
- 'Nutcracker' oesophagus
  Very high peristaltic amplitude—mean of 10 wet swallows >120 mmHg (16 kPa)—in distal oesophagus with normal peristalsis sequence
- Hypersensitive LOS
  High lower oesophageal sphincter pressure—mean >25 mmHg (3.3 kPa)—but normal relaxation and normal peristalsis in the body of the oesophagus

OESOPHAGEAL CANCER

SQUAMOUS CELL CARCINOMA

Predisposing factors
1. Smoking, alcohol
2. Lye stricture (>25 years later)
3. Plummer-Vinson syndrome (cervical oesophageal web and iron deficiency anaemia)
4. Tylosis (see Table 15.2)

ADENOCARCINOMA

1. Incidence increasing
2. Barrett's oesophagus (≥3 cm intestinal metaplasia in oesophagus) major predisposing factor

STOMACH AND DUODENUM

CLINICAL CLUES

DYSPEPSIA

Definition: Chronic or recurrent pain or discomfort centered in the upper abdomen (should be distinguished from classical biliary colic due to gallstones).

CAUSES

1. Non-ulcer (functional) dyspepsia (50%)
2. Chronic peptic ulcer
3. Gastro-oesophageal reflux disease (with or without oesophagitis)
4. Gastric cancer
5. Chronic pancreatitis
6. Mesenteric angina (presents with postprandial pain, fear of eating and weight loss)

7. Metabolic e.g. hypercalcaemia, uraemia, diabetes mellitus, thyroid disease, porphyria
8. Drugs e.g. non-steroidal anti-inflammatory drugs (NSAIDs), theophylline, digitalis, iron, alcohol

NAUSEA AND VOMITING

CAUSES

1. Intestinal obstruction
   Anatomical
   - Small bowel obstruction e.g. adhesions
   - Gastric outlet obstruction e.g. pyloric ulcer
   Functional
   - Diabetic gastroparesis
   - Idiopathic gastroparesis
   - Chronic intestinal pseudo-obstruction
2. Infections
   - Food poisoning (especially *Staph. aureus*, *B. cereus)*
   - Viral or bacterial diarrhoea
   - Acute viral hepatitis
3. Central nervous system disorders
   - Migraine
   - Meningitis
   - Increased intracranial pressure
   - Meniere's disease
   - Motion sickness
4. Metabolic disorders
   - Hypercalcaemia
   - Renal failure
   - Diabetic ketoacidosis
   - Adrenal insufficiency
   - Hyperthyroidism
5. Drugs and radiation therapy
   - Alcohol
   - Digitalis
   - Theophyllines
   - Opioids
   - Chemotherapeutic agents
6. Visceral pain
   - Peritonitis
   - Cholecystitis
   - Pancreatitis
7. Psychiatric disorders
   - Anorexia or bulimia nervosa
8. Other
   - Pregnancy
   - Conditioned reflexes
   - Panic attacks

PATHOPHYSIOLOGY

Table 5.1 *Gastrointestinal peptide hormones with physiological roles*

Peptide hormone	Cell and organ	Action	Releasers
Gastrin	G cell in antrum and duodenum	Increases gastric acid	Gastric distension Protein Calcium
Cholecystokinin	I cell in duodenal mucosa	Increases pancreatic enzyme secretion, gallbladder contraction	Protein Fat
Secretin	S cell in duodenal mucosa	Increases pancreatic bicarbonate secretion	Acid? Fat?

OTHER GASTROINTESTINAL PEPTIDE HORMONES

Other peptides or hormones with probable physiological roles include:

- Neurotensin—released from ileum and right colon; may mediate the 'ileal brake' (reduction in gastric acid secretion and upper gut motility when fats and carbohydrates reach the distal small bowel).
- Motilin—released from duodenum—involved in the regulation of the migratory motor complex ('intestinal housekeeper').
- Vasoactive intestinal polypeptide (VIP)—modulates inhibition of smooth muscle, e.g. lower oesophageal sphincter, intestinal fluid secretion.
- Somatostatin—modulates general inhibition of gastrointestinal smooth muscle.

DISEASE STATES

CHRONIC GASTRITIS

Table 5.2 *Features of chronic gastritis*

Feature	Type A	Type B
Autoimmune disease	Yes	No (*H. pylori* infection)
Pernicious anaemia	10%	No
Parietal cell antibody	90%	Absent
Intrinsic factor antibody	15%	Absent
Area usually affected	Gastric body	Gastric antrum
Serum gastrin (fasting)	Elevated	Low to normal

DIAGNOSIS OF *HELICOBACTER PYLORI* INFECTION

- **Serology** (IgG): cheap, sensitive and specific (>90%), *not* useful to follow-up success of treatment.
- **Urea breath test:** highly sensitive and specific (>95%), ^{13}C non-radioactive, ^{14}C radioactive.
- **Histology:** highly sensitive and specific (>90%).
- **Culture:** lower sensitivity but 100% specific; useful to document antibiotic resistance in those who have repeatedly failed treatment.

H. PYLORI INFECTION AND DISEASE

Associated with:
1. Chronic duodenal ulcer (>95%)
2. Gastric ulcer (80%)
3. Gastric adenocarcinoma (80%)
4. Mucosa associated lymphoid tissue (MALT) lymphoma (100%)

NON-STEROIDAL ANTI-INFLAMMATORY DRUG (NSAID) INDUCED ULCERS

Chronic NSAID users are at a 3–6 times increased risk of ulcer bleeding, perforation or death. This risk is increased with the simultaneous use of glucocorticoids.
Risk of peptic ulcer complications increased by:
1. Advanced age (≥60 years) and female gender
2. Past history of peptic ulcer
3. High dose
4. First three months of treatment
5. Presence of other severe illnesses

Effective prophylaxis in high-risk patients requiring long term NSAIDs:
1. Misoprostol
2. High-dose H_2 antagonist (standard dose only reduces duodenal, not gastric ulcer)
3. Proton pump inhibitor
4. *H. pylori* eradication

N.B. Enteric coated or rectal NSAIDs do *not* reduce the risk. Specific cyclo-oxygenase(cox)II inhibitors have a much lower risk of ulceration.

CAUSES OF UPPER GASTROINTESTINAL BLEEDING

More common
1. Chronic peptic ulcer (duodenal ulcer 40%, stomach ulcer 20%)
2. Acute peptic ulcer (erosions) (5%)
3. Mallory-Weiss tear (10%).

Less common
1. Oesophageal and gastric varices
2. Erosive oesophagitis, carcinoma (gastric, oesophageal)

3. Aortoenteric fistula (rare, but always consider this if the patient has had an abdominal aortic graft)
4. Dieulafoy's ulcer (localised defect that involves an ectatic submucosal artery)
5. Arteriovenous malformations
6. Hereditary telangiectasia, pseudoxanthoma elasticum, Ehlers-Danlos syndrome, blue rubber bleb naevus syndrome, vasculitis, amyloid
7. Watermelon stomach (gastric antral vascular ectasias)
8. Bleeding diathesis (e.g. disseminated intravascular coagulopathy)
9. Cameron ulcers (in a large hiatus hernia)
10. Portal hypertensive gastropathy

GIANT GASTRIC FOLDS

Causes
1. Zollinger-Ellison syndrome
2. Ménétrièr's disease (associated with hypoalbuminaemia and oedema)
3. Hypertrophic gastropathy (hyperchlorhydric)
4. Lymphoma (the giant gastric folds cross into the duodenum)
5. Carcinoma
6. Chronic renal failure
7. Normal variant
8. Cronkhite-Canada syndrome

SMALL AND LARGE INTESTINE

CLINICAL CLUES

DIARRHOEA: CLINICAL FRAMEWORK

A useful clinical framework is to distinguish between colonic ('left sided') and small bowel ('right sided') diarrhoea. With colonic diarrhoea (often due to inflammation) there is typically blood, mucus, tenesmus, urgency and frequent small volume stools. With small bowel diarrhoea there is no blood, mucus, tenesmus or urgency; the stools are of large volume with only a modest increase in stool frequency.

Evaluate the clinical features—they can provide clues to the likely diagnosis.

History
1. Youth—consider coeliac disease, inflammatory bowel disease, lactase deficiency
2. Oil droplets or muscle fibres in stool—pancreatic insufficiency
3. Recent travel—parasites, *E. coli* etc
4. Previous surgery—bacterial overgrowth, dumping, postvagotomy diarrhoea, ileal resection, short bowel syndrome, previous cholecystectomy
5. Recurrent or severe peptic ulcer disease—Zollinger-Ellison syndrome

6. Medications—laxatives, magnesium antacids, antibiotics, lactulose, colchicine
7. Frequent infections—immunoglobulin deficiency
8. Family history of diarrhoea—coeliac disease, inflammatory bowel disease, lactase deficiency, familial polyposis coli

Physical examination
1. Marked weight loss—thyrotoxicosis, cancer, malabsorption, inflammatory bowel disease
2. Arthritis—inflammatory bowel disease, Whipple's disease
3. Hyperpigmentation—Whipple's disease, Addison's disease, coeliac disease, Cronkhite-Canada syndrome
4. Fever—inflammatory bowel disease, amoebiasis, lymphoma, tuberculosis, Whipple's disease
5. Chronic lung disease—cystic fibrosis
6. Postural hypotension—diabetes mellitus, Addison's disease
7. Neuropathy—diabetes mellitus, amyloidosis
8. Onycholysis—Cronkhite-Canada

Laboratory screen
1. Abnormal liver function tests—inflammatory bowel disease, colonic cancer with metastases, coeliac disease with autoimmune chronic hepatitis
2. Lymphopenia (and hypoproteinaemia)—lymphangiectasia
3. Eosinophilia—parasites, eosinophilic gastroenteritis

Faecal leucocytes
1. Increased—infectious colitis, pseudomembranous colitis, inflammatory bowel disease
2. Absent—viral causes, enterotoxigenic diarrhoea, hormonal causes, laxative abuse, coeliac disease

PATHOPHYSIOLOGY OF DIARRHOEA—Mechanisms and causes

1. SECRETORY (net secretion exceeds absorption)

Characteristics
a) High volume (commonly >1 L/day)
b) Stool osmolality = 2 [stool (Na) and (K)]; the osmotic gap is normal, i.e. <30–40 mmol/L
c) Persists with fasting
d) Watery diarrhoea: no pus, blood or steatorrhoea

Causes
a) Associated with an adenylate-cyclase mechanism
   i) Infection with enterotoxin-producing bacteria, e.g. *Vibrio cholera, E. coli*
   ii) Hormonal, e.g. vasoactive intestinal polypeptide (VIP)oma

   iii) Methylxanthines, e.g. theophylline, caffeine
   iv) Bile acids, e.g. post-ileal resection or disease
b) Not associated with an adenylate-cyclase mechanism
   i) Infections, e.g. *Staphylococcus aureus, Shigella, Clostridium perfringens*, viral
   ii) Hormonal, e.g. gastrin (Zollinger-Ellison syndrome), calcitonin (medullary carcinoma of thyroid), serotonin (carcinoid syndrome)
   iii) Villous adenoma

2. OSMOTIC (diarrhoea due to solvent drag)

Characteristics
a) Disappears with fasting
b) Stool osmolality >2 [stool (Na and K)]; usually the osmotic gap is >100 mmol/L
c) Large frothy stools related to ingestion of food

Causes
a) Carbohydrate malabsorption, e.g. disaccharide deficiency
b) Ingestion of poorly absorbed solute, e.g. magnesium antacids, mannitol, sorbitol, lactulose
c) Postsurgical, e.g. vagotomy and pyloroplasty, gastrojejunostomy

3. ABNORMAL INTESTINAL MOTILITY

Causes
a) Laxative abuse
b) Thyrotoxicosis
c) Diabetic diarrhoea with visceral neuropathy
d) Irritable bowel syndrome?

4. EXUDATIVE

Characteristics
a) Small volume and frequent stools
b) Blood, mucus (suggests left-sided colonic disease)

Causes
a) Colonic cancer
b) Inflammatory bowel disease
c) Infection, e.g. invasive *E. coli, Shigella*

INFECTIOUS DIARRHOEA

Table 5.3 Non-invasive bacteria: characteristics

Bacteria	Onset (hours)	cAMP	Fever	Intestinal fluid	Comment
Staphylococcus aureus	1 to 6	+	−	+	Vomiting predominant
Clostridium perfringens	8 to 12	−	+/−	+ + + +	Precooked foods, rewarmed: diarrhoea >vomiting
Escherichia coli (toxin)	12	+	+/−	+	Travellers' diarrhoea
Vibrio cholera	12	+	+	+ + + +	Antibiotics shorten course (unlike others)
Bacillus cereus	a. 1 to 6	+	−	+	Resembles *Staph aureus:* in fried rice typically
	b. 12 to 24	+	−	+ + + +	Resembles *C. perfringens*

Table 5.4 Invasive bacteria: characteristics

Bacteria	Fever	Bloody diarrhoea	Bacteraemia	Antibiotic therapy	Comment
*Shigella**	+	+	+	Ampicillin or fluoroquinolones	Increasing resistance to trimethoprim-sulfamethoxazole
*Salmonella** (non-typhi)	+	−	−	Nil (unless blood culture +ve or HIV/AIDS patient)	
Vibrio parahaemolyticus	+	+	−	Questionable value	Shellfish ingestion
Campylobacter jejuni	±	+	±	Erythromycin or fluoroquinolones	Mimics *Salmonella*
Escherichia coli	+	−	−	Nil	Rare
*Yersinia***	+	±	±	Aminoglycosides or trimethoprim-sulfamethoxazole	Acute disease similar to *Shigella*

*May cause a terminal ileitis.
*Extraintestinal manifestations include erythema nodosum, erythema multiforme, non-suppurative arthritis, thyroiditis, liver granuloma and liver abscess.

Table 5.5 *Gastrointestinal infections in patients with AIDS (see also Table 12.4)*

Pathogen	Clinical features	Diagnostic tests
Cryptosporidium	Enteritis, weight loss	Stool acid-fast stain or phase contrast microscopy
Isospora belli	Enteritis	Fresh stool (trichrome stain), duodenal aspirate
Shigella, Salmonella, E. histolytica, Yersinia, etc	Colitis (blood, diarrhoea, fever)	Stool examination
N. gonorrhoea	Proctitis (anorectal pain, discharge, tenesmus)	Proctoscopy, rectal Gram stain, culture
C. trachomatis	Proctitis, haematochezia, diarrhoea	Proctoscopy, culture
T. pallidum	Anorectal chancre or polyp	Proctoscopy, VDRL, rectal biopsy
Mycobacterium avium intracellulare (MAI)	Malabsorption (may resemble Whipple's disease)	Culture, small bowel biopsy (PAS positive macrophages: distinguish from Whipple's on electron microscopy)
Giardia lamblia	Enteritis (intermittent watery, foul-smelling diarrhoea)	Stool examination (50% false negative), duodenal aspirate (10% false negative)
Candida	Oesophagitis	
Herpes simplex virus	Oesophagitis, proctitis, discrete vesicles, neurological signs	Endoscopy, Tzanck preparation, culture
Cytomegalovirus	GI ulceration anywhere, e.g. giant oesophageal ulcers, diarrhoea	'Owl eye' intranuclear inclusion bodies

AIDS = acquired immunodeficiency syndrome.

MALABSORPTION

The most common causes of malabsorption are coeliac disease, chronic pancreatitis, post-gastrectomy, Crohn's disease and lactose deficiency.

CLINICAL CLUES

1. History of pale, greasy, foul smelling stools that are difficult to flush away (steatorrhoea).

2. Chronic diarrhoea and
   a) weight loss
   b) iron deficiency anaemia (e.g. coeliac disease)
   c) metabolic bone disease (proximal small bowel disease)
   d) oedema and hypoproteinaemia (protein-losing enteropathy)
3. Evidence of nutritional deficiency, e.g. glossitis (B vitamins, folate, iron), anaemia (megaloblastic, iron deficiency, etc), bruising (vitamin K), night blindness (vitamin A), peripheral neuropathy (B_{12}, B_1), tetany (calcium, magnesium), weakness or nocturia (potassium).

CAUSES

1. Lipolytic phase defects
   a) Chronic pancreatitis, pancreatic carcinoma
   b) Cystic fibrosis
2. Micellar phase defects
   a) Bacterial overgrowth
   b) Terminal ileal disease or resection: <100 cm—bile salt diarrhoea; ≥100 cm—steatorrhoea
   c) Extrahepatic biliary obstruction or chronic liver disease
3. Mucosal phase defects
   a) Coeliac disease
   b) Tropical sprue
   c) Lymphoma, Whipple's disease, small bowel ischaemia or resection, hypogammoglobulinaemia, amyloidosis, HIV infection.
4. Delivery phase defects
   a) Intestinal lymphangectasia
   b) Tumour infiltration of lymphatics.

DIFFERENTIAL DIAGNOSIS OF SUBTOTAL VILLOUS ATROPHY (a 'flat biopsy')

1. Coeliac disease
2. Tropical sprue
3. Giardiasis
4. Immunodeficiency (hypogammoglobulinaemia)
5. Bacterial overgrowth
6. Lymphoma
7. Drugs, e.g. colchicine, neomycin
8. Radiation or ischaemia
9. Microsporidiosis
10. Viral infection
11. Zollinger-Ellison syndrome (occasionally)

Table 5.6 Typical results of investigations in malabsorption

Investigation	Coeliac disease	Bacterial overgrowth	Whipple's disease	Terminal ileal disease	Chronic pancreatitis
Stool fat (or C^{14} triolein breath test)	High-normal	High	High	High	Very high
D-xylose*	Low	Low	Low	Normal	Normal
Schilling's test with or without IF†	Normal (rarely abnormal due to ileal involvement)	Abnormal	Normal	Abnormal	Abnormal occasionally
Folate (serum)	Low (>50%)	High-normal	Low	Normal	Normal
Small bowel biopsy‡ (proximal)	Flat biopsy (subtotal or total villous atrophy)	Normal	Clubbing and flattening of villi; PAS positive inclusions	Normal	Normal
C^{14}-glycine breath test	Normal	Abnormal (early peak)**	Normal	Abnormal (late peak)	Normal

*This is a test of proximal small bowel function. Falsely low values occur in chronic renal failure, dehydration, ascites, hyperthyroidism and in the elderly.

†While pernicious anaemia corrects with intrinsic factor (IF), ileal disease does not correct. Bacterial overgrowth corrects with antibiotics and pancreatic insufficiency with pancreatic supplements. False-negative results occur with incomplete urinary collections, decreased extracellular volume and renal disease.

‡Small bowel series are abnormal in severe mucosal disease (e.g. dilatation, flocculation of barium, loss of fine mucosal pattern) but this is not specific. It should be ordered to exclude anatomical abnormalities (e.g. diverticula, Crohn's disease).

PAS = periodic acid-Schiff technique.

**20–30% false negative results occur.

DISEASE STATES

COELIAC DISEASE

Patients typically present with diarrhoea and weight loss in the third or fourth decade. Also consider this diagnosis with folate or iron deficiency (especially if both are present), osteomalacia (and osteoporosis) or hypoalbuminaemia, and in the presence of Howell-Jolly bodies on blood smear (autosplenectomy); steatorrhoea is often *not* present.

Diagnosis
1. Evidence of malabsorption.
2. Abnormal small bowel biopsy.
3. Clinical, biochemical and histological improvement after institution of a gluten-free diet. (Rarely symptom response may take 24–36 months; up to 50% of patients do not have complete resolution of histological changes on a gluten free diet).
4. Antigliadin antibody—inaccurate; antiendomysial antibody—sensitive screening test.

Treatment
1. No response to a gluten-free diet—consider poor dietary compliance, incorrect diagnosis, other concurrent disease (e.g. lactose or pancreatic insufficiency), development of intestinal lymphoma or diffuse ulceration, and collagenous sprue.
2. Up to 50% of patients with refractory coeliac disease respond to steroids.

THE COLON

CLINICAL CLUES

LOWER ABDOMINAL PAIN

CAUSES

Common
Irritable bowel syndrome
Gynaecological disease
Lactase deficiency
Diverticulitis
Inflammatory bowel disease
Intestinal obstruction

Uncommon
Chronic intestinal pseudo-obstruction
Mesenteric ischaemia
Malignancy (e.g. ovarian carcinoma)
Spinal disease

Testicular disease
Abdominal wall pain
Metabolic diseases: diabetes mellitus, familial Mediterranean fever, C1 esterase deficiency (angioneurotic oedema), porphyria, lead poisoning, tabes dorsalis, renal failure

CLINICAL CLASSIFICATION OF CONSTIPATION IN ADULTS

1. Simple constipation (no gross structural abnormality)
Inadequate fibre intake
Faulty defaecation
Pregnancy
Old age or infirmity
Drug side effects: aluminium antacids, iron, anticholinergics, opiates

2. Structural colonic disease
Colonic cancer
Anal fissure, infection or stenosis
Colonic stricture
Aganglionosis and/or abnormal myenteric plexus
  Hirschsprung's disease
  Chagas' disease
  Neuropathic pseudo-obstruction
Abnormal colonic muscle
  Myopathy
  Dystrophia myotonica
  Systemic sclerosis

3. Neurological causes
Diabetic autonomic neuropathy
Spinal cord damage or disease: e.g. multiple sclerosis, anterior sacral meningocele
Parkinson's disease

4. Endocrine or metabolic causes
Hypothyroidism
Hypercalcaemia
Diabetes mellitus
Uraemia, hypokalaemia
Porphyria

5. Slow transit constipation
Documented delayed colonic transit of unknown cause

6. Obstructed defaecation
Pelvic floor dysfunction

7. Irritable bowel syndrome

CHRONIC INTESTINAL PSEUDO-OBSTRUCTION

A syndrome characterised by clinical features of mechanical small bowel obstruction but no luminal occlusion.

CLINICAL CLUES

Abdominal pain—continuous or episodic
Bloating and visible distension—continuous or episodic
Vomiting—continuous or episodic
Constipation (if predominant colonic involvement)
Diarrhoea (if bacterial overgrowth from small bowel motor involvement)
Dysphagia, chest pain (if oesophageal involvement)
Weight loss (if reduced food intake or malabsorption)
Palpable bladder (if megacystitis)
Symptoms and signs of underlying cause (e.g. neurological, endocrine, connective tissue disease)

DIAGNOSIS

Imaging studies (plain films, barium contrast studies, endoscopy)
Functional studies (gastric and small bowel transit, oesophageal manometry, gastroduodenal manometry, cystometrogram)
Diagnostic laparotomy (plus full thickness biopsy)
Evaluate for underlying cause

DISEASE STATES CAUSING CHRONIC INTESTINAL PSEUDO-OBSTRUCTION

1. Myenteric plexus disease
    Familial visceral neuropathies
    Sporadic visceral neuropathies, e.g. paraneoplastic (small-cell lung cancer)
    Hirschsprung's disease
2. Smooth muscle disease
    Familial and sporadic visceral myopathies
    Scleroderma
    Polymyositis
    Amyloid
3. Endocrine disease
    Hypothyroidism
    Hypoparathyroidism
    Phaeochromocytoma
4. Drugs
    e.g. phenothiazines, tricyclic antidepressants, clonidine, vinca alkaloids
5. Neurological disease
    Parkinson's disease
    Progressive muscular dystrophy
    Myotonic dystrophy
    Familial autonomic dysfunction

MEGACOLON

<small>CAUSES</small>

1. Congenital—Hirschsprung's disease
2. Acquired
   a) Drugs e.g. opioids
   b) Disease affecting the nervous system, e.g. diabetes mellitus, Parkinson's disease, lead poisoning, porphyria
   c) Hypothyroidism
   d) Hypokalaemia
   e) Idiopathic
3. Toxic megacolon (see below)

LAXATIVES AND CATHARTICS

1. Bulk-forming laxatives, e.g. psyllium, bran, cellulose are slow-acting natural and semisynthetic polysaccharides and cellulose derivatives. With a low fluid intake they may cause intestinal obstruction.
2. Emollient laxatives, e.g. mineral oil, glycerine, are stool softeners. They may cause mineral oil aspiration and pneumonia.
3. Stimulant cathartics, e.g. phenolphthalein, anthraquinones (senna, danthron) may act directly on the neural plexus or smooth muscle. Rapidly acting, they may cause myenteric plexus damage ('cathartic colon'), electrolyte imbalance or, in the long term, melanosis coli.
4. Saline cathartics, e.g. magnesium citrate, sodium phosphate, may cause electrolyte imbalance.
5. Osmotic laxatives, e.g. lactulose.

DISEASE STATES

INFLAMMATORY BOWEL DISEASE (IBD)

<small>CHRONIC ULCERATIVE COLITIS</small> (CUC)

Aetiology
1. Susceptibility loci on chromosomes 3, 7, 12 and within the histocompatibility complex on chromosome 6.
2. Smoking protective

Classification
1. Clinical
   a) Mild: <4 motions daily, minimal bleeding (most have proctosigmoiditis—10% progress to more extensive disease)
   b) Moderate: 4 to 6 motions daily, blood, pain, malaise, low grade fever
   c) Severe (fulminant colitis): >6 motions daily, profuse bleeding, high fever, hypoalbuminaemia, toxic megacolon
2. Extent of disease, e.g. proctitis, left-sided colitis, pancolitis

Exclude other causes of colitis
1. Infectious: amoebiasis, *Shigella, Yersinina, Campylobacter, E. coli* 0157: H7, antibiotic associated e.g.pseudo-membranous colitis, HIV infection.

2. Crohn's disease
3. NSAIDs
4. Ischaemia
5. Radiation
6. Heavy metals

Treatment

In principle, mild distal disease can be treated with topical rectal preparations. Severe disease or more proximal disease is treated with systemic medications.

1. Mild: topical steroids or 5-aminosalicylic acid (ASA) enemas (distal colonic disease) and sulfasalazine (or oral 5-ASA) for diffuse disease. 5-ASA inhibits the lipoxygenase pathway (and thereby reduces production of leukotriene B4).
2. Moderate: oral prednisone and sulfasalazine or oral 5-ASA (long-term steroids do not reduce relapse rates).
3. Severe: bowel rest, parenteral steroids and nutrition. Avoid hypokalaemia, barium enema, opiates and anticholinergics. In refractory disease there may be a place for steroid-sparing medications such as azathioprine.

Side effects of sulfasalazine (due to the sulfapyridine moiety) include malaise, nausea, diarrhoea (in slow acetylators); rash, fever, Stevens-Johnson syndrome (allergy); haemolysis (Heinz body), pancreatitis, neutropenia, aplastic anaemia, impaired folate absorption; oligospermia and dys-spermia.

Olsalazine (two molecules 5-ASA joined by an azobond)—induces diarrhoea (8%).

Mesalazine (5-ASA protected by acrylic coating) releases 5-ASA in the terminal ileum and colon (use cautiously in those with renal disease). Note that it can sometimes cause diarrhoea.

Sulfasalazine or 5-ASA is also useful for *maintenance of remission.* Azathioprine reduces relapse rates.

Cyclosporin (intravenously) may provide a prompt medium-term remission in fulminant colitis but side effects (e.g. hypertension, renal disease, cholestasis, gum hypertrophy, seizures) and relapse remain problems.

Methotrexate is not effective.

Complications of ulcerative colitis

1. Local
   a) Toxic megacolon—acute colonic dilatation (transverse diameter >6 cm)—requires intensive supportive therapy with intravenous fluids, steroids and antibiotics, and careful daily abdominal examinations, girth measures and abdominal X-rays in the first critical 72 hours.
   b) Massive bleeding.
   c) Perforation.
   d) Carcinoma—often multicentric and related to disease extent and duration: risk begins to increase (by 1–2% per year) 7 years after diagnosis in those with pancolitis, and after 15 years in those with left-sided disease (no increased risk with proctitis alone).
   e) Strictures.

Screening annually by colonoscopy and multiple biopsies 7 years after diagnosis of pancolitis is recommended. If high-grade dysplasia is found and confirmed, colectomy is indicated.

2. Extracolonic
   a) Liver disease (10%)
      i) Sclerosing cholangitis
      ii) Fatty liver
      iii) Chronic hepatitis
      iv) Cirrhosis
      v) Bile duct cancer (cholangiocarcinoma)
   b) Haematological disorders
      i) Anaemia (due to chronic disease, iron deficiency, haemolysis from sulfasalazine or microangiopathy)
      ii) Thomboembolism
   c) Arthropathy
      i) Peripheral (large joints)
      ii) Ankylosing spondylitis (HLA-B27 positive)
   d) Skin and mucous membranes
      i) Erythema nodosum (coincides with active disease but not more severe disease)
      ii) Pyoderma gangrenosum
      iii) Apthous ulcers in the mouth
   e) Ocular disease
      i) Uveitis, conjunctivitis, episcleritis

Colectomy cures the disease but does not cure the following extracolonic complications: ankylosing spondylitis, sclerosing cholangitis and other liver disease, and pyoderma gangrenosum.

CROHN'S DISEASE

Aetiology
1. Susceptibility loci on chromosomes 3, 7, 12 and 16
2. Smokers at increased risk

Classification
1. Small bowel disease alone 30%
2. Small and large bowel disease 50%
3. Large bowel disease alone 20%

Complications
1. Local

   The entire GI tract can be affected

   a) Anorectal disease (75% with small bowel and 95% with large bowel disease are affected)
   b) Bowel obstruction (usually terminal ileum)
   c) Fistulas
   d) Toxic megacolon and perforation (uncommon)
   e) Carcinoma of small and large bowel—risk slightly increased; screening is not indicated

2. Extracolonic

Similar to ulcerative colitis, but note particularly the following:

a) Liver disease (less common)
b) Cholesterol gallstones increased
c) Renal disease—stones (urate, oxalate, calcium), pyelonephritis, hydronephrosis
d) Malabsorption
e) Osteomalacia
f) Amyloid (typically renal involvement—always consider this if the patient has proteinuria)

Treatment

Generally similar to CUC. Sulfasalazine is more effective in colonic disease, while steroids are more effective in small bowel disease. Controlled-release oral budesonide is useful for ileo-colonic disease (only a small proportion of active drug reaches systemic circulation after first-pass metabolism in the liver). 5-ASA reduces relapse. Metronidazole is useful for perianal disease. Methotrexate but not cyclosporin is useful in refactory Crohn's disease.

PREGNANCY AND IBD

Fertility is reduced and the risk of spontaneous abortion is greater in Crohn's disease. Although prognosis is unaffected by pregnancy, in ulcerative colitis if exacerbations occur these are more likely in the first trimester. In Crohn's disease exacerbations are more likely in the third trimester.

COLONIC POLYPS AND COLORECTAL CANCER

COLONIC POLYPS

1. Hyperplastic—no malignant potential
2. Adenomatous—only premalignant polyp and three types: tubular, villous (may induce hypokalaemia, profuse mucus), tubulo-villous.

Table 5.7 Risk of cancer with colonic polyps

Size of polyp	% with carcinoma	
	Tubular adenoma	Villous adenoma
<1cm	1%	10%
>2cm	25%	50%

Juvenile polyps are hamartomas that may cause bleeding, intussusception and obstruction. While the polyps are not malignant, patients with familial juvenile polyposis have a slightly increased risk of carcinoma.

HEREDITARY POLYPOSIS SYNDROMES

• **Familial adenomatous polyposis (FAP):** >95% develop colorectal cancer; colectomy for prevention is indicated; explains 1% of new colon cancers.

Genetic defect (autosomal dominant): mutation of adenomatous polyposis coli (APC) gene on long arm of chromosome 5.

- **Hereditary non-polyposis colon cancer (HNPCC or Lynch syndrome):**
  Lynch syndrome I—no family history of other cancers
  Lynch syndrome II—increased familial occurrence of other cancers (e.g. ovary, uterus)
  Family history helps to identify the syndrome: ≥3 relatives with documented colon cancer, one of whom is a first-degree relative of the other two; or ≥1 family member <50 years of age develops colon cancer; or colon cancer involving ≥2 generations.
  Genetic defects (autosomal dominant with incomplete penetrance): mutations on chromosomes 2, 3 and 7 associated with 70–80% of cases.
- **Gardener's syndrome:**
  Autosomal dominant: variant of FAP
  Skin: cysts, fibromas, lipomas (multiple).
  Other: bone osteomas, supernumerary teeth, epidermoid and sebaceous cysts, thyroid and adrenal tumours, retinal pigment epithelial hypertrophy.
- **Turcot-Despres syndrome:**
  Variant of FAP.
  Polyps (adenomatous) of colon plus malignant glioma (or other brain tumours).
- **Peutz-Jeghers syndrome:**
  Autosomal dominant.
  Skin: pigmented macules on hands, feet, lips.
  Gastrointestinal tract: hamartomas (and rarely adenocarcinoma) in stomach, small and large bowel.
  Other: sex cord tumours.

NON-HEREDITARY POLYPOSIS SYNDROME

- **Cronkhite-Canada syndrome**
  (See below, 'THE SKIN AND THE GUT: ASSOCIATIONS', page 127)

COLORECTAL CANCER

RISK FACTORS

1. Age ≥50 years—increases sharply, doubles each decade until age 60, peaks at age 80.
2. Family history of colon cancer—2x increased risk in first-degree relatives.
3. Hereditary polyposis syndromes.
4. Inflammatory bowel disease.
5. History of female genital or breast cancer—2x increased risk.
6. Previous resection of colon cancer—2–6% have a synchronous cancer and 1–5% metachronous cancer.

PRESENTING FEATURES

Right-sided (e.g. caecal): iron deficiency anaemia, abdominal mass.
Left-sided (narrower): symptoms of obstruction, rectal bleeding.

The staging of colonic cancer is confusing, with many systems in use. A convenient system is outlined.

Table 5.8 Staging of colonic cancer

Stage	Pathological description	Treatment
Dukes' A	Tumour in the mucosa, submucosa or lamina but not reaching the muscularis	Surgical excision
Dukes' B	Into muscularis B1 not to the level of the serosa	Surgery and chemotherapy for tumours with bad prognostic features
	B2 including the serosa	B2 adjuvant chemotherapy probably of benefit
Dukes' C	Local lymph nodes involved	Surgical excision and adjuvant chemotherapy recommended
Dukes' D	Metastatic disease	Systemic chemotherapy

Chemotherapy (based on 5-fluorouracil) has a role in improving quality of life in patients with advanced metastatic disease and a good level of function. There are limited data to support small increases in survival in this setting.

RECTUM

Mobile tumours more than 5 cm from the anal verge can be excised and an anastomosis formed.

Because the rectum is fixed, radiotherapy has a greater role to play in treatment of inoperable or recurrent disease in the rectum. Adjuvant chemotherapy and irradiation is recommended after resection of Dukes' B2 and Dukes' C rectal carcinoma. Radiotherapy reduces the risk of local recurrence.

POSTOPERATIVE MANAGEMENT (NO EVIDENCE OF METASTASES)

- Follow-up colonoscopy in 6–12 months, then at 3 years, and if normal every 5 years.
- Adjuvant chemotherapy: 5-fluorouracil and levamisole decrease recurrence by 40% and mortality by one-third in Duke stage C (regional node involvement).

SCREENING RECOMMENDATIONS

- Average risk individuals ≥50 years: annual faecal occult blood ± flexible sigmoidoscopy 5 yearly (or colonoscopy 10 yearly). If faecal occult blood test is positive, evaluate entire colon e.g. by colonoscopy.

- Colon cancer in one or two first-degree relatives, or an adenomatous polyp in a first degree relative under age 60: same screening procedures as 'average risk' but screening should begin at age 40.

LOWER GASTROINTESTINAL BLEEDING

CAUSES

Haemorrhoids commonly bleed, but more sinister causes (especially colonic cancer) must always be excluded. If bleeding is substantial, consider the following:
More common
1. Angiodysplasia.
2. Diverticular disease (often from the right colon).

Less common
1. Massive upper gastrointestinal bleeding.
2. Colonic cancer or polyp.
3. Inflammatory bowel disease.*
4. Meckel's diverticulum.*
5. Ischaemic colitis.
6. Solitary colonic ulcer.
7. Other: small bowel tumour, haemobilia, pancreatic disease, vascular anomalies, elastic tissue diseases, vasculitis, amyloid, bleeding diathesis.

Table 5.9 *Acute intestinal ischaemia*

Feature	Acute mesenteric ischaemia	Colonic ischaemia
Age	Elderly usually	>60 years of age (90%)
Clinical	Looks ill	Do not appear ill
	Severe abdominal pain	Mild abdominal pain
	Minimal abdominal signs early *i.e. pain out of proportion to signs*	Minimal abdominal signs
	Rectal bleeding late	Moderate rectal bleeding or bloody diarrhoea
Precipitating cause	Common, e.g. atrial fibrillation, myocardial infarct	Rare; early colonoscopy often helpful

*very important to exclude in young adults.

THE PANCREAS

PATHOPHYSIOLOGY

HYPERAMYLASAEMIA

CAUSES

Pancreatic disease
1. Acute pancreatitis, chronic pancreatitis.
2. Pancreatic pseudocyst or abscess (persistent amylase elevation is a clue).
3. Neoplasm.
4. Trauma.

Non-pancreatic disease
1. Macroamylasaemia (2-hour urinary amylase normal or low).
2. Renal failure.
3. Parotitis (isoenzyme identification will differentiate).
4. Intestinal perforation, obstruction, infarction.
5. Ruptured ectopic pregnancy.
6. Drugs, e.g. morphine.
7. Diabetic ketoacidosis.
8. Tumours, e.g. oesophagus, lung, ovary (serum lipase normal, unlike with pancreatic disease).
9. Burns.

DISEASE STATES

ACUTE PANCREATITIS

CAUSES

1. Gallstones (50–60%)
2. Alcohol (30–40%)
3. Idiopathic (10%)
4. Other
   a) Traumatic—after ERCP, penetrating peptic ulcer, trauma.
   b) Inflammatory—mumps, infectious mononucleosis.
   c) Duct obstruction—carcinoma, roundworms.
   d) Metabolic—hypercalcaemia (and MEN I), hyperlipidaemia, haemochromatosis, diabetes mellitus, uraemia, porphyria, pregnancy.
   e) Vascular.
   f) Drugs—thiazides, steroids, the contraceptive pill, azathioprine.
   g) Pancreas divisum (congenital anomaly).

Table 5.10 *Worsening prognostic criteria for acute pancreatitis (Ranson's criteria)*

At admission or diagnosis	During initial 48 hours
1. Age > 55 years	1. Haematocrit fall >10%
2. White blood cell count >16 000/mm³	2. Blood urea nitrogen >5 mg/100 mL (1.8 mmol/L), after IV fluids
3. Blood glucose >200 mg/100 mL (11 mmol/L)	3. Serum calcium <8 mg/100 mL (1.9 mmol/L)
4. Serum lactate dehydrogenase >400 IU/100 mL	4. PaO₂ <60 mmHg
5. AST (SGOT) >250 IU/L	5. Albumin <32 g/L
	6. Fluid deficit >4 L

Note: <3 criteria: mild pancreatitis (mortality 1%).
3–4 criteria: moderate pancreatitis (mortality 15%).
5–6 criteria: severe pancreatitis (mortality 40%).
7–8 criteria: very severe pancreatitis (mortality approaches 100%).
The amylase level is not of prognostic value.

CHRONIC PANCREATITIS

CAUSES

1. Chronic alcoholism
2. Idiopathic
3. Hypertriglyceridaemia
4. Hypercalcaemia
5. Trauma
6. Hereditary (autosomal dominant)
7. Cystic fibrosis
8. Tropical (nutritional)
9. Haemochromatosis
10. Prolonged parental hyperalimentation
11. Obstruction
    — Benign, e.g. pancreas divisum with obstruction of the accessory ampulla
    — Cancer, e.g. of the ampulla or duct (short history)

Causes of pancreatic calcification
1. Alcoholic pancreatitis (25–50%)
2. Hyperparathyroidism
3. Hereditary pancreatitis

N.B. 2 and 3 are rare.

PANCREATIC ISLET CELL TUMOURS

A. ZOLLINGER-ELLISON SYNDROME

Clinical manifestations suggestive of a gastrinoma
1. Multiple peptic ulcers, peptic ulcer in an unusual location (e.g. post-

bulbar), peptic ulcer resistant to medical therapy, ulcer recurrence after operation, or frequent or early ulcer recurrence.
2. Extensive family history of duodenal ulcer, or a family history of MEN I (page 241).
3. Unexplained prolonged diarrhoea or steatorrhoea (due to mucosal damage by acid, inactivation of lipase or bile acids and increased intestinal secretion).
4. Hypercalcaemia associated with ulcer disease (MEN I).
5. Enlarged duodenal or gastric folds associated with ulcer disease.

Diagnosis
1. Fasting serum gastrin >300 pg/mL suggestive, >1000 pg/mL likely.
2. Acid hypersecretion (two-thirds have a basal acid output (BAO) >15 mEq/h), (15 mmol).
3. Secretin test is the provocative test of choice (paradoxical increase in gastrin >200 pg/mL over basal level is highly specific). Calcium infusion, but not a protein meal, causes a rise in gastrin in 90% of patients.
4. Localise tumour (ultrasound, CT scan of the abdomen, angiography, venous sampling) if possible.

Differential diagnosis of hypergastrinaemia and acid hypersecretion

a) Retained gastric antrum after ulcer surgery.
b) Massive small bowel resection.
c) Gastric outlet obstruction.
d) Thyrotoxicosis.
e) Antral G cell hyperplasia (gastrin increases after a protein meal).

Differential diagnosis of hypergastrinaemia and hypochlorhydria

a) Type A atrophic gastritis and pernicious anaemia.
b) Previous vagotomy.
c) Renal failure.
d) Drugs—proton pump inhibitors (e.g. omeprazole).

B. WATERY DIARRHOEA, HYPOKALAEMIA AND ACHLORHYDRIA (WDHA)

Vasoactive intestinal polypeptide (VIP) secreting tumours produce these characteristic manifestations.

C. GLUCAGONOMA

A slow growing pancreatic tumour results in diabetes mellitus, stomatitis, anaemia and necrolytic migratory erythema.

D. MULTIPLE ENDOCRINE NEOPLASIA (MEN)

(See Chapter 9)

THE SKIN AND THE GUT: ASSOCIATIONS

1. Peutz-Jeghers syndrome: see above
2. Gardener's syndrome: see above
3. Ataxia-telangiectasia
   Skin: telangiectases on face, ears, conjunctiva, antecubital fossa

    GI: stomach carcinoma

    Other: seizures

4. Acanthosis nigricans and adenocarcinoma
5. Carcinoid syndrome
    Skin: telangiectases (face, neck), flushing (episodic, often involving the face)
    GI: watery diarrhoea, irregular hepatomegaly (there are often hepatic metastases from e.g. terminal ileum, small bowel, lung, gonads)
    Other: wheeze, right heart murmurs
6. Osler-Weber-Rendu or hereditary haemorrhagic telangiectasia (autosomal dominant)
    Skin: telangiectases (nail beds, palms, feet especially)
    GI: haemorrhage from bowel, buccal mucosa
    Other: nasopharyngeal haemorrhage, pulmonary arteriovenous fistula, high output cardiac failure
7. Pseudoxanthoma elasticum (autosomal recessive)
    Skin: yellow plaques and papules in flexural areas ('chicken fat') and angioid streaks in the fundi
    GI: bowel ischaemia and bleeding
8. Blue rubber bleb syndrome
    Skin: haemangiomas, e.g. on the tongue
    GI: haemorrhage into bowel or liver
9. Systemic mastocytosis
    Skin: telangiectases, flushing, pigmented papules, pruritus (severe), dermographism
    GI: peptic ulcer (histamine release), diarrhoea, malabsorption, infiltration of the bowel by mast cell leukaemia or lymphoma
10. Pyoderma gangrenosum
    Skin: tender red area that becomes bullous and ulcerates, often on the legs
    GI: inflammatory bowel disease (does not coincide with disease activity)
11. Dermatitis herpetiformis (coeliac disease)
12. Glucagonoma
    Skin: migratory necrolytic rash (on flexural and friction areas)
    GI: glossitis, weight loss, diabetes mellitus
13. Zinc deficiency
    Consider this diagnosis in the setting of Crohn's disease with fistulas, cirrhosis, parenteral nutrition, or in alcoholic pancreatitis
    Skin: red, scaly and crusting lesions around mouth, eyes and genitalia, and white patches on the tongue
    GI: diarrhoea
14. Systemic sclerosis and reflux oesophagitis
15. Degos' disease (malignant atrophic papulosis—very rare)
    Skin: dome-shaped red papule (early); small porcelain white atrophic papule (late)
    GI: intestinal perforation and infarction, primarily in young men

16. Tylosis (very, very rare)
    Skin: hyperkeratosis of palms and soles
    GI: oesophageal cancer
17. Cronkhite-Canada Syndrome
    Skin: onycholysis, pigmentation, alopecia
    GI: gastric, small bowel and colonic polyps, hypertrophic gastric
            folds, villous atrophy, protein losing enteropathy

NUTRITION

Table 5.11   *Clinical findings associated with vitamin and mineral deficiencies*

Physical examination	Associated vitamin deficiencies
Mucocutaneous	
Dermatitis/cheilosis/glossitis	Riboflavin (B_2), pyridoxine (B_6), niacin
Bleeding/swollen gums	Vitamin C
Petechiae/ecchymoses	Vitamins C & K
Perifollicular haemorrhages/keratitis	Vitamin C
Rash (face/body: pustular, bullous, vesicular, seborrhoeic, acneiform), skin ulcers, alopecia	Zinc
Neurological	
Peripheral neuropathy	Thiamine, vitamin B_{12}, chromium, vitamin E
Dementia/confusion	Thiamine, niacin, zinc, manganese
Night blindness	Vitamin A
Ophthalmoplegia	Thiamine
Haematological	
Pallor (anaemia)	Vitamin B_{12}, folic acid, iron, copper
Miscellaneous	
Dysgeusia	Zinc
Fractures	Vitamin D
Loosening of teeth, periostial haemorrhages	Vitamin C
Cardiac failure/cardiomyopathy	Thiamine, selenium
Hypothyroidism	Iodine

TOTAL PARENTERAL NUTRITION

INDICATIONS

1. Postoperative (bowel surgery, protracted recovery)
2. Severe acute pancreatitis

Internal Medicine

3. Severe inflammatory bowel disease (complicated ulcerative colitis, severe Crohn's with malabsorption)
4. Acute radiation enteritis or chemotherapy enteritis
5. Enterocutaneous fistula involving the small bowel
6. Short gut syndrome
7. Preoperative (severely malnourished patients only)
8. Severe malabsorption syndromes

COMPLICATIONS

Local (central vein catheter)
1. Pneumothorax/haemothorax
2. Venous thrombosis
3. Air embolus
4. Infection
5. Thrombophlebitis

Systemic
1. Hyper/hypoglycaemia
2. Electrolyte disturbances
3. Azotaemia and hyperosmolarity
4. Liver dysfunction (hepatocellular or cholestatic), and fatty liver
5. Acalculous cholecystitis
6. Cholelithiasis (long-term therapy)
7. Vitamin or mineral deficiency (rare)
8. Metabolic bone disease (rare)

Hepatology

CLINICAL CLUES

SYMPTOMS

Fatigue, pruritus, bleeding, abdominal pain, nausea, anorexia, myalgia, jaundice, dark urine, pale stools, fever, weight loss; may be no symptoms.

SIGNS

PERIPHERAL SIGNS OF CHRONIC LIVER DISEASE, HEPATOCELLULAR DYSFUNCTION

Spider naevi, palmar erythema, white nails, gynaecomastia, body hair loss, testicular atrophy, hepatomegaly

SIGNS OF PORTAL HYPERTENSION

Splenomegaly, ascites, peripheral oedema

SIGNS OF POOR HEPATOCELLULAR SYNTHETIC FUNCTION

Bruising, peripheral oedema (reflecting depleted coagulation factors and albumin levels)

SIGNS OF END-STAGE LIVER DISEASE

Wasting, progressive severe fatigue, encephalopathy (asterixis, foetor, coma)

OTHER SIGNS

Hepatic rub—peritoneal inflammation from underlying infarction or malignancy
Right upper quadrant bruit—intrahepatic shunting, alcoholic hepatitis, malignancy, large haemangioma

HEPATOMEGALY

CAUSES

1. Diffusely enlarged and smooth

Massive
    Metastatic disease
    Alcoholic liver disease with fatty infiltration
    Myeloproliferative diseases (e.g. polycythaemia rubra vera, myelofibrosis)

Moderate
    The above causes
    Haemochromatosis
    Haematological disease (e.g. chronic myeloid leukaemia, lymphoma)
    Fatty liver (e.g. diabetes mellitus)

Mild
    The above causes
    Hepatitis (viral, drugs)
    Cirrhosis
    Biliary obstruction
    Granulomatous disorders (e.g. sarcoid)
    Infiltrative disorders (e.g. amyloid)
    HIV infection

2. Diffusely enlarged and irregular

Metastatic disease
Cirrhosis
Hydatid disease
Polycystic liver disease

3. Localised swelling

Riedel's lobe (a normal variant—the lobe may be palapable in the right
    lumbar region)
Metastasis
Large simple hepatic cyst
Hydatid cyst
Hepatoma
Liver abscess (e.g. amoebic abscess)

4. Hepatosplenomegaly

Chronic liver disease with portal hypertension
Haematological disease (e.g. myeloproliferative disease, lymphoma)
Infection (e.g. acute viral hepatitis, infectious mononucleosis)
Infiltration (e.g. amyloid, sarcoid)
Connective tissue disease (e.g. systemic lupus erythematosus (SLE))

CAUSES OF A PALPABLE GALLBLADDER

With jaundice
1. Carcinoma of the head of the pancreas
2. Carcinoma of the ampulla of Vater
3. In-situ gallstone formation in the common bile duct (rare)
4. Mucocele of the gallbladder due to a stone in Hartmann's pouch and a stone in the common bile duct (rare)

Without jaundice
1. Mucocele of the gallbladder
2. Carcinoma of the gallbladder

PATHOPHYSIOLOGY

LIVER FUNCTION TESTS

TRANSAMINASES

1. Alanine aminotransferase (ALT or SGPT)—found predominantly in liver
2. Aspartate aminotransferase (AST or SGOT)—found in liver, muscle, heart, kidney, brain

Table 6.1 Transaminases in acute viral and alcoholic hepatitis

Acute viral hepatitis	Acute alcoholic hepatitis
ALT and AST often >1000 IU/L	ALT and AST < 500 IU/L usually
ALT > AST	AST > ALT 2:1
Gamma GT+	Gamma GT + + +

- Transaminases >1000 IU/L—consider viral hepatitis, shock liver, acute drug-induced hepatitis or occasionally acute cardiac failure.
- Transaminases do not correlate with the severity of hepatic disease in general—they may be normal in cirrhosis.
- Transaminases >400 U/L are *not* a feature of alcoholic liver disease—consider paracetamol (acetaminophen) co-ingestion.

SERUM ALKALINE PHOSPHATASE (SAP)

Found in liver, bone, intestine, kidney, placenta.

Elevated liver fraction in intrahepatic and extrahepatic biliary obstruction (in the latter, usually proportionally to the degree of obstruction). If isolated elevation of SAP is detected, first exclude non-hepatic origin, e.g. pregnancy, adolescence, bone disease, alpha chain disease. If of hepatic origin, perform an ultrasound, followed by ERCP if duct disease is likely, or liver biopsy if intrahepatic disease is likely.

GAMMA GLUTAMYL TRANSPEPTIDASE (GGT)

Widely distributed enzyme that can be induced, e.g. by alcohol, phenytoin, barbiturates, tricyclic antidepressants.

ALBUMIN

Hypoalbuminaemia suggests chronic liver disease ($t^1/_2$ albumin, 20 days).

GLOBULINS

Increased IgM occurs in primary biliary cirrhosis, while increased IgA occurs in alcoholic cirrhosis and primary biliary cirrhosis. Decreased alpha$_1$-globulin suggests alpha$_1$ antitrypsin deficiency.

PROTHROMBIN TIME (PT) OR INTERNATIONAL NORMALISED RATIO (INR)

Vitamin K dependent factors are II, VII, IX and X. The INR is abnormal in parenchymal and obstructive liver disease, but returns to normal (or improves by 30%) within 24 hours of vitamin K injection in extrahepatic obstruction. More severe liver disease will have a more abnormal INR.

BILIRUBIN METABOLISM (see Figure 6.1)

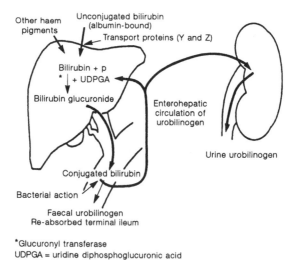

*Glucuronyl transferase
UDPGA = uridine diphosphoglucuronic acid
P = intracellular binding proteins

Figure 6.1 *Normal bilirubin metabolism.*

132

Unconjugated
1. Haemolysis
2. Impaired conjugation (decreased activity of glucuronyl transferase)
   a) Gilbert's syndrome (diagnosed by exclusion of haemolysis, the presence of normal liver function, and by a rise in the bilirubin level after fasting)
   b) Crigler-Najjar syndrome (types I and II)

Conjugated
1. Familial

Feature	Dubin-Johnson syndrome	Rotor's syndrome
Inheritance	Autosomal recessive	Autosomal recessive
Oral cholecystography	Gallbladder not visualised	Gallbladder visualised
BSP test	Secondary rise at 90 minutes	Normal at 90 minutes but abnormal at 45 minutes
Liver biopsy	Greenish black pigment	No pigment
Urinary coproporphyrin	Normal	Increased

BSP = bromsulphthalein

2. Hepatocellular disease
   i. Hepatitis—viral, autoimmune, alcoholic
   ii. Cirrhosis
   iii. Drugs and toxins
   iv. Venous obstruction
3. Cholestatic disease
   i. Intrahepatic cholestasis—drugs, recurrent jaundice of pregnancy, primary biliary cirrhosis, benign recurrent intrahepatic cholestasis (BRIC)
   ii. Extrahepatic biliary obstruction—stones, carcinoma of the pancreas or bile duct, strictures of the bile duct

Table 6.2 *Clinical features and liver function test profiles in hepatic (hepatocellular) and cholestatic (obstructive) jaundice*

	Suggests hepatocellular jaundice	Suggests obstructive jaundice
Clinical features	Nausea, anorexia, fatigue, myalgia, known infectious exposure, IV drug use, blood transfusions, alcohol, medication abuse, positive family history of liver disease or jaundice	Pain, pruritus, dark urine, pale stools, fever, past biliary surgery, weight loss, older age

Table 6.2 Continued

	Suggests hepatocellular jaundice	Suggests obstructive jaundice
Transaminases (AST, ALT)	+ + (>3x normal)	+ (<3x normal)
Alkaline phosphatase	Normal to increased (<3x normal)	+ + (>3x normal)
INR or prothrombin time after vitamin K	Does not correct	Corrects if extrahepatic obstruction relieved

AST = aspartate aminotransferase; ALT = alanine aminotransferase; INR = international normalised ratio

DISEASE STATES

VIRAL HEPATITIS

TESTS FOR VIRAL HEPATITIS

Table 6.3 Tests for hepatitis B (HB)

Condition	HBsAg	Anti-HBc*	Anti-HBs	HBeAg
Acute hepatitis B	+ + (may be −)	± (IgM)	−	+ if high infectivity
Early convalescence ('window period')	−	+ IgM ± IgG	−	+ or −
Recent recovery from acute hepatitis B	−	± IgG ± IgM	+	−
Infection in remote past	−	+IgG or −	+ or −	−
Chronic carrier	+	+ + IgG	−	−
Vaccination (successful)	−	−	+ +	−
Chronic hepatitis	+	−	−	+
Some core-mutant chronic hepatitis B	+	−	−	−**

HBsAg = hepatitis B surface antigen; anti-HBc = anti-hepatitis B core antibody; anti-HBs = anti-hepatitis B surface antibody; HBeAg = hepatitis B e antigen.
*present for only a short time.
**HBV DNA positive.
N.B. If HBsAg is persistent for longer than 6 months, and liver function tests are normal, the chance of chronic liver disease being present is <5%. However, if liver function tests (ALT, AST) are abnormal, 20–40% will have chronic liver disease. (See Figure 6.2 for pathophysiology).

Chronic hepatitis (reversible)   Cirrhosis (irreversible)

Chronic hepatitis
(mild)

Chronic hepatitis
(severe)

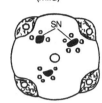

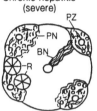

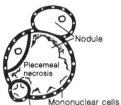

Pattern of histological charges in chronic
hepatitis
PZ = portal zone, SN = spotty necrosis;
PN = piecemeal necrosis: BN = bridging
necrosis: R = rosettes

In chronic hepatitis the zonal architecture
of the liver is preserved. In cirrhosis,
nodular regeneration leads to loss of the
essential hepatic architecture. Chronic
hepatitis is essentially reversible,
cirrhosis is not.

Figure 6.2 *Chronic hepatitis and cirrhosis.*
Reproduced, with permission, from Sherlock S and Dooley J.
Diseases of liver and biliary system. 10th ed. Oxford: Blackwell,
1997.

Table 6.4 *Tests for other viruses causing hepatitis*

Test	Meaning of a positive result	Comment
Hepatitis A virus (HAV)		
Anti-HAV IgM	Recent acquisition of HAV	Acute hepatic illness likely to be hepatitis A
Anti-HAV IgG	Past infection/ vaccination	Immunity
Hepatitis C virus (HCV)		
Anti-HCV	Exposure to HCV	Interpret in conjunction with other clinical and laboratory data. Likely to be infected
HCV RNA by qualitative PCR[1]	Presence of virus	Positive test indicates infection and viraemia
HCV RNA by quantitative PCR[1]	Presence of virus and level of viraemia	Useful for following response to treatment
Hepatitis D virus (HDV)		
Anti-HDV IgG/IgM	Exposure to HDV	Acute or chronic hepatitis D
Delta antigen	HDV present	Acute or chronic hepatitis D

Table 6.4 Continued

Test	Meaning of a positive result	Comment
Hepatitis E virus (HEV)		
Anti-HEV IgM	Recent acquisition of HEV	Acute hepatitic illness likely to be hepatitis E
Other infections		
Cytomegalovirus (CMV) IgM	Recent acquisition of CMV	Acute hepatitic illness likely to be due to CMV
Epstein-Barr virus (EBV) IgM	Recent acquisition of EBV	Acute hepatitic illness likely to be due to EBV
Anti-HIV	HIV-AIDS	Opportunistic hepatobiliary infections
Toxoplasmosis serology	—	Consider toxoplasmosis
Q fever serology	—	Consider Q fever

[1]PCR = polymerase chain reaction.

N.B. Hepatitis G is a flavivirus transmitted by blood transfusion that causes persistent infection. Serological tests are available. This virus does not cause serious or significant chronic liver disease.

TREATMENT

INTERFERON THERAPY FOR VIRAL HEPATITIS

1. Hepatitis B

Success rate: 40% seroconversion from replicative (HBeAg and HBV DNA detectable in serum) to non-replicative (anti-HBe); 10% lose HBs-Ag; relapse following successful treatment 1–2%.

Indications for therapy: ↑ALT, HBeAg and HBV DNA positive, not 'pre-core' mutants, not immunosuppressed and compensated liver disease (N.B. successful therapy induces acute hepatitis-like elevation in transaminases)

2. Hepatitis C

Success rate: 35% response at 6 months and 25% sustained response at 12 months after initiating therapy. Response reduced in those with advanced liver disease, disease of long duration, high levels of HCV RNA and genotype Ib.

Indications for therapy: ↑ALT, HCV RNA present, and chronic hepatitis on histology.

3. Complications

'Flu like' symptoms, depression, marrow suppression, autoimmune reactions (e.g. thyroiditis—may not be reversible), other (alopecia, rashes, diarrhoea, paraesthesias). No established benefit after failure of a previous course of interferon, or if normal ALT levels. Benefit in hepatitis C-associated essential mixed cryoglobulinaemia unclear.

OTHER THERAPIES FOR VIRAL HEPATITIS

Hepatitis B	lamivudine
	famciclovir
Hepatitis C	ribavirin

POSTOPERATIVE JAUNDICE

Table 6.5 *Distinguishing features that help to determine the cause of postoperative jaundice*

Aetiology	Feature
Hypotension	ALT > 1000 U/L, LDH elevated
Drugs e.g. halothane	None
Infection	Increased white cell count, fever
Total parenteral nutrition (TPN)	Liver function test profiles rise 1–4 weeks after TPN commenced
Haematoma resorption	↑ Unconjugated bilirubin
Cardiac failure	Elevated jugular venous pressure, enlarged pulsatile liver
Haemolysis	↑ Unconjugated bilirubin, ↑ LDH, ↓ haptoglobin, abnormal blood smear
Renal failure	↑ Creatinine
Bile duct injury, retained gallstone	↑ SAP

ALT = alanine aminotransferase; LDH = lactate dehydrogenase; SAP = serum alkaline phosphatase.

Table 6.6 *Common causes of jaundice in immunosuppressed patients*

Aetiology	Examples
Hepatitis—infectious	*Mycobacterium avium intracellulare*, tuberculosis, cytomegalovirus
Hepatitis—drugs	Isoniazid, AZT, sulfonamides
AIDS cholangiopathy	Cytomegalovirus, cryptosporidia
Veno-occlusive disease	Antineoplastic drugs (e.g. busulfan)
Neoplasm	Lymphoma, Kaposi's sarcoma

AZT = azidothymidine or zidovudine.

CIRRHOSIS

This is characterised by disorganised lobular architecture, loss of liver cells, nodular regeneration of remaining liver cells with surrounding fibrosis, and collapse and fibrosis of the reticulin network.

CAUSES

1. Alcohol
2. Viral hepatitis (B, C, delta)
3. Cryptogenic (idiopathic)
4. Drugs causing chronic hepatitis
5. Primary sclerosing cholangitis
6. Primary biliary cirrhosis
7. Haemochromatosis
8. Wilson's disease
9. Cardiac disease—chronic constrictive pericarditis
10. Alpha$_1$-antitrypsin deficiency
11. Other, e.g. inflammatory bowel disease, secondary biliary obstruction, cystic fibrosis

SEQUALAE OF CIRRHOSIS

1. Portal hypertension and ascites
2. Portal vein thrombosis
3. Spontaneous bacterial peritonitis
4. Hepatic encephalopathy
5. Hepatorenal syndrome
6. Hepatocellular carcinoma

The Child-Pugh (Table 6.7) score is useful for assessing the severity of cirrhosis and the prognosis.

Table 6.7 Child-Pugh score

Score	Serum albumin (g/L)	Serum bilirubin (μmol/L)	Prothrombin time seconds prolonged	Ascites	Encephalopathy
1	>35	<34	1–3	Nil	Nil
2	28–35	34–51	4–6	Slight	Grade 1–2
3	<28	>51	>6	Moderate	Grade 3–4

A = <7 (one year survival 100%)
B = 7–9 (one year survival 80%)
C = >9 (one year survival 45%).

FULMINANT HEPATIC FAILURE

This is defined as hepatic failure with encephalopathy developing <8 weeks after the onset of jaundice in a patient with no history of prior liver disease.

CAUSES

Infection (hepatitis A, B, D or E but rarely C); drugs e.g. paracetamol (acetaminophen); ischaemia; acute Budd-Chiari syndrome; Wilson's disease; fatty liver of pregnancy; and Reye's syndrome.

POOR PROGNOSTIC FEATURES

Older age, grade 3 or 4 encephalopathy, prothrombin time >50 seconds, drug-induced cause except paracetamol (acetaminophen).

CHRONIC HEPATITIS (Figure 6.2)

This is defined as at least 6 months of a chronic inflammatory infiltration.

CAUSES

1. Hepatitis C
2. Hepatitis B, Delta
3. Idiopathic autoimmune hepatitis
   a) Type I: usually young women, hyperglobulinaemia, positive ANA and anti-smooth muscle antibody diagnostic
   b) Type IIa: typically young women, hyperglobulinaemia, high titres of anti-liver/kidney microsomal (anti-LKM1) antibody, steroid responsive
   c) Type IIb: often older men, hepatitis C present, normal globulins, low titres of anti-LKM1, interferon responsive
   d) Type III: often women, lack ANA and anti-LKM1, antibodies to soluble liver antigen
4. Drugs, e.g. alpha-methyldopa, chlorpromazine, isoniazid, nitrofurantoin, propylthiouracil, methotrexate
5. Alpha$_1$-antitrypsin deficiency
6. Wilson's disease

PORTAL HYPERTENSION

Over 60% of patients with cirrhosis have clinically significant portal hypertension (>30 cm of saline at surgery, or >4 mmHg (0.53 kPa) wedged hepatic venous pressure (WHVP) above inferior vena caval pressure). Clinically, this can result in the development of collaterals and variceal bleeding, ascites and hepatic encephalopathy, as well as splenomegaly and hypersplenism.

CLASSIFICATION

1. *Intrahepatic sinusoidal*—cirrhosis (commonest cause)
2. *Presinusoidal*—(the portal vein end: liver function is largely unimpaired)
   a) Extrahepatic, e.g. neonatal sepsis, hypercoaguable blood disease
   b) Intrahepatic, e.g. lymphoma, schistosomiasis
3. *Postsinusoidal*—(the hepatic vein end)
   a) Budd-Chiari syndrome and inferior vena caval obstruction

b) Veno-occlusive disease (small hepatic veins injured by bush teas, drugs, e.g. azathioprine, 6-thioquanine, dacarbazine, DTIC, glycyrhyzin)

DIAGNOSIS

1. *Indirect evidence*—the presence of varices at endoscopy
2. *Direct evidence* (rarely required for diagnosis)
    a) Angiography (portal vascular bed not seen as clearly but hepatic arterial system can be seen) or portal venography undertaken when extrahepatic portal venous obstruction suspected
    b) Wedged hepatic venous pressure: increased in cirrhosis, but normal ($\approx$5 mmHg (0.67 kPa)) in presinusoidal portal hypertension, e.g. portal vein thrombosis

ASCITES

Most commonly cirrhosis (80%) and malignancy (10%) cause ascites; right heart failure is also important (5%).

Classification of ascites using the protein content is not specific. Currently the serum-ascites albumin gradient (SAAG) is the most useful measure: a value $\geq$11 g/L usually indicates portal hypertension.

Table 6.8 *Classification of ascites by serum-ascites albumin gradient (SAAG)*

SAAG: high ($\geq$11 g/L)	SAAG: low (<11 g/L)
Cirrhosis	Peritoneal carcinomatosis
Alcoholic hepatitis	Tuberculous peritonitis
Cardiac ascites	Pancreatic ascites
Massive liver metastases	Bile leak
Fulminant hepatic failure	
Cirrhosis plus another cause	

Table 6.9 *Characteristics of paracentesis fluid*

Aetiology	Colour	SAAG (g/L)	RBC	WBC (10%/L)	Cytology	Other
Cirrhosis	Straw	$\geq$11	Few	<250	–	Protein <25 g/L
Infected ascites	Straw	$\geq$11	Few	$\geq$250 polymorphs or $\geq$500 cells	–	+ve culture
Neoplastic	Straw/ haemorrhagic/ mucinous	<11	Variable	Variable	Malignant cells	Protein >25 g/L

Table 6.9 *Continued*

Aetiology	Colour	SAAG (g/L)	RBC	WBC (10%/L)	Cytology	Other
Tuberculosis	Clear/turbid/ haemorrhagic	<11	+ + +	>1000 70% lymphocytes	–	Acid-fast bacilli + culture Protein >25 g/L
Cardiac failure	Straw	≥11	0	<250	–	Protein >25 g/L
Pancreatic	Turbid/ haemorrhagic	<11	Variable	Variable	–	Amylase increased
Lymphatic obstruction or disruption	White	<11	0	0	–	Fat globules on staining

RBC = red blood cells; WBC = white blood cells.

BUDD-CHIARI SYNDROME

1. Hepatic vein thrombosis presents acutely with pain, hepatomegaly and ascites, usually in young adults.
2. Causes include the contraceptive pill, myeloproliferative disease, malignancy (e.g. renal, adrenal, testicular, thyroid), paroxysmal nocturnal haemoglobinuria, a fibrous membrane, hepatic amoebiasis, schistosomiasis, and drugs (e.g. azathioprine, adriamycin).
3. Ultrasound with Doppler flow studies followed by liver biopsy can identify the problem. Angiography is useful to confirm the diagnosis and exclude a surgically correctable cause, e.g. a fibrous membrane.

SPONTANEOUS BACTERIAL PERITONITIS

This is not uncommon, particularly in alcoholics. Clinical features may be minimal early on. The diagnosis is made by examining and culturing the ascitic fluid: ≥500 cells, or ≥250 polymorphs per cubic millilitre is suggestive. A low pH and high lactate are helpful but insensitive indicators. Empirical therapy should be begun before the results of culture are available—e.g. with cefotaxime.

HEPATIC ENCEPHALOPATHY

This is a complex organic brain syndrome characterised by disturbances in consciousness and personality, fluctuating neurological signs, flapping tremor and a distinctive EEG (symmetrical high voltage slow waves 2 to 5 per second). It occurs in the setting of advanced hepatocellular disease with acute or chronic liver failure, or with extensive portosystemic shunting. The mechanisms are uncertain, but there is a rough correlation with arterial ammonia levels.

141

PRECIPITATING FACTORS IN ACUTE-ON-CHRONIC LIVER FAILURE

1. Gastrointestinal bleeding (increases ammonia load)
2. High dietary protein intake or constipation (increases ammonia)
3. Electrolyte disturbances (hypokalaemia increases the renal production of ammonia, while alkalosis increases the amount of ammonia that crosses the blood-brain barrier)
4. Infection
5. Deteriorating liver function, e.g. alcoholic binge, development of hepatoma
6. Drugs, e.g. sedatives
7. Metabolic, e.g. hypoglycaemia, hypoxia, hypercapnia, anaemia, myxoedema

GRADES OF SEVERITY OF HEPATIC ENCEPHALOPATHY

Grade	Clinical features
I	Personality and mood changes, disturbed sleep pattern, poor hand writing, foetor, asterixis
II	Mild disorientation, inappropriate behaviour, slurred speech, ataxia, hyporeflexia
III	Disorientation, amnesia, somnolent but rousable, incoherent speech, marked asterixis, hyper-reflexia, clonus, rigidity
IV	A. Responsive to painful stimuli, hypotonia, hyporeflexia, hyperventilation
	B. Unresponsive, decorticate/decerebrate posture

HEPATORENAL SYNDROME

This is defined as advanced liver disease (usually alcoholic cirrhosis) with ascites complicated by functional acute prerenal failure. The onset of renal failure is typically slow, tubular function is good (urinary sodium <20 mEq/L (20 mmol/L), urine to plasma osmolality >1.5) and there is no sustained benefit from increasing intravascular volume.

OTHER CAUSES OF RENAL DISEASE IN PATIENTS WITH LIVER DISEASE

1. Acute tubular necrosis may occur in hepatocellular disease (e.g. following infection, bleeding) or cholestasis (e.g. postoperatively, sepsis)
2. The liver and kidneys may be damaged by one disease process
   a) Toxins and drugs, e.g. carbon tetrachloride, paracetamol (acetaminophen) overdose, methoxyflurane
   b) Infection, e.g. Weil's disease
   c) Polycystic kidney disease
   d) Shock from any cause
   e) Amyloid
   f) Vasculitis
3. Chronic autoimmune hepatitis may be associated with nephrotic syndrome and underlying glomerulonephritis

HEPATOCELLULAR CARCINOMA

Patients with cirrhosis from viral hepatitis (B, delta or C) or haemochromatosis are at the highest risk. Alpha-fetoprotein is elevated in 50%.

Table 6.10 *Primary sclerosing cholangitis (PSC) and primary biliary cirrhosis (PBC)*

Feature	PSC	PBC
Age	Young	Middle aged and elderly
Sex	Typically men (70%)	Typically women (90%)
Clinical	Pain	Pruritus
	Cholangitis	Xanthomas, xanthelasma
	Hepatosplenomegaly	Hyperpigmentation
		Hepatosplenomegaly
Liver function tests	SAP + + +	SAP + +
	Bilirubin fluctuates	
Antimitochondrial antibody	Negative	Positive 90% (also elevated in chronic hepatitis, connective tissue disease)
pANCA	Positive (up to 90%)	Negative
Cholangiography	Irregular and beaded ducts	Pruned ducts
Associated diseases	Ulcerative colitis (70%)	CREST syndrome
	Crohn's disease (rare)	
	Sjögrens syndrome (rare)	Sjögrens syndrome
	Thyroiditis (rare)	Thyroiditis
	Hypothyroidism (rare)	Renal tubular acidosis
	Pancreatitis (rare)	
	Retro-orbital and retroperitoneal fibrosis (rare)	
Complications	Portal hypertension	Osteomalacia
	Liver failure	Steatorrhoea (due to bile acid deficiency, associated pancreatic insufficiency or coexistent coeliac disease)
	Bile duct carcinoma	Portal hypertension, liver failure (late)

SAP = serum alkaline phosphatase; pANCA = peri-nuclear anti-neutrophil cytoplasmic antibody. CREST = calcinosis, Raynaud's syndrome, oesophageal dysmotility, sclerodactyly and telangiectasia.

Table 6.11 Haemochromatosis and Wilson's disease

Feature	Haemochromatosis	Wilson's disease
Age	Typically 40–60 years	Typically 10–20 years, but up to 60 years
Sex	Usually males (10:1)	Males and females
Inheritance	Autosomal recessive	Autosomal recessive
Liver diseases	Chronic hepatitis, cirrhosis, hepatoma	Hepatitis, fulminant hepatitis, chronic hepatitis
Other manifestations	Diabetes mellitus Pigmentation of skin Cardiac disease Arthropathy Testicular atrophy (pituitary iron deposits)	Kayser-Fleischer rings* Neurological signs Haemolysis Renal tubular disease
Diagnosis	Serum iron, TIBC,[†] ferritin,[‡] transferrin saturation[§] Liver biopsy to measure hepatic iron index,** and to document cirrhosis as this predisposes to hepatocellular carcinoma	Serum caerulopasmin low Urinary copper increased
Therapy	Venesection (arthropathy, hypopituitarism do not respond)	D-pencillamine
Relatives	Serially follow first degree relatives >10 years of age[‡]	Serially follow first-degree relatives until >30 years of age

*May also be seen on slit-lamp examination in primary biliary sclerosis and primary sclerosing cholangitis sometimes.
[†]TIBC = total iron binding capacity.
[‡]Haemochromatosis gene assay documents heterozygous and homozygous disease.
[§]Transferrin saturation >62% in males (>50% in females) identifies >90% of homozygotes; calculated by iron/TIBC × 100.
**Hepatic iron index = liver iron concentration (μmol/g drug weight/age in years: >2 indicative of haemochromatosis).

Table 6.12 Drugs and the liver

Liver disease	Drug examples
Acute hepatitis	Halothane, phenytoin, chlorothiazide Drugs causing chronic hepatitis
Cholestasis	Hypersensitivity reaction:* chlorpromazine, other phenothiazines, sulfonamides, sulfonylureas, phenylbutazone, rifampicin, nitrofurantoin, flucloxacillin

Table 6.12 Continued

Liver disease	Drug examples
	Dose related:[†] anabolic steroids, the contraceptive pill
Mixed cholestasis/hepatitis	Amoxycillin/clavulanic acid
Fatty liver	Tetracycline, valproic acid, salicylate, amiodarone, perhexiline (microvesicular); methotrexate, alcohol (macrovesicular)
Peliosis hepatitis (large blood-filled cavities)	Anabolic steroids, the contraceptive pill, tamoxifen
Cyotoxic (liver cell necrosis)	Paracetamol (acetaminophen), carbon tetrachloride (zone 3)
Angiosarcoma	Vinyl chloride, thorotrast, arsenic

Amoxycillin/clavulanic acid can cause acute cholestatic hepatitis.
*Canalicular bile plugs ± portal tract inflammatory infiltrate with eosinophils.
[†]No inflammatory infiltrate or necrosis.

Reye's syndrome
Usually children and adolescents are affected 1 to 3 days following an upper respiratory tract infection; aspirin ingestion is strongly associated.

Persistent vomiting is followed by stupor and coma. Jaundice is absent or minimal. The ALT and arterial ammonia are high, and hypoglycaemia is profound and persistent. Raised intracranial pressure is common. Jamaican vomiting sickness is similar, but is caused by ingestion of a local plant.

THE CONTRACEPTIVE PILL AND THE LIVER: ASSOCIATIONS

1. Hepatic adenoma (and very rarely hepatocellular carcinoma)
2. Focal nodular hyperplasia
3. Peliosis hepatis
4. Budd-Chiari syndrome
5. Cholestasis
6. Cholesterol gallstones
7. Unmasking of the Dubin-Johnson syndrome

CAUSES OF HEPATIC GRANULOMAS

1. Sarcoidosis
2. Infection, e.g. tuberculosis, atypical mycobacteria, leprosy, brucellosis, histoplasmosis, schistosomiasis, Q fever
3. Primary liver disease, e.g. primary biliary cirrhosis
4. Idiopathic granulomatous hepatitis
5. Miscellaneous, e.g. drugs (sulfonamides, penicillin, allopurinol, quinidine, phenytoin, phenylbutazone, halothane), berylliosis, silicosis, lymphoma

DIAGNOSTIC HINTS: LIVER AND OTHER SYSTEMIC DISEASE

1. Liver and cardiac disease—consider underlying cardiac failure, constrictive pericarditis, haemochromatosis, alcoholism, amyloidosis
2. Liver and lung disease—consider underlying alpha$_1$-antitrypsin deficiency
3. Liver and neurological disease—consider underlying Wilson's disease, hepatic encephalopathy, alcohol
4. Liver disease and photosensitivity—consider underlying porphyria cutanea tarda
5. Liver and renal disease (see hepatorenal syndrome)

LIVER TRANSPLANTATION

Disease-specific indications for transplantation include: end stage cirrhosis (any cause), primary sclerosing cholangitis, Caroli's disease (intrahepatic biliary tree: multiple cystic dilatations), Budd-Chiari syndrome, and fulminant hepatic failure. Hepatitis C patients do as well as others despite recurrent infection in the graft usually occurring; in active hepatitis B graft survival is reduced up to 20%, but prophylactic hepatitis B immune globulin increases the success rate, as does pretreatment with lamivudine.

Absolute contradictions include: active sepsis outside the biliary tract, metastatic hepatobiliary malignancy, HIV infection and advanced cardiopulmonary disease.

Relative contradictions include: advanced age (>60 years), biliary infection, unreformed alcoholism, a blocked portal vein, previous major upper abdominal surgery, major renal impairment, and other medical disease (e.g. poorly controlled diabetes).

PREGNANCY AND THE LIVER

Table 6.13 Liver disease in pregnancy

Disease	Cause	Comment
Incidental to pregnancy	Viral hepatitis	Most common cause of liver disease in pregnancy
	Alcohol related	—
	Autoimmune chronic hepatitis	Most prevalent in females of reproductive age
Related to pregnancy (possibly influenced by hormones present in pregnancy)	Complicated gallstone disease	Bile ducts enlarge in pregnancy, tend to regress after delivery
	Hepatic adenoma	May enlarge and bleed, rare
	Focal nodular hyperplasia	May enlarge
	Budd-Chiari syndrome	Hepatic venous outflow obstruction

Table 6.13 Continued

Disease	Cause	Comment
Specific to pregnancy	Benign intrahepatic Cholestasis	Pruritus, jaundice in 3rd trimester
	Acute fatty liver	Vomiting, pain, jaundice, liver failure— deliver immediately
	HELLP	In pre-eclampsia (page 318)

COMPLICATIONS OF ALCOHOLISM

GASTROINTESTINAL TRACT

1. Chronic liver disease (alcoholic hepatitis, cirrhosis)
2. Hepatomegaly (fatty liver, chronic liver disease)
3. Diarrhoea (watery due to alcohol, or steatorrhoea due to chronic alcoholic pancreatitis or rarely liver disease)
4. Pancreatitis (although acute attacks occur, usually there is underlying chronic disease)
5. Acute gastritis (erosions)
6. Parotitis/parotidomegaly

CARDIOVASCULAR SYSTEM

1. Hypertension
2. Cardiomyopathy
3. Arrhythmias

NERVOUS SYSTEM

1. Nutrition related problems:
   Wernicke's encephalopathy, Korsakoff's psychosis (thiamine deficiency), pellagra (dermatitis, diarrhoea, dementia due to niacin deficiency)
2. Withdrawal syndromes
   Tremor, hallucinations, 'rum fits', delirium tremens
3. Dementia (cerebral atrophy, Marchiafava-Bignami disease, nutrition deficiency)
4. Cerebellar degeneration
5. Central pontine myelinosis (causing pseudobulbar palsies, spastic quadriparesis)
6. Autonomic neuropathy
7. Proximal myopathy
8. Acute intoxication

HAEMATOLOGICAL SYSTEM

1. Megaloblastic anaemia (dietary folate deficiency, rarely B_{12} deficiency due to chronic pancreatitis with failure to cleave B_{12}-R protein complex)
2. Iron deficiency anaemia due to bleeding erosions or varices

3. Aplastic anaemia (direct toxic effect on the bone marrow)
4. Thrombocytopenia (bone marrow suppression, hypersplenism)

METABOLIC ABNORMALITIES

1. Acidosis (lactic, ketoacidosis)
2. Hypoglycaemia
3. Hypocalcaemia, hypomagnesaemia
4. Hypertriglyceridaemia, hyperuricaemia

GALLSTONES

Association with an increased incidence of cholesterol gallstones:
1. Increasing age
2. Female gender, oestrogen therapy, the contraceptive pill (more lithogenic bile)
3. Race, e.g. American Indians
4. Obesity (lithogenic bile)
5. Intrahepatic cholestasis of pregnancy
6. Pancreatitis
7. Ileal resection or disease
8. Drugs, e.g. clofibrate (lithogenic bile)

Association with an increased incidence of calcium bilirubinate (pigment) stones:
1. Chronic haemolysis
2. Cirrhosis
3. Biliary infection

Natural history of asymptomatic gallstones: 80% remain asymptomatic, and cholecystectomy is not recommended unless symptoms occur. Fewer than 20% who experience symptoms will develop complications, but cholecystectomy is indicated.

At increased risk of complications are the elderly, diabetics, those with large stones (>2.5 cm), and those with a non-functioning or calcified gallbladder.

PORPHYRIAS

There are 5 major syndromes in adults (all autosomal dominant).

HEPATIC PORPHYRIA

ACUTE INTERMITTENT PORPHYRIA (AIP)

1. Defect: partial deficiency of porphobilinogen deaminase.
2. Clinical features (similar to lead poisoning)
   a) Abdominal pain, vomiting, constipation.
   b) Peripheral neuropathy (motor).
   c) Skin *never* affected.
   Attacks may be precipitated by drugs (alcohol, barbiturates, sulfonamides, the contraceptive pill).

3. Investigation
   a) Acute attacks—increased urinary porphobilinogen (PBG) and delta-aminolevulinic acid (ALA) (thus the urine is dark); faecal porphyrins normal.
   b) Remission—findings as above.

VARIEGATE PORPHYRIA (VP)

1. Defect: protoporphyrinogen oxidase deficiency
2. Clinical features
   a) Acute attacks
      i) Similar to AIP except for the skin
      ii) Skin is photosensitised, resulting in fragility, pigmentation and hypertrichosis in light-exposed areas.
3. Investigations
   a) Acute attacks—similar to AIP except faeces contain excess copro-porphyrins and protoporphyrins
   b) Remission—urine may be normal.

Treatment of AIP/VP
- Avoid drugs which precipitate it in patients known to have it.
- Treat acute attacks with haematin.

PORPHYRIA CUTANEA TARDA

1. Defect: uroporphyrinogen decarboxylase deficiency.
2. Clinical features
   a) No acute attacks and not usually drug related.
   b) Skin—bullae and hyperpigmentation on exposed areas (like VP).
   c) Underlying alcoholic liver disease or hepatitis C common; may be a history of toxin exposure, e.g. hexachlorobenzene.
3. Investigations
   a) Normal PBG and ALA in urine and normal porphyrins in stools.
   b) Greatly increased uroporphyrin in urine (red urine).

HEREDITARY COPROPORPHYRIA (VERY RARE)

Clinically like VP with raised faecal and sometimes urinary coproporphyrin.

ERYTHROPOIETIC PORPHYRIA

ERYTHROPOIETIC PROTOPORPHYRIA

1. Defect: ferrochelatase deficiency.
2. Clinical feature: skin photosensitivity.
3. Investigations: free protoporphyrin in red blood cells (urine normal).

Nephrology

IMPORTANT CLINICAL CLUES

HAEMATURIA

- May be glomerular or non-glomerular.
- Glomerular bleeding responsible for <5% of haematuria at age >40, but roughly one quarter of cases in young adults.
- Glomerular bleeding results in dysmorphic erythrocytes or red cell casts in the urine.
- Mesangial or glomerular basement membrane damage is usually responsible for haematuria arising from the glomerulus.

CAUSES

GLOMERULAR BLEEDING	NON-GLOMERULAR BLEEDING
IgA nephropathy	Renal cell carcinoma
Thin basement membrane disease	Bladder or ureteric tumour
Nephritic syndrome (glomerulonephritis)	Cystitis
	Calculi
	Prostatic disease (e.g. carcinoma)
	Urethritis
	Polycystic kidneys
	Pyelonephritis
	Analgesic nephropathy
	Bleeding disorders

PROTEINURIA

- Dipstick urinalysis is relatively specific for albumin.
- Total protein excretion over 24 hours is a more specific measure for proteinuria. Upper limit of normal is 100 mg per day.
- >3.5 g proteinuria per day indicates nephrotic syndrome.

CAUSES

- Tubular injury, resulting in defective resorption of small molecular-weight proteins, e.g. $\beta 2$ microglobulin.

- Primary glomerular injury >2 g/day of proteinuria indicates a poorer prognosis.
- Bence-Jones proteinuria, which is overproduction of free immunoglobulin light chains.
- Haemodynamic stress, for example due to heavy exercise or severe illness (such as congestive heart failure, burns, fever, severe hypertension). Protein leakage through the glomerulus results from action of vasoactive hormones.
- Orthostatic proteinuria is only present when the patient stands. Benign prognosis.

Table 7.1 *Causes of false positive tests for proteinuria*

Cause of false +ve	Dipstick test	Protein precipitation test
High urine pH (>8 due to urea-splitting bacteria)	+	−
Antiseptics	+	−
Gross haematuria	+	+
Very concentrated urine	+	+
Antibiotics (penicillin, cephalosporins)	−	+
Radiocontrast	−	+

POLYURIA AND POLYDIPSIA

CAUSES

- Diuretics
- Chronic renal failure
- Diuretic phase of acute renal failure or postoperative diuresis
- Diabetes mellitus (uncontrolled)
- Diabetes insipidus (nephrogenic, central) or compulsive water drinking
- Hypokalaemia
- Hypercalcaemia

ANURIA (<50 mL urine/day)

CAUSES

- Obstruction
- Bilateral renal artery occlusion
- Rapidly progressive glomerulonephritis
- Cortical necrosis

Note that acute tubular necrosis does not cause anuria, but commonly causes oliguria (<400 mL/day).

CHANGES IN KIDNEY SIZE

ENLARGED KIDNEYS

Unilateral	Bilateral
Renal cell carcinoma	Polycystic kidneys
Hydronephrosis or pyonephrosis	Bilateral hydronephrosis or pyonephrosis
Acute renal vein thrombosis	Bilateral renal cell carcinoma
Solitary kidney (rarely palpable)	Diabetic nephropathy (early)
Unilateral duplex kidney	Acute bilateral renal vein thrombosis
(rarely palpable)	Nephrotic syndrome
	Amyloid or other infiltration
	Acromegaly

SMALL KIDNEYS

Unilateral	Bilateral
Congenital hypoplasia	Chronic renal failure (except if caused by
Reflux nephropathy	polycystic kidneys, diabetes, amyloidosis,
Renal artery stenosis	obstructive uropathy, lymphoma)
Post infarction	

Table 7.2 Causes of urine discoloration

Colour	Cause
Dark yellow, brown	Bilirubin
Brown-black	Homogentisic acid (ochronosis)
	Melanin (melanoma)
	Metronidazole
	Methyldopa/levodopa
	Phenothiazine
Red	Beets
	Rifampicin
	Porphyria
	Haemoglobinuria/myoglobinuria
	Phenazopyridine hydrochloride (Pyridium)
	Urates
Blue-green	Indomethacin
	Amitriptyline
Turbid white	Pyuria
	Chylous fistula
	Crystalluria

CLINICAL FACTORS SUGGESTIVE THAT RENAL FAILURE IS CHRONIC RATHER THAN ACUTE

- Small kidneys
- Renal bone disease
- Peripheral neuropathy
- Anaemia

Table 7.3 *Urinary casts*

Type	Appearance	Composition	Cause
Hyaline	Clear cylinders	Tamm-Horsfall mucoprotein	Normal
Red cell	Cells with no nucleus in clear cylinders	Tamm-Horsfall mucoprotein combined with red cells	Acute proliferative GN, SLE, IE
White cell	Cells with lobulated nuclei in clear cylinders	Tamm-Horsfall mucoprotein combined with white cells	IN, SLE Pyelonephritis Renal vasculitis Renal infarction
Granular	Cylindrical granular structures	? degeneration of cellular casts	Renal parenchymal disease
Waxy	Cylindrical smooth structures	? degeneration of cellular casts	Renal parenchymal disease
Fatty	Oval fat bodies in clear cylinders	Cholesterol ester and Tamm-Horsfall mucoprotein	NS, and diabetic glomerulosclerosis
Epithelial	Epithelial cells in clear cylinders	Renal epithelial cells and Tamm-Horsfall mucoprotein	Tubular diseases Recovery from ATN

GN = glomerulonephritis
SLE = systemic lupus erythematosus
IE = infective endocarditis
IN = interstitial nephritis
NS = nephrotic syndrome
ATN = acute tubular necrosis

HAEMOPTYSIS AND RENAL FAILURE

DIFFERENTIAL DIAGNOSIS

- Goodpasture's syndrome
- Systemic vasculitis, e.g. SLE, Wegener's granulomatosis, polyarteritis nodosa, cryoglobulinaemia
- Renal vein thrombosis causing pulmonary emboli

- Concurrent renal and cardiac failure
- Legionnaire's disease

HELPFUL SKIN SIGNS IN RENAL DISEASE

1. **Post-streptococcal glomerulonephritis**
- Erythema nodosum
- Impetigo
2. **Purpura in renal disease**
- Henoch-Schönlein purpura
- Cryoglobulinaemia—may be associated ulceration and gangrene
- Amyloidosis—post-proctoscopic periorbital purpura is a classical sign
- Any form of systemic vasculitis can cause palpable purpura

PATHOPHYSIOLOGY

DISORDERS OF SODIUM METABOLISM

HYPERNATRAEMIA (serum sodium >3.56 g/L [150 mmol/L])

CLINICAL FEATURES

1. Neurological—confusion, seizures, coma
2. Neuromuscular irritability—hyperreflexia, twitching muscles, ataxia

CAUSES

A. *With extracellular fluid volume depletion*, i.e. loss of proportionately more water than salt
- Diuretics
- Osmotic purgatives, e.g. lactulose
- Osmotic diuresis, e.g. with hyperglycaemia
- Renal failure or tubular dysfunction
- Excessive sweating, e.g. heavy sustained exercise without replenishment, cystic fibrosis
B. *With euvolaemia,* due to loss of water only
- Unreplenished losses from skin and urine in individuals unable to drink, e.g. hospitalised patients
- Diabetes insipidus, which is either central where there is a failure to synthesise or secrete antidiuretic hormone (and an inappropriate lack of thirst), or nephrogenic, where there is renal tubular resistance to the hormone
C. *With extracellular volume expansion*, i.e. retention of proportionately more salt than water
- Administration of hypertonic saline
- Primary hyperaldosteronism
- Cushing's syndrome

HYPONATRAEMIA (serum sodium <3.1 g/L [135 mmol/L])

CLINICAL FEATURES

1. Neurological—lethargy, agitation, altered consciousness at serum sodium <2.76 g/L (120 mmol/L), seizures
2. Muscular—cramps

CAUSES

A. *With extracellular fluid volume depletion*, i.e. salt and water loss, but proportionately greater loss of salt
- Renal losses, e.g. diuretics, mineralocorticoid deficiency, renal tubular acidosis, salt-losing nephropathy, osmotic diuresis
- Gastrointestinal losses, e.g. vomiting, diarrhoea, peritonitis, pancreatitis
- Third space losses, e.g. ascites, pleural effusion
B. *With euvolaemia*, i.e. pure excess of total body water. Usually there is no accompanying oedema
- Syndrome of inappropriate antidiuretic hormone secretion (SIADH)
- Addison's disease
- Hypothyroidism
C. *With extracellular volume expansion*, i.e. retention of sodium with disproportionately greater amounts of water
- Cardiac failure
- Cirrhosis
- Nephrotic syndrome
- Renal failure
D. *Pseudohyponatraemia*
- Severe hyperlipidaemia
- Hyperglycaemia
- Myeloma

SYNDROME OF INAPPROPRIATE SECRETION OF ANTIDIURETIC HORMONE (SIADH)

CAUSES

1. Ectopic ADH production
   a) Lung carcinoma (especially small cell), pancreatic carcinoma, mesothelioma
   b) Pulmonary tuberculosis
2. Excess pituitary ADH production
   a) Central nervous system tumour, trauma, infection, or haemorrhage
   b) Myxoedema
   c) Acute intermittent porphyria
3. Drugs—chlorpropamide, tricyclic antidepressants, monoamine oxidase inhibitors, vincristine, tolbutamide, haloperidol, phenothiazines, carbamazepine, cyclophosphamide, clofibrate, thiazide diuretics
4. Idiopathic

- Low serum osmolality without oedema
- Urinary sodium matches sodium intake, i.e. is inappropriately high
- Urine less than maximally dilute (in most cases, urine osmolarity is higher than is appropriate for serum osmolality and intravascular volume status)
- Serum sodium level improves with water restriction
- Plasma creatinine is normal
- Absence of Addison's disease and hypothyroidism
- Hypouricaemia is usual

TREATMENT

- Restrict fluid to between 800 and 1000 mL intake per 24 hours
- Induce nephrogenic diabetes insipidus with demeclocycline

DISORDERS OF POTASSIUM METABOLISM

HYPERKALAEMIA

CLINICAL FEATURES

- Cardiac arrhythmias
- Muscle weakness

CAUSES

1. Increased total body potassium
   a) Renal failure
   b) Distal renal tubular disease
   c) Potassium-sparing diuretics: spironolactone, triamterene, amiloride
   d) Hypoaldosteronism, due to hyporeninaemic hypoaldosteronism, ACE inhibitors, NSAIDs, Addison's disease
2. Redistribution of potassium to extracellular space
   a) Acidosis
   b) Haemolysis, rhabdomyolysis
   c) Periodic paralysis
   d) Drugs, e.g. succinylcholine in renal failure, β-blockers, digitalis poisoning
3. Pseudohyperkalaemia
   a) Haemolysis of blood sample
   b) Very high leucocyte or platelet numbers

TREATMENT OF HYPERKALAEMIA

Therapy	Onset of action	Mechanism
Intravenous calcium	Minutes	Antagonises membrane effects
Sodium bicarbonate	15–30 minutes	Redistributes potassium
Glucose with insulin	15–30 minutes	Redistributes potassium
Intravenous salbutamol	15–30 minutes	Redistributes potassium
Cation exchange resins	60–120 minutes	Removes potassium
Dialysis	Minutes	Removes potassium

HYPOKALAEMIA

- Peripheral muscle weakness
- Renal tubular dysfunction (polyuria, polydipsia)
- Cardiac arrhythmias
- Paralytic ileus

CAUSES

1. Decreased total body potassium
   a) Gastrointestinal losses, e.g. vomiting, diarrhoea, villous adenoma
   b) Renal losses
      i) Associated with metabolic acidosis, e.g. diabetic ketoacidosis, renal tubular acidosis, carbonic anhydrase inhibitors
      ii) Associated with metabolic alkalosis, e.g. diuretics, mineralocorticoid excess, Bartter's syndrome
   c) Skin losses
2. Redistribution
   a) Alkalosis (acute: metabolic or respiratory)
   b) Periodic paralysis
   c) Insulin excess
   d) B2 agonists

DISORDERS OF MAGNESIUM BALANCE

HYPERMAGNESAEMIA

CLINICAL FEATURES

- Altered mentation
- Decreased deep tendon reflexes
- Hypopnoea
- Hypotension

CAUSES

- Renal failure
- Excessive intake of laxatives containing magnesium

HYPOMAGNESAEMIA

CLINICAL FEATURES

1. Neuromuscular—lethargy, weakness, irritability
2. Gastrointestinal—anorexia, nausea, vomiting, paralytic ileus
3. Cardiovascular—increased sensitivity to digitalis, possible tachyarrhythmias
4. Hypocalcaemia and hypokalaemia

CAUSES

1. Decreased intake
   a) Starvation
   b) Alcoholism
   c) Prolonged intravenous fluids
2. Decreased absorption secondary to malabsorption syndromes
3. Increased output
   a) Diarrhoea
   b) Diuretics
   c) Diuretic phase of recovery from acute tubular necrosis
   d) Drugs—cisplatin, cyclosporin, aminoglycosides
   e) Hyperaldosteronism
   f) Phosphorus depletion
   g) Bartter's syndrome

METABOLIC ACID-BASE DISORDERS

Look at the pH, $PaCO_2$ and HCO_3^-.

METABOLIC ACIDOSIS

- If the pH and HCO_3^- are reduced, determine if this is a metabolic or mixed disturbance:
  a) Calculate the expected $PaCO_2$ in normally compensated metabolic acidosis, i.e. $PaCO_2$ in mmHg only should equal $1.5\,(HCO_3^-) + 8\,(\pm 2)$ (or $PaCO_2$ in mmHg should only approximately equal the last 2 digits of the pH)
  b) If the $PaCO_2$ is lower than calculated, the patient has respiratory alkalosis and metabolic acidosis; if the pH is higher than calculated, the patient has respiratory acidosis and metabolic acidosis
  c) Next calculate the anion gap to aid in determining the cause of the metabolic acidosis (see below)

METABOLIC ALKALOSIS

- If the pH and HCO_3^- are elevated, determine if this is a metabolic or mixed disturbance:
  a) Calculate the expected $PaCO_2$ in normally compensated metabolic alkalosis, i.e. $PaCO_2$ should increase 6 mmHg (0.8 kPa) for every 10 mEq/L (10 mmol/L) increase in HCO_3^-
  b) $PaCO_2$ lower than calculated equals respiratory alkalosis and metabolic alkalosis; $PaCO_2$ higher than calculated equals respiratory acidosis and metabolic alkalosis
     Next, determine the spot urinary chloride to aid in determining the cause of the metabolic alkalosis
- HCO_3^- can be calculated from the arterial blood gases:

$$HCO_3^- = \frac{24\,(PaCO_2)}{[H^+]}$$

H^+ is determined (approximately) by subtracting the last 2 digits of the pH from 80.

ANION GAP

Calculate as follows: $Na^+ - (Cl^- + HCO_3^-) = 12 (\pm 4)$ normally

CAUSES OF A *HIGH* ANION GAP ACIDOSIS (MNEMONIC MUDPALES)

Cause	Suggestive clinical/laboratory features
M—Methanol	Increased osmolar gap; abdominal pain (increased amylase), hyperaemic optic disc (blindness late)
U—Uraemia	Elevated serum urea and creatinine
D—Diabetic (or alcoholic)	Raised blood sugar, acetone breath, ketoacidosis
PA—Paraldehyde	Distinctive smell on breath
L—Lactate	Serum lactate
E—Ethylene glycol	Oxalate crystalluria
S—Salicylates	History; serum salicylate

- Calculated serum osmolality =

$$\frac{2\,Na^+K^+(mmol/L) + Glucose\,(mmol/L)}{18} + \frac{Urea\,(mmol/L)}{2.8}$$

- Measured serum osmolality (280–300 mOsm/kg) normally does not exceed calculated osmolality by >10 mOsm/kg H_2O
- If measured osmolality is elevated, this indicates that increased measured osmoles are present, e.g. the 'ols' (mannitol, ethanol, methanol); isoniazid
- Elevated lactate occurs with primary circulatory failure and secondary to ethanol, methanol, biguanides, or acute liver failure
- In a vomiting patient with chronic renal failure and a normal pH and $PaCO_2$, always check the anion gap. If increased, this suggests **metabolic acidosis** *and* **metabolic alkalosis** are present.

CAUSES OF A *NORMAL* ANION GAP ACIDOSIS

A) With hypokalaemia
   i) Bicarbonate loss from the renal tract or gastrointestinal tract (diarrhoea or pancreatic fistula)
   ii) Hyperchloraemic acidosis (e.g. renal tubular acidosis)
B) With hyperkalaemia
   i) Hyporeninaemic hypoaldosteronism
   ii) Adrenal failure
   iii) Aldosterone resistance, e.g. interstitial nephritis, amyloid, spironolactone
   iv) Acid load, e.g. cholestyramine

Internal Medicine

CAUSES OF A *LOW* ANION GAP ACIDOSIS (MNEMONIC RULO)

R—Reduced unmeasured anions
U—Underestimation of sodium (e.g. hyperviscosity states) or unmeasured cations (e.g. calcium, magnesium, lithium)
L—Laboratory error
O—Overestimation of chloride, e.g. bromism

CAUSES OF METABOLIC ALKALOSIS

a) Chloride unresponsive (urinary spot chloride >15 mEq/L [15 mmol/L])
    i) Severe potassium depletion
    ii) Cushing's syndrome, hyperaldosteronism
    iii) Bartter's syndrome
b) Chloride responsive (urinary spot chloride <10 mEq/L [mmol/L])
    i) Renal loss of acid, e.g. diuretics, magnesium deficiency
    ii) Gastrointestinal loss of acid, e.g. vomiting, villous adenoma
    iii) Administration of alkali, e.g. sodium bicarbonate, citrate

ACUTE RENAL FAILURE

CAUSES

PRERENAL

1. Decreased circulating volume—haemorrhage, dehydration
2. Hypotension—shock due to sepsis, pump failure, drugs, liver failure
3. Increased renal vascular resistance—hepatorenal syndrome
4. Renovascular disease—atheroma, embolus, dissection

RENAL

1. Acute glomerular disease—glomerulonephritis
2. Acute tubular necrosis—secondary to hypovolaemia, drugs (e.g. radio-contrast media, aminoglycosides), rhabdomyolysis, haemoglobinuria, crystal deposition
3. Acute-on-chronic renal failure—precipitated by infection, dehydration, obstruction or nephrotoxic drugs
4. Tubulointerstitial disease—due to drug hypersensitivity (e.g. antibiotics), NSAIDs, cyclosporin, urate or calcium deposition; infectious causes
5. Vascular disease—vasculitides, thrombotic microangiopathy, malignant hypertension, use of angiotensin converting enzyme inhibitors in the setting of renal artery stenosis or nephrosclerosis, atheroembolic disease

POSTRENAL

1. Bilateral ureteric obstruction
    a) Intraureteric—clot, pyogenic debris, calculi, shed papillae
    b) Extraureteric—retroperitoneal fibrosis (due to radiation, idiopathic, methysergide), pelvic tumour, surgery
2. Bladder neck obstruction—prostatic hypertrophy, prostatitis, tumour, calculus, clot

3. Urethral obstruction—calculus, clot trauma, phimosis, paraphimosis
4. Neurogenic bladder

Suspect obstructive uropathy if a patient with renal failure has:

- Symptoms of renal colic, anuria, poor stream, incontinence, gross haematuria, or repeated or refractory urinary tract infection
- Abdominal mass and fluctuating urine output
- Hyperchloraemic metabolic acidosis and hypokalaemia

Table 7.4 Laboratory findings in acute renal failure

Abnormality in urine	Likely cause
Proteinuria	Glomerulonephritis
Red blood cell casts	Glomerulonephritis, vasculitis
White blood cell casts	Interstitial nephritis
Eosinophiluria	Interstitial nephritis
Crystals	Urate or oxalate nephropathy

Laboratory finding	Prerenal cause	Acute tubular necrosis
Urinary sodium	<20 mEq/L (20 mmol/L)	>40 mEq/L (40 mmol/L)
Urine specific gravity	>1.020	<1.020
Urine osmolality	≥500 mOsm	≤350 mOsm
Urine/plasma osmolality	>1.5	<1.1
Fractional excretion of sodium (FE Na)	<1%	≥1%
$FE\,Na = \dfrac{U\,Na}{P\,Na} \times \dfrac{P\,Creatinine}{U\,Creatinine} \times 100$		
Renal failure index	<1	>1
$Renal\ failure\ index = \dfrac{Urinary\ sodium}{Urine/Plasma\ creatinine}$		

Causes of an increased urea: creatinine ratio
1. Increased urea output—upper gastrointestinal tract bleed, high protein diet, sepsis, corticosteroids
2. Hypovolaemia
3. Obstructive uropathy
4. Cardiac failure

CHRONIC RENAL FAILURE

COMMON CAUSES

1. Chronic glomerulonephritis
2. Reflux nephropathy

3. Analgesic nephropathy
4. Polycystic kidneys
5. Diabetes mellitus
6. Hypertensive nephrosclerosis
7. Lupus nephritis
8. Obstruction
9. Systemic vascular disease

ELECTROLYTE ABNORMALITIES IN CHRONIC RENAL FAILURE

1. Acute hyperkalaemia
   a) Medication—ACE inhibitors, potassium-sparing diuretics, NSAIDs, β-blockers
   b) Hyporeninaemic hypoaldosteronism (usually in diabetic nephropathy)
2. Hypokalaemia
   a) Renal tubular acidosis
   b) Excessive diuretic use
   c) Diarrhoea
   d) Secondary hyperaldosteronism
   e) Correction of acidosis without potassium supplementation
3. Hypercalcaemia
   a) Tertiary hyperparathyroidism
   b) Excess vitamin D supplementation
   c) Aluminium osteomalacia (low parathyroid hormone and 1,25 vitamin D)
   d) Hypophosphataemia
   e) Myeloma kidney
   f) Sarcoidosis
   g) Thiazide diuretics
   h) Metastatic carcinoma

DISEASE STATES

URINARY TRACT INFECTION (UTI)

SIMPLE URINARY TRACT INFECTION

- Refers to bacterial cystitis
- Commonly caused by *E. coli* and *Staphylococcus saprophyticus*
- If positive urinalysis accompanies typical clinical history, treat with either trimethoprim, cephalexin, or amoxycillin-clavulanate
- 3 days of treatment is usually adequate

RISK FACTORS FOR COMPLICATED URINARY TRACT INFECTION

- Male sex
- Pregnancy

- Catheterisation
- Recent instrumentation
- Hospital-acquired infection
- Known anatomical urological abnormality
- UTI occurring in individual <12 years of age
- 3 or more UTIs in one year
- Symptoms lasting longer than 7 days
- Recent antibiotic use
- Diabetes mellitus
- Immunosuppression
- Lower socioeconomic status

INDICATIONS TO PERFORM UROLOGICAL INVESTIGATION IN PATIENTS WITH UTI

(Cystoscopy and retrograde pyelography)
- Multiple relapses
- Painless haematuria
- Childhood UTI
- Renal stones
- Recurrent pyelonephritis
- Symptoms suggestive of urinary tract obstruction

TREATMENT OF COMPLICATED UTI

- Likely organisms are *E. coli*, other Gram-negative organisms, enterococci
- First-line therapy with 3rd generation cephalosporin
- If enterococcus is causative, use ampicillin and gentamicin
- 10–14 days of treatment

UTI IN PREGNANCY

- Women are predisposed in pregnancy because of collecting system dilatation, glycosuria, and aminoaciduria
- Highest risk is in 3rd trimester
- Bacteriuria should always be treated during pregnancy

CAUSES OF STERILE PYURIA

- Tuberculosis
- Analgesic nephropathy
- Renal stones
- Interstitial nephritis
- Renal abscess
- Urethritis, prostatitis
- Partially treated bacterial UTI, or viral infection

Xanthogranulomatous pyelonephritis may cause a flank mass with chronic UTI

Table 7.5 Urolithiasis

Type of stone	Radio-opacity	Frequency	Medical therapy
Calcium (oxalate, phosphate)	Opaque	70%	Correct underlying cause Increase urine output Orthophosphates Allopurinol if hyperuricosuria Alkali if distal renal tubular acidosis (RTA) Potassium and citrate if idiopathic hypercalciuria Thiazides
Uric acid These are dissolvable stones May cause staghorn calculi	Lucent	5%	Increase fluid intake Alkalinise urine with citrate Allopurinol
Struvite (magnesium ammonium phosphate)	Opaque	15%	Surgical removal Long-term antibiotics Urease inhibitor
Oxalate	Opaque	Rare	Correct underlying cause Decrease dietary oxalate Increase dietary calcium Cholestyramine Vitamin B6
Cystine May cause staghorn calculi	Mildly opaque	Rare	Increase fluid intake Alkalinise urine (pH >7) D-penicillamine (with pyridoxine)
Xanthine (low serum & urine uric acid associated)	Lucent	Rare	Increase fluid intake Alkalinise urine Allopurinol

Pure calcium phosphate stones may be caused by distal tubular acidosis or hyper vitaminosis D

GLOMERULAR DISEASE

CLINICAL FEATURES OF GLOMERULAR DISEASE

1. Persistent proteinuria
2. Nephrotic syndrome
3. Haematuria
4. Acute nephritic syndrome

5. Rapidly progressive glomerulonephritis
6. Chronic glomerulonephritis and chronic renal failure

NEPHROTIC SYNDROME

This is defined by the following criteria:

a) Proteinuria >3.5 g/24 hours
b) Hypoalbuminaemia (serum albumin <30 g/L (<35 mmol/L)
c) Oedema
d) Hyperlipidaemia (increased LDL and cholesterol)

CAUSES

1. *Primary glomerulonephritis (GN)*—especially membranous in adults and minimal change disease in children
2. *Secondary glomerulonephritis*, due to:
   a) Drugs—Angiotensin converting enzyme inhibitors, gold salts, D-penicillamine, heroin, probenecid
   b) Systemic autoimmune disease—SLE, Sjögren's syndrome
   c) Infection—infective endocarditis, HIV, hepatitis B
   d) Malignancy, resulting in membranous glomerulonephritis, especially lymphoma
   e) Serum sickness reaction, e.g. as a result of insect sting or medication

NEPHRITIC SYNDROME

CLINICAL FEATURES

1. Hypertension
2. Haematuria
3. Oedema
4. Oliguria
5. Proteinuria may be present

CAUSES

1. Primary glomerulonephritis
   a) With nephritic syndrome alone
      i) Post-infective GN
      ii) Crescentic GN
      iii) IgA nephropathy
      iv) Alport's syndrome
      v) Haemolytic uraemic syndrome
   b) Nephritic and nephrotic syndromes combined
      i) Mesangiocapillary GN
      ii) Mesangioproliferative GN
2. Secondary glomerulonephritis
   a) SLE
   b) Infective endocarditis
   c) Cryoglobulinaemia

d) Shunt nephritis
e) Polyarteritis nodosa
f) Wegener's granulomatosis
g) Henoch-Schönlein purpura

CLASSIFICATION OF GLOMERULONEPHRITIS

PRIMARY

Diffuse
1. Minimal change lesion
2. Membranous
3. Proliferative
   a) Post-infective, including post-streptococcal
   b) Mesangiocapillary
   c) Crescentic
   d) Mesangioproliferative

Focal
1. IgA nephropathy
2. Focal glomerulosclerosis

SECONDARY TO SYSTEMIC DISEASE

e.g. SLE, Henoch-Schönlein purpura, polyarteritis nodosa, Goodpasture's syndrome, Wegener's granulomatosis, infective endocarditis

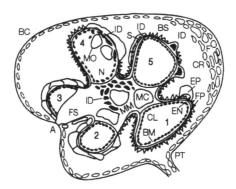

Figure 7.1 *A highly schematised illustration of a cross-section of a single glomerulus showing normal glomerular architecture and some of the characteristic changes seen in glomerular disease. One lobule with 5 capillary loops is illustrated within Bowman's capsule (BC). The capillary loops are supported by the intercapillary mesangium, containing mesangial cells (MC) and mesangial matrix (MM). Note that the normal glomerular capillary wall (loop 1) is composed of 3 layers:*

GLOMERULAR DISEASE WITH ACUTE REVERSIBLE RENAL FAILURE

Post-streptococcal GN

1. Follows Group A, β-haemolytic pharyngeal infection after 6–21 days
2. Laboratory features include proteinuria <3 g/day, low serum total and C3 complement, and granular subepithelial deposits of IgG and C3 on renal biopsy (lumpy-bumpy pattern)

TREATMENT

- Is supportive, with generally full recovery

CRESCENTIC GLOMERULONEPHRITIS WITH PROGRESSIVE RENAL FAILURE

DEFINITION

- Deteriorating renal function over weeks to months, often with oliguria
- Active urinary sediment with >50% crescents, and fibrinoid necrosis on renal biopsy
- Further defined by immunofluorescence:

◀ ───

Figure 7.1 *Continued   endothelial cells (EN), basement membrane (BM) and epithelial cells (EP) with epithelial cell foot processes (FP).*

Loop 2 illustrates minimal change nephrotic syndrome with only diffuse effacement or 'fusion' of epithelial cell foot processes. Foot process effacement is also seen in other areas where increased capillary permeability with proteinuria would occur. In loop 3 a focal sclerotic lesion (FS) is seen with collapse of the capillary loop and adhesion (A) to Bowman's capsule. Immune complex deposits (ID) are shown in black at 3 sites: within the mesangial matrix (loop 4); as subendothelial deposits between endothelial cells and basement membrane as seen in SLE and mesangioproliferative glomerulonephritits (loop 4); and as the diffuse finely granular subepithelial deposits of membranous nephropathy (left, loop 5) with intervening 'spikes' (S) of basement membrane, or the larger more widely spaced epithelial humps (right, loop 5) seen in post-streptococcal glomerulonephritis. Mesangial and subendothelial deposits usually elicit an infiltrate of neutrophils (N) and monocytes (MO) that may displace endothelial cells and directly injure basement membrance, as shown in loop 4. With severe injury, fibrin (F) leakage into Bowman's space (BS) may induce formation of a cellular crescent (CR) composed of proliferating parietal epithelial cells and circulating mononuclear cells as shown from 1 to 3 o'clock. CL = capillary lumen; PT = proximal tubule.

Reproduced, with permission, from Wyngaarden JB, Smith LH, editors. Cecil's Textbook of Medicine. 18th ed. Philadelphia: WB Saunders, 1988: 583.

1. Linear IgG deposits on capillary loop—due to deposition of antiglomerular basement membrane antibodies. This is known as Goodpasture's syndrome if co-existent lung haemorrhage is present, characterised by haemoptysis, bilateral pulmonary infiltrates on chest X-ray, increased diffusing capacity for carbon monoxide and iron deficiency
2. Granular immune complex deposition
3. Minimal or negative immunofluorescence

TREATMENT
- High-dose intravenous corticosteroids
- Plasmapheresis for antiglomerular basement membrane disease

PROGNOSIS
- 25% mortality
- 40% or more progress to end-stage renal disease

GLOMERULAR DISEASE WITH HAEMATURIA AND VARIABLE PROTEINURIA AND RENAL FUNCTION

CAUSES

1. **IgA nephropathy**
   - Haematuria and erythrocyte casts occur, frequently in conjunction with pharyngitis.
   - Renal biopsy shows mesangial proliferation, with IgA deposition on immunofluorescence.
   - May result from excessive mucosal IgA production. Serum IgA is elevated in 50%.
   - Secondary causes include chronic liver disease, dermatitis herpetiformis, and ankylosing spondylitis.
   - Proteinuria and hypertension may occur, and are poor prognostic indicators.
   - 20% progress to end-stage renal disease.
2. **Membranoproliferative glomerulonephritis**
   - Presents with either nephrotic syndrome (50%), nephritic syndrome (20%), or non-nephrotic proteinuria.
   - Hypocomplementaemia is present, as may be the C3 nephritic factor.
   - May be idiopathic or due to secondary causes such as chronic infection, shunt nephritis, SLE, sickle cell disease, congenital C2 or C3 deficiency, or mixed cryoglobulinaemia.
   - Renal biopsies demonstrate duplication of the glomerular basement membrane on electron microscopy.
   - Type II disease may be associated with partial lipodystrophy.
   - Treatment is basically supportive.
   - If hypertension and heavy proteinuria are present, may progress to end-stage renal disease.
3. **Henoch-Schönlein purpura**
   - Haematuria and erythrocyte casts.
   - Purpura, typically on the buttocks and lower limbs.

- Abdominal pain and bloody diarrhoea may occur.
- Renal biopsy findings resemble IgA nephropathy.
- Treatment is supportive.
- Usually runs a benign course in children, but may cause chronic renal failure in adults.

GLOMERULAR DISEASE WITH HEAVY PROTEINURIA AND VARIABLE RENAL FAILURE

CAUSES

1. Minimal change nephropathy
  - Abrupt onset of nephrotic syndrome.
  - Primary cause of nephrotic syndrome in children.
  - Renal function normal, except if caused by NSAIDs.
  - Secondary cases may be due also to Hodgkin's disease.
  - Renal biopsy normal, except electron microscopy shows fusion of the foot processes of glomerular epithelial cells.
  - Responds to immunosuppression, but rate of relapse is high.

2. Membranous glomerulonephritis
  - Proteinuria is the predominant feature, but hypertension and renal insufficiency may occur.
  - Renal vein thrombosis is a not uncommon complication.
  - Primary cause of nephrotic syndrome in adults.
  - Multiple secondary causes include chronic infection, systemic autoimmune diseases, malignancies (e.g. lymphoma, carcinoma of the breast, lung or gut) and drugs (including captopril, gold salts and D-penicillamine).
  - Renal biopsy shows epithelial deposits and thickened capillary loops, and granular IgG and C3 on immunofluorescence.
  - May spontaneously remit without treatment.
  - May respond to corticosteroids.
  - 20% progress to end-stage renal disease.

3. Focal glomerular sclerosis
  - Presents with hypertension, proteinuria, haematuria and renal failure.
  - Secondary causes include reflux nephropathy, HIV infection, morbid obesity, heroin abuse.
  - Renal biopsy shows focal and segmental glomerular sclerosis, with mesangial IgM and C3 deposits on immunofluorescence.
  - Immunosuppression may be helpful, as may angiotensin converting enzyme inhibitors for heavy proteinuria.

OTHER GLOMERULAR DISORDERS

DIABETIC NEPHROPATHY (see also page 209)

- Most common cause of end-stage renal disease.
- Results from glycosylation of glomerular basement membranes, hypertension and renal vascular changes.

Stages of diabetic nephropathy

I. Glomerular hyperfiltration. Glomerular filtration rate (GFR) 20–50% above normal. Microalbuminuria (>300 mg/24 hours).
II. GFR returns toward normal, but there is early structural damage.
III. Hypertension develops.
IV. Increasing proteinuria (>500 mg/day), falling GFR. This phase lasts 10–15 years.
V. Progression to end-stage renal disease. Heavy proteinuria. This phase lasts 5–7 years.

Pathological changes

- Nodular and diffuse glomerular sclerosis.
- Capsular drops and fibrin caps are pathognomonic.
- Basement membrane thickening.

Treatment

- Careful monitoring and control of blood pressure (with ACE inhibitors) and blood glucose levels retard progression of disease.

SYSTEMIC LUPUS ERYTHEMATOSUS (SLE)

See Chapter 12 (page 314).

TUBULOINTERSTITIAL DISEASE

ACUTE INTERSTITIAL NEPHRITIS

CLINICAL FEATURES

- Fever
- Pyuria
- Haematuria
- Proteinuria
- Renal insufficiency
- Arthralgias
- Rash
- Eosinophilia

CAUSES (MNEMONIC SOLID)

S— stones
O—obstruction
L— electrolyte disorders; hypokalaemic, hypercalcaemic, uric acid, or oxalate nephropathy
I— infection, e.g. streptococcus, EBV, CMV
D—drugs

DRUGS CAUSING ACUTE INTERSTITIAL NEPHRITIS

- Antibiotics, especially methicillin, penicillin, sulfonamides
- NSAIDs
- Diuretics, e.g. thiazides, frusemide

- Cimetidine
- Anticonvulsants, e.g. phenytoin, phenobarbitol

CHRONIC INTERSTITIAL NEPHRITIS

CLINICAL FEATURES

- Hypertension
- Proteinuria
- Insidious renal failure

CAUSES

- Analgesic nephropathy
- Transplant rejection
- Vesicoureteric reflux
- Autoimmune disease, e.g. Sjögren's, SLE
- Lymphoma
- Granulomatous disease
- Lead or cadmium poisoning
- Sickle cell disease
- Myeloma
- Alport's syndrome

Analgesic nephropathy
- Presents with sterile pyuria, renal colic secondary to papillary necrosis, hypertension, renal failure, or transitional cell carcinomas of the urinary tract.
- Due to past excessive use of phenacetin (total intake of 3 kg or 1 g/day for 3 years).
- Patients will often complain of chronic pain, and have a history of peptic ulcer, anaemia and headaches.

PAPILLARY NECROSIS

CLINICAL FEATURES

- Recurrent renal colic
- Fluctuating urine output secondary to obstruction

CAUSES (MNEMONIC POSTCARD)

P— Pyelonephritis
O—Obstruction
S— Sickle cell disease
T— Tuberculosis
C—Chronic alcoholism with cirrhosis
A—Analgesics
R—Renal vein thrombosis
D—Diabetes mellitus

POLYCYSTIC KIDNEY DISEASE

Hereditary—autosomal dominant

Clinical features

- Haematuria
- Urinary tract infection
- Hypertension
- Polycythaemia
- Progressive renal failure
- Responsible for 10% of end-stage renal disease

Associations

- Cysts in liver, spleen, pancreas
- Berry aneurysms and subarachnoid haemorrhage
- Cardiac valve myxomatous degeneration
- Diverticulosis

RENAL TUBULAR ACIDOSIS (RTA)

Should be suspected in hyperchloraemic acidosis with a normal anion gap and hypokalaemia.

Table 7.6 *Causes of renal tubular acidosis (RTA)*

Distal (Type I) RTA	Proximal (Type II) RTA
Hereditary	Dysproteinaemias, e.g. myeloma, amyloid
Hypercalcaemia	Heavy metal toxicity, e.g. lead, Wilson's
Hyperglobulinaemia	disease, cadmium, cobalt
Drugs, e.g. lithium, toluene, analgesics, amphotericin B	Drugs, e.g. carbonic anhydrase inhibitors
	Amino acid disorders, e.g. cystinosis
Amyloid	Carbohydrate disorders, e.g. glycogen storage
Hydronephrosis (chronic)	disease (Type I)
Autoimmune disease, e.g. Sjögren's, primary biliary cirrhosis	Renal transplant
	Idiopathic
Idiopathic	

Table 7.7 *Laboratory and clinical findings*

Finding	Distal RTA	Proximal RTA
Serum potassium	Decreased	Decreased
Serum bicarbonate (usually)	<15 mEq/L (15 mmol/L)	>15 mEq/L (15 mmol/L)
Urine pH	Inappropriately alkaline	Inappropriately alkaline
Morning urine pH	Never <6	Commonly <6
After acid load (urine pH)	Never <5.3	<5.3
Stones and nephrocalcinosis	Common	Rare
Bicarbonate therapy	Sensitive	Resistant

N.B.

- Type III RTA is a rare mixture of distal and proximal RTA.
- Type IV RTA is characterised by acid urine during severe periods of acidosis, a low urine bicarbonate and a high serum potassium; they do not form stones. It is associated with hyporeninaemic hypoaldosteronism (e.g. due to diabetes mellitus or interstitial nephritis).

FANCONI SYNDROME

CAUSES

- Inherited in autosomal recessive fashion
- Acquired secondary to Wilson's disease, amyloidosis, cystinosis, Type I glycogen storage disease, Lowe's (oculocerebrorenal) syndrome

CLINICAL AND LABORATORY FEATURES

A variety of proximal tubular transport defects results in:

- Proximal RTA
- Aminoaciduria
- Glycosuria
- Hyperuricosuria
- Hypophosphataemic rickets

BARTTER'S SYNDROME

CAUSE

- Very rare autosomal recessive disorder
- Results in juxtaglomerular hyperplasia

LABORATORY AND CLINICAL FINDINGS

It presents as if the patient has taken a large dose of frusemide

- Hypokalaemia and alkalosis
- High urinary potassium and chloride
- Volume contraction and high renin-aldosterone, but normal blood pressure

TREATMENT

- Electrolyte supplements
- Spironolactone

THERAPEUTICS

SITE OF ACTION OF DIURETICS (Figure 7.2)

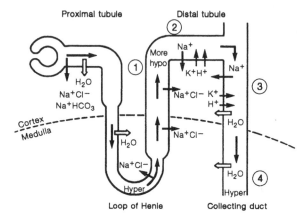

Figure 7.2 *Sites of action of various diuretics. 1. Frusemide and other loop diuretics act on the thick ascending limb of the loop of Henle. 2. Thiazides act on the early portion of the distal convoluted tubule. 3. Aldosterone antagonists, triamterene and amiloride act primarily on the collecting ducts. 4. Antagonists to V2 vasopressin receptors act on the collecting ducts.*
Reproduced, with permisssion, from: Ganong WF. Medical Physiology. 17th ed. Los Altos: Appleton & Lange, 1995.

KEY FACTORS IN THE CONSERVATIVE MANAGEMENT OF CHRONIC RENAL FAILURE

- Exclude and treat any reversible compounding problems, e.g. obstruction, infection
- Control blood pressure closely
- Use phosphate binders to prevent renal osteodystrophy
- Give vitamin D supplements for hypocalcaemia as necessary
- Monitor for metabolic acidosis and treat
- Monitor for hyperkalaemia and restrict potassium intake
- Monitor for anaemia and treat with erythropoietin
- Avoid antiplatelet agents
- Fluid restriction may be required

DIALYSIS

INDICATIONS

- Uraemic symptoms not responding to conservative measures
- Volume overload despite diuretics and salt and fluid restriction

- Resistant hyperkalaemia
- Progressive decline in renal function
- Haemorrhagic pericarditis
- Intractable metabolic acidosis
- Neuropathy
- Treatment of overdose with methanol, aspirin, ethylene glycol, lithium, mannitol, and theophylline

Table 7.8 *Peritoneal versus haemodialysis*

	Peritoneal	Haemodialysis
Advantages	Greater freedom of fluid and diet Removes larger fluid volumes Maintains better haematocrit	Less time each week No protein loss
Disadvantages	Large protein loss Peritonitis Pulmonary collapse, hydrothorax Abdominal hernias Hyperglycaemia Catheter displacement, bowel or bladder perforation Peritoneal membrane failure	Circulatory access problems Vascular access infections Increased bleeding (heparin) Osteodystrophy Dialysis dementia (dyspraxia, myoclonus, abnormal gait, ?due to aluminium toxicity) Infection risk, e.g. hepatitis Dialysis dysequilibrium, due to brain oedema and osmolar shifts

RENAL TRANSPLANTATION

Remains the treatment of choice for end-stage renal disease.

CAUSES OF RECURRENT ALLOGRAFT RENAL DISEASE

- Type II membranoproliferative GN
- Focal glomerulosclerosis
- Diabetes mellitus
- Primary hyperoxaluria
- Haemolytic-uraemic syndrome
- IgA nephropathy
- Scleroderma
- Anti-GBM disease

CAUSES OF GRAFT FAILURE

1. Rejection
   a) Hyperacute (minutes to hours)—necessitates graft removal.
   b) Acute (days to years)—manifested by fever, hypertension, graft tenderness, oliguria, and leucocytosis.

    c) Chronic (months to years)—manifests by increasing proteinuria, decreasing GFR and worsening hypertension. Requires graft removal.
2. Acute tubular necrosis—20–50% of cases, secondary to ischaemia.
3. Surgical complications (e.g. renal artery stenosis, outflow obstruction)

DISADVANTAGES OF RENAL TRANSPLANTATION

- Lifelong immunosuppression
- Cushing's syndrome from steroids
- Opportunistic infections (primary cause of early death), e.g. cytomegalovirus
- Increased risk of malignancy, especially skin cancer, non-Hodgkin's lymphoma due to immunosuppressive therapy
- Increased cardiovascular mortality (primary cause of death)

CYCLOSPORIN A

Has become the mainstay of treatment for graft rejection. It acts by blocking the production of interleukin 2 by CD4+ lymphocytes (T helper cells), but has a number of serious side effects:

- Renal—chronic interstitial nephritis, hypertension, acute renal failure (probably through causing arteriolar vasoconstriction), haemolytic uraemic syndrome
- Hepatic cholestasis
- Neurological—tremor, seizures, pseudotumour cerebri
- Hirsutism
- Gum hypertrophy
- Opportunistic infection
- Lymphoma
- Drug interactions—erythromycin markedly impairs hepatic secretion of cyclosporin, phenytoin markedly increases it

8

Neurology

CLINICAL CLUES ON EXAMINATION

HEAD, NECK AND CRANIAL NERVES

I (OLFACTORY) NERVE

CAUSES OF ANOSMIA

Bilateral upper respiratory tract infection
meningioma of the olfactory groove (late)
ethmoid tumours; head injury (including cribriform plate fracture)
meningitis
hydrocephalus
Kallman's syndrome (hypogonadotrophic hypogonadism).
Unilateral head trauma; meningioma of the olfactory groove (early).

II OPTIC NERVE

Table 8.1 *Causes of blindness*

Rapid onset		Gradual onset
Bilateral	**Unilateral**	**Bilateral & unilateral**
Bilateral occipital lobe infarction	Retinal artery embolism	Cataracts
Ischaemia or trauma	Retinal vein thrombosis	Glaucoma
Severe bilateral papilloedema	Vitreous haemorrhage	Diabetic retinopathy
	Temporal arteritis	Bilateral optic nerve or chiasmal compression
	Retinal detachment	
Rapidly progressive optic chiasmal compression	Optic neuritis	Bilateral optic nerve inflammation or ischaemia
	Ischaemic optic neuropathy	
Bilateral optic nerve damage (e.g. methyl alcohol poisoning)		Bilateral retinal disease
Hysteria		

Table 8.2 *Distinguishing features of papilloedema and retrobulbar neuritis*

Papilloedema	Retrobulbar neuritis
Optic disc swollen without venous pulsation	Optic disc appearance acutely is normal*
Normal acuity (early)	Poor acuity
Large blind spot	Large central scotoma
Normal pupillary light reflex	Afferent pupillary defect
Peripheral constriction of fields	Pain on eye movement
	Onset usually sudden and unilateral

*In papillitis (anterior optic nerve disease) the disc is swollen.

CAUSES OF PAPILLOEDEMA

1. Space-occupying lesions causing raised intracranial pressure. Note that in the Foster-Kennedy syndrome, a unilateral anterior fossa tumour causes raised intracranial pressure and optic nerve compression simultaneously, resulting in papilloedema in the contralateral eye and optic atrophy in the ipsilateral eye.
2. Any cause of cerebral oedema (e.g. head trauma).
3. Acute hydrocephalus (associated with large ventricles).
4. Benign intracranial hypertension (pseudotumour cerebri, associated with small ventricles)—idiopathic; drugs (e.g. the contraceptive pill, nitrofurantoin, tetracycline, vitamin A, steroids); Addison's disease; venous sinus thrombosis; trauma; obesity in young women.
5. Hypertension (grade IV).
6. Central retinal vein thrombosis.
7. Retro-orbital mass.

VISUAL FIELD DEFECTS (Figure 8.1)

III (OCULOMOTOR), IV (TROCHLEAR) AND (VI) ABDUCENS NERVES

Table 8.3 *Pupils: causes of constriction and dilatation*

Constriction	Dilatation
Horner's syndrome	Mydriatic drops or atropine poisoning
Argyll Robertson pupils	Third nerve lesion
Pontine lesion (often bilateral)	Adie's pupil (decreased reactivity)*
Opioids	Post trauma, deep coma, cerebral death
Pilocarpine drops	Amphetamine or glutethamide overdose
Elderly	Cocaine, anxiety
	Iritis (if synechiae form)
	Anticholinergic drugs

*Holmes-Adie syndrome refers to a dilated pupil with virtually no reaction to light, a slow reaction to accommodation, absent ankle reflexes. Other tendon reflexes may also be absent.

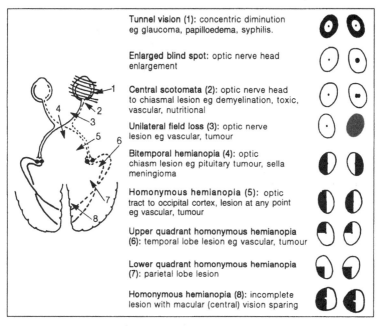

Tunnel vision (1): concentric diminution eg glaucoma, papilloedema, syphilis.

Enlarged blind spot: optic nerve head enlargement

Central scotomata (2): optic nerve head to chiasmal lesion eg demyelination, toxic, vascular, nutritional

Unilateral field loss (3): optic nerve lesion eg vascular, tumour

Bitemporal hemianopia (4): optic chiasm lesion eg pituitary tumour, sella meningioma

Homonymous hemianopia (5): optic tract to occipital cortex, lesion at any point eg vascular, tumour

Upper quadrant homonymous hemianopia (6): temporal lobe lesion eg vascular, tumour

Lower quadrant homonymous hemianopia (7): parietal lobe lesion

Homonymous hemianopia (8): incomplete lesion with macular (central) vision sparing

Figure 8.1 *Visual field defects associated with lesions of the visual system. As a general rule, if one eye is affected the lesion is anterior to the optic chiasm; bitemporal field defects are due to chiasmal disease; and homonymous field defects result from disease of the opposite optic tract or radiation.*

HORNER'S SYNDROME

Clinical clues
Partial ptosis; constricted pupil; apparent enophthalmos; decreased sweating over the ipsilateral face (but only when the lesion is below the carotid bifurcation); elevation of the lower lid; conjunctival injection.

Causes
Interruption of sympathetic innervation due to:
1. Brainstem lesions, e.g. lateral medullary syndrome; syringobulbia; tumour.
2. Lower brachial plexus lesions, e.g. carcinoma of the apex of the lung (usually squamous cell carcinoma).
3. Neck lesions, e.g. thyroid malignancy; trauma; carotid artery injury or inflammation.
4. Intracranial lesions, e.g. carotid aneurysm or dissection; pericarotid tumour; cluster headache.

Internal Medicine

This syndrome is due to vertebral or posterior inferior cerebellar artery thrombosis. The patient presents with vertigo, Horner's syndrome, ipsilateral V (pain and temperature loss), IX and X nerve palsies, ipsilateral cerebellar signs, and contralateral loss of pain and temperature over the trunk and limbs.

III NERVE PALSY

Clinically
- complete ptosis (if lesion complete)
- eye 'down and out'
- dilated pupil unreactive to light (consensual response intact in the unaffected pupil) or accommodation

Causes
Central lesion: brainstem infarct, tumour.
Peripheral lesion: aneurysm (usually on posterior communicating artery), tumour causing raised intracranial pressure (dilated pupil occurs early);
infarction (typically in diabetics—pupil is spared).

IV NERVE PALSY

This produces diplopia maximum when the eye looks 'down and in'; tilting the head to the side of the lesion results in a failure of the affected eye to intort. The most common cause is head injury, although it is often idiopathic.

This may be associated with a III nerve palsy, but rarely may occur as an isolated defect with a lesion of the contralateral cerebral peduncle. (The IV nerve crosses after exiting the brainstem.)

VI NERVE PALSY

This produces failure of lateral eye movement and diplopia.

Bilateral   Wernicke's encephalopathy, mononeuritis multiplex, trauma and raised intracranial pressure.
Unilateral Central (vascular, tumour).
Peripheral disease (e.g. trauma), idiopathic.
N.B. Myasthenia gravis and thyroid eye disease can cause 'pseudo' sixth nerve palsies.

NYSTAGMUS

Types and causes
Jerk nystagmus
Horizontal

Conjugate
1 Brainstem lesions especially in the medulla
2 Vestibular lesion
3 Cerebellar lesion
4 Phenytoin and other drugs
5 Alcohol intoxication

Dysconjugate
1 Internuclear ophthalmoplegia (nystagmus of the abducting eye with failure of adduction of the eye on the affected side, due to a medial longitudinal fasciculus lesion: in young adults with bilateral involvement, multiple sclerosis is almost always the cause; in the elderly consider brainstem infarction).

Vertical
1 Brainstem lesion
   a) Upgaze nystagmus suggests a lesion in the midbrain or upper pons, or Wernicke's encephalopathy.
   b) Downgaze nystagmus suggests a foramen magnum lesion, cerebellar degeneration or Wernicke's encephalopathy.
2 Toxic, e.g. alcohol, phenytoin.

Pendular nystagmus
1. Decreased macular vision, e.g. albinism.
2. Congenital.

Table 8.4 Causes of ptosis and proptosis

Ptosis	Proptosis
Normal pupils	**Bilateral**
Senile ptosis	Graves' disease
Myasthenia gravis	**Unilateral**
Myotonic dystrophy	Graves' disease
Fascioscapulohumeral dystrophy	Cavernous sinus thrombosis
Ocular myopathy	(associated with chemosis and painful
Thyrotoxic myopathy	ophthalmoplegia)
Botulism; snake bite	Carotid-cavernous fistula
Constricted pupil	Tumour (benign, e.g. dermoid, or
Horner's syndrome	malignant)
Tabes	Capillary haemangioma
Dilated pupil	Cellulitis of the eye
III nerve palsy	Sarcoidosis
Bilateral	Neurofibromatosis
Midbrain lesion	

V (TRIGEMINAL) NERVE

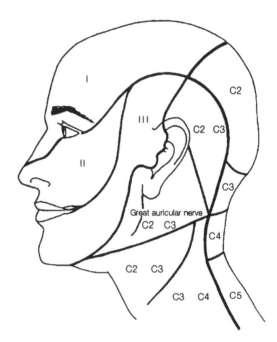

Figure 8.2 *Dermatomes of the head and neck.*
Reproduced, with permission, from: Talley NJ, O'Connor S. Clinical Examination. A Systematic Guide to Physical Diagnosis. 3rd ed. Sydney: MacLennan & Petty, 1996.

CAUSES OF A TRIGEMINAL NERVE PALSY

1. Central (pons, medulla* and upper cervical cord*): vascular, tumour, syringobulbia (increasing cavitation of the central pons and medulla).
2. Peripheral (posterior fossa): aneurysm, skull base tumour.
3. Trigeminal ganglion (petrous temporal bone): meningioma, fracture of the middle fossa.
4. Cavernous sinus (associated with III, IV and VI palsies): aneurysm, thrombosis, tumour.
5. Other systemic problems: Sjögren's syndrome; SLE.

CAUSES OF FACIAL PAIN

1. Trigeminal neuralgia (N.B. exclude multiple sclerosis, meningioma) and post-herpetic neuralgia.

---

*Sensory loss only

2. Paratrigeminal syndrome (severe retro-orbital pain with ipsilateral ptosis and meiosis).
3. Superior orbital fissure syndrome (retro-orbital boring pain with cranial nerve paresis of III, IV, V and VI).
4. Cluster headaches (severe, focal pain of rapid onset, usually in males, with tearing and rhinorrhoea).
5. Temporal arteritis (usually in patients >50 years with an elevated ESR, anaemia, fevers and fatigue). Strong association with polymyalgia rheumatica.
6. Temporomandibular arthritis, and diseases of the sinuses, teeth and ears.
7. Glaucoma.
8. Aneurysm of internal carotid or posterior communicating arteries.
9. Atypical facial pain (psychiatric disease).

VII (FACIAL) NERVE

CAUSES OF FACIAL NERVE PALSY

Unilateral
Upper motor neurone palsy; vascular, tumour etc.

Lower motor neurone palsy:
   a) Pontine—vascular, tumour, syringobulbia, multiple sclerosis.
   b) Posterior fossa—acoustic neuroma, meningioma.
   c) Petrous temporal bone—Bell's palsy, Ramsay Hunt syndrome (facial nerve palsy, vesicular involvement of pharynx and external auditory canal), otitis media, fracture.
   d) Parotid—tumour, sarcoidosis.

Bilateral
Lower motor neurone palsies:
   a) Guillain-Barré syndrome (associated with ascending lower motor neurone lesions, normal sensation and an increased CSF protein with a normal cell count).
   b) Bilateral parotid disease (including sarcoidosis).

VIII (ACOUSTIC) NERVE

CAUSES OF DEAFNESS

Nerve (sensorineural) deafness
1. Tumour, e.g. acoustic neuroma (which may also cause ipsilateral V and VII lesions and cerebellar signs: neurofibromatosis may be associated with bilateral acoustic neuromas).
2. Trauma, noise exposure.
3. Toxic, e.g. streptomycin.
4. Infection, e.g. congenital rubella syndrome, congenital syphilis.
5. Degeneration, e.g. presbycusis.
6. Ménière's disease.
7. Brainstem lesions; vascular disease of the internal auditory artery (rare).

Conduction deafness
1. Wax.
2. Otitis media.

3. Otosclerosis.
4. Paget's disease of bone.

1. Degeneration in the organ of Corti (e.g. aspirin).
2. Ménière's disease.
3. Diseases causing conduction or nerve deafness.
4. Temporal lobe disease occasionally.
5. Intracranial vascular lesions, e.g. glomus tumours, arteriovenous fistulas (pulsatile tinnitus).
6. Idiopathic.

CAUSES OF VERTIGO

Vertigo is an hallucination of motion, e.g. the room spinning around.

Peripheral lesions (no central nervous system (CNS) signs)
Associated with no deafness or tinnitus:
1. Benign paroxysmal positional vertigo (Hallpike manoeuvre is positive).
2. Vestibular neuronitis.
3. Acute labyrinthitis.
Associated with deafness and tinnitus:
4. Ototoxic drugs, e.g. aminoglycosides.
5. Ménière's disease (occurs usually in those >50 years with the triad of vertigo, tinnitus and deafness).
6. Acoustic neuroma (early signs include tinnitus, deafness and dizziness; later loss of the corneal reflex, facial weakness and cerebellar signs evolve).
7. Internal auditory artery occlusion.

Central lesions
CNS signs present: vertigo and nystagmus are commonly associated.
1. Brainstem ischaemia (e.g. vertebrobasilar insufficiency), demyelination (e.g. multiple sclerosis).
2. Tumours, e.g. cerebellum, fourth ventricle.
3. Temporal lobe lesions, e.g. epilepsy, ischaemia.
4. Basilar migraine.
5. Encephalitis or abscess.
6. Subclavian steal syndrome.
7. Drugs, e.g. aspirin, alcohol, phenytoin, quinine.

IX (GLOSSOPHARYNGEAL) AND X (VAGUS) NERVES

CAUSES OF IX AND X NERVE PALSIES

Central
1. Vascular (e.g. lateral medullary syndrome).
2. Tumour.
3. Syringobulbia.
4. Motor neurone disease (not ninth cranial nerve).

Peripheral (posterior fossa)
1. Aneurysm.
2. Tumour (usually metastatic).
3. Chronic meningitis.
4. Guillain-Barré syndrome.

XII (HYPOGLOSSAL) NERVE

CAUSES OF XII NERVE PALSY

Upper motor neurone lesions
1. Vascular.
2. Motor neurone disease.
3. Tumour.
4. Multiple sclerosis.

Lower motor neurone lesions
1. Unilateral
   Central
   a) thrombosis of the vertebral artery
   b) motor neurone disease
   c) syringobulbia
   Peripheral
   a) posterior fossa aneurysm
   b) tumour
   c) chronic meningitis
   d) trauma
   e) Arnold-Chiari malformation
2. Bilateral
   Motor neurone disease
   Arnold-Chiari malformation
   Guillain-Barré syndrome

N.B. It may be difficult to detect unilateral lesions as tongue muscles (except the genioglossus) are bilaterally innervated. Weakness will be apparent on protrusion (tongue deviates to weak side) as the main protruder is genioglossus.

MULTIPLE CRANIAL NERVE LESIONS

- Malignancy: nasopharyngeal carcinoma, brainstem malignancies, posterior fossa mass
- Infection: chronic meningitis, tuberculosis
- Sarcoidosis
- Diabetes
- Paget's disease (basilar invagination)
- Arnold-Chiari malformations (lower cranial nerve signs)
- Inflammation of the superior orbital fissure
- Cavernous sinus syndrome
- Idiopathic polyneuritis cranialis

PSEUDOBULBAR AND BULBAR PALSIES

Pseudobulbar palsy refers to upper motor neurone lesions of IX, X and XII, and can be caused by bilateral cerebrovascular disease (e.g. both internal capsules), multiple sclerosis, motor neurone disease and the Steele-Richardson syndrome (or progressive supranuclear palsy: a syndrome which resembles Parkinson's disease except that there is often no resting tremor and supranuclear gaze palsy occurs).

Bulbar palsy refers to lower motor neurone lesions of IX, X and XII, and can be caused by motor neurone disease, Guillain-Barré syndrome, brainstem infarction or polio.

Table 8.5 *Upper and lower motor neurone lesions*

Upper motor neurone lesion (UMN)	Lower motor neurone lesion (LMN)
Lesion has interrupted a neural pathway above anterior horn cell, e.g. at cerebral cortex, internal capsule, cerebral peduncles, brainstem, spinal cord	Lesion has interrupted a spinal reflex arc, e.g. spinal motor neurones, motor root, peripheral nerve
Weakness *extensors* and *abductors* in upper limb, *flexors* and *adductors* in lower limb	Weakness of muscles innervated. Tends to be more distal than proximal
Muscle wasting absent (or slight)	Muscle wasting prominent
Hyper-reflexia and clonus	Absent or reduced reflexes
Spasticity	Hypotonicity
No fasciculations	Fasciculations (prominent in anterior horn cell diseases usually)
Extensor plantar response	

REFLEX ROOT LEVELS

Table 8.6 *Tendon reflexes*

Reflex	Root	Muscle
Biceps	C5, C6	Biceps
Triceps	C7, C8	Triceps
Supinator	C5, C6	Brachioradialis
Finger	C8	Finger flexors
Knee	L3, L4	Quadriceps
Ankle	S1	Gastrocnemius, soleus
Plantar	S1	Plantar
Abdominal	T8–T12	Anterior abdominal
Anal	S3, S4	Anal sphincter
Cremasteric	T12, L1	Cremaster

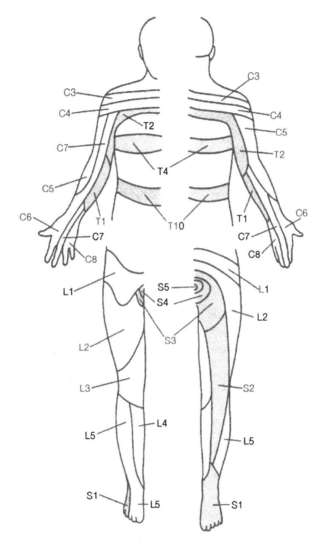

Figure 8.3 *Dermatomes of the upper limb and trunk. Dermatomes of the lower limb.*

Table 8.7 *Neuropathies and myopathies*

Features	Neuropathy	Myopathy
Muscle weakness	+	+
Muscle atrophy	+	±
Pattern of weakness	Distal, or nerve or root distribution	Proximal and symmetrical usually
Reflexes	Decreased (as neuropathy implies lower motor neurone)	Spared
Fasciculations	±	–
Sensory loss	Usually	–
Muscle enzymes	Usually normal	Usually elevated

NEUROPATHY

Peripheral neuropathy may be sensory ('glove and stocking') and/or motor, and/or autonomic. Predominant sensory neuropathy resulting in sensory ataxia and pseudoathetosis is unusual (termed sensory neuronopathy).

Table 8.8 *Peripheral neuropathy: aetiology*

Timing	Sensory	Sensorimotor	Motor
Acute (days)	B6 intoxication Diabetes*	Arsenic Diabetes*	Guillain Barré Porphyria* Diphtheria Organophosphates Diabetes
Subacute (weeks to months)	Cisplatin Paclitaxel Sjögrens Paraneoplastic Amyloid* Paraproteins Diabetes Antiretrovirals	Diabetes Low B_1, B_6, B_{12}* Hypothyroidism Uraemia* Paraneoplastic HIV Isoniazid Vincristine Vasculitis (e.g. SLE, PAN*)	Subacute idiopathic, demyelinating polyneuropathy Heavy metals (e.g. lead*) n-hexane (glue sniffing) Paraproteinaemias Diabetic amyotrophy
Chronic (months to years)	Hereditary sensory neuropathy Diabetes*	Alcohol* Diabetes* Charcot-Marie Tooth[†]	Chronic idiopathic demyelinating polyneuropathy (CIDP) Diabetes

*Painful peripheral neuropathy.
[†]Charcot-Marie-Tooth disease (now termed hereditary motor and sensory neuro-pathy—HMSN): characterised by pes cavus, distal muscle atrophy below elbows and thighs, absent reflexes and thickened nerves.

MONONEURITIS MULTIPLEX

This refers to separate involvement of more than one peripheral and/or very rarely cranial nerve.

CAUSES

- Vasculitis, e.g. polyarteritis nodosa
- Diabetes mellitus
- Carcinoma
- SLE, rheumatoid arthritis
- Sarcoidosis
- Acromegaly, hypothyroidism
- Leprosy
- Idiopathic

MYOPATHIES

CLASSIFICATION

1. Congenital
2. Muscular dystrophies
   a) Duchenne's dystrophy (pseudohypertrophic)—sex-linked recessive, affecting males only; the calves and deltoids are hypertrophied early and weak later; proximal weakness is early; dilated cardiomyopathy is common. Patients usually die in the second or third decade.
   b) Becker (sex-linked recessive)—same as Duchenne's disease but much less severe.
   c) Limb girdle (autosomal recessive or dominant).
   d) Facioscapulohumeral (autosomal dominant or recessive).
   e) Myotonic dystrophy (autosomal dominant)—percussion and post-contraction myotonia is characteristic with frontal baldness, dull triangular facies, partial ptosis, sternomastoid atrophy, testicular atrophy, cardiac conduction defects and often mild mental retardation; the EMG is distinctive ('dive bomber' effect).
3. Acquired myopathy (mnemonic PACE PODIS)
   P—Polymyositis (females more often affected than males; EMG is distinctive with small fibrillation motor unit action potentials), or dermatomyositis (associated with malignancy)
   A—Alcohol
   C—Carcinoma
   E—Endocrine disease, e.g. hyperthyroidism or hypothyroidism, Cushing's syndrome, acromegaly, metabolic myopathies (e.g. McArdle's syndrome)
   P—Periodic paralysis (late)
   O—Osteomalacia
   D—Drugs, e.g. clofibrate, chloroquine
   I— Inclusion body myositis
   S— Sarcoidosis

N.B. Other causes of proximal muscle weakness that are not myopathies include myasthenia gravis and other myasthenic syndromes.

Table 8.9 Myasthenia gravis and the Lambert Eaton syndrome

Feature	Myasthenia gravis	Lambert Eaton syndrome
Defect	Postsynaptic	Presynaptic
Associations	Other autoimmune diseases; thymoma (25% malignant)	Malignancy especially small cell lung cancer in 50%; other autoimmune diseases
Anti-acetylcholine receptor antibodies	80% positive	Negative (anticalcium channel antibodies are found)
Historically	Patients notice fatigue with repetitive action	Decreasing fatigue with repeated actions
Clinically	Ptosis, fatiguability, proximal weakness	Proximal weakness common, absent reflexes; autonomic changes; eyes usually spared
Treatment	Acetylcholinesterase inhibitors; immunosuppression; thymectomy and plasmapheresis	Plasmapheresis and immunosuppression if the underlying malignancy cannot be treated; 3,4 diaminopyridine

SPINAL CORD LESIONS

MOTOR LOSS

A spinal cord lesion causes a lower motor neurone lesion at the level of the lesion, and upper motor neurone signs below that level.

SENSORY LOSS

Patterns of sensory loss depend on the level and type of lesion. Transection of the cord causes a loss of all modalities bilaterally below the level involved, while extrinsic compression of the cord spares the perineum ('sacral sparing').

Dissociated sensory loss often indicates spinal cord disease, although this may sometimes occur in peripheral neuropathy.

DIFFERENTIAL DIAGNOSIS OF DISSOCIATED SENSORY LOSS

Pain and temperature (spinothalamic) loss
1. Syringomyelia.*
2. Brown-Séquard syndrome† (contralateral leg)

---

*Progressive cavitation of the spinal cord especially in the cervical spine leading to dissociated sensory loss in a 'cape' distribution and wasting of the muscles in the lower neck, shoulders, arms, and hands. Loss of upper limb tendon reflexes.

† A hemi-cord lesion with ipsilateral loss of power, joint position and vibration, and contralateral loss of pain and temperature.

3. Anterior spinal artery thrombosis
4. Lateral medullary syndrome (contralateral to other signs)
5. Peripheral neuropathy (small fibre) due to diabetes mellitus, amyloid, Fabry's disease

Vibration and proprioception (dorsal column) loss
1. Vitamin B_{12} (cobalamin) deficiency (subacute combined degeneration of the cord—spastic and ataxic paraparesis, and peripheral neuropathy). B_{12} deficiency may also result in upper motor neurone signs in the legs symmetrically, but absent reflexes due to peripheral neuropathy; optic atrophy and dementia can occur.
2. Brown-Séquard syndrome (ipsilateral leg).[†]
3. Spinocerebellar degeneration (e.g. Friedreich's ataxia).
4. Multiple sclerosis.
5. Tabes dorsalis.
6. Peripheral neuropathy (large fibre) e.g. diabetes mellitus, hypothyroidism, sensory neuronopathies.

CAUDA EQUINA LESIONS

1. Leg/buttock pain
2. Lower limb weakness
3. Loss of sphincter control
4. Saddle sensory loss

DYSPHASIA

This is defined as a dominant cortical disorder of the use of written and verbal symbols for communication.

Table 8.10 *Dysphasia: classification and clinical features*

Feature	Receptive	Expressive	Conductive	Nominal
Site	Wernicke's area (dominant temporal lobe)	Broca's area (third frontal convolution)	Arcuate fasciculus and/or conducting fibres	Angular gyrus (temporal lobe)
Comprehension	Impaired	Normal	Normal	Normal
Naming objects	Poor	Poor	Poor	Poor
Repetition	Poor	May be possible with great effort	Poor	Normal
Fluency and prosody	Preserved but uses jargon, paraphasias and neologisms	Decreased to anarthria	Preserved but paraphasic	Normal except for naming objects

DYSARTHRIA

Disordered articulation with normal speech content.
Test by asking the patient to say 'British constitution' etc.
Causes can include

- Cerebellar disease—arrhythmic or explosive speech or speech broken into syllables.
- Bilateral upper motor neurone disease—trying to squeeze words out; described as a harsh or strained quality.
- Bilateral lower motor neurone damage—nasal speech; a 'hot potato' in the mouth.
- Bilateral facial nerve palsies—slurred speech secondary to labial weakness.
- Extrapyramidal—monotonous, low volume, mumbled.

DYSPHONIA

Laryngeal nerve problems—husky voice, decreased volume, bovine cough.

CLINICAL FEATURES OF ANY PATHOLOGY BY CEREBRAL LOBE

Focal symptoms and signs are helpful to define the site.

FRONTAL LOBE

Personality change
Primitive reflexes, e.g. grasp, pout
Anosmia
Optic nerve compression (atrophy)
Gait apraxia
Leg weakness (parasagittal)
Loss of micturition control
Dysphasia (expressive)
Seizures
Proverb interpretation lost

PARIETAL LOBE

Dysphasia (dominant)
Acalculia,* agraphia,* left-right disorientation,* finger agnosia*

---

*Gerstmann's syndrome: dominant hemisphere parietal lobe only.

Sensory and visual inattention,[†] construction and dressing apraxia,[†] spatial neglect and inattention
Lower quadrantic hemianopia,[‡] astereognosis[‡]
Seizures

TEMPORAL LOBE

Memory loss
Upper quadrantic hemianopia
Epilepsy

OCCIPITAL LOBE

Homonymous hemianopia
Alexia
Epilepsy (flashing light aura)

DISEASE STATES

GUILLAIN-BARRÉ SYNDROME

Widespread demyelination which occurs rapidly over days to weeks. In fulminant disease axonal degeneration can occur, making full recovery of premorbid function less likely.

PREDISPOSING FACTORS

- Majority postinfectious—*Campylobacter jejuni* gastroenteritis, herpes viruses—Epstein Barr virus, cytomegalovirus
- Other predisposing factors or known associations include lymphoma, Hodgkin's disease, SLE, surgery, vaccination, insect stings.

CLINICAL CLUES

- Ascending motor weakness (eyes are spared)
- Progressive areflexia
- Some sensory disturbances
- Pain can be prominent especially once recovery starts

PHARMACOLOGY/THERAPY

Intravenous immunoglobulin is equal to plasmapheresis in efficacy.
Weakness of the respiratory muscles often needs support with mechanical ventilation.

MOTOR NEURONE DISEASE

A group of diseases which have loss of motor neurone function throughout the central and peripheral nervous systems: cortex, brainstem and spinal cord.

[†]Non-dominant parietal lobe.
[‡]Non-localising.

Internal Medicine

Amyotrophic lateral sclerosis (ALS): upper and lower motor neurone involvement. 10% of cases are familial. Forms of ALS include primary lateral sclerosis (predominantly UMN).

CLINICALLY

LMN form
Insidious onset of asymmetrical weakness with wasting, atrophy and often cramping. Chewing and swallowing can also be affected early.

UMN form
Hyper-reflexia and hypertonicity occur early.
Symptomatically stiffness is prominent.
Speech and swallowing may be affected early (pseudobulbar variant).

PHARMACOLOGY/THERAPY

Both upper and lower motor neurones are almost always involved eventually. Median survival 3–5 years.
Survival prolonged by the use of riluzole.
Multifocal motor block (predominantly LMN) may mimic motor neurone disease.

MULTIPLE SCLEROSIS (MS)

PATHOPHYSIOLOGY

MS is a chronic demyelinating disease of the central nervous system characterised by demyelination, gliosis and changes of chronic inflammation predominantly in the white matter of the brain and spinal cord with relative axonal sparing. It is most likely an autoimmune disease. Plaques are demyelinated nerves with surrounding gliosis. There are clear risks including: higher socioeconomic status; familial clusters; immune markers, suggesting that they influence and may drive the course of the disease; viral markers, the significance of which is unknown; and higher rates in cooler climates.

CLINICALLY

Clinically this disease affects both sensory and motor function as well as cerebellar, brainstem and visual function, and occasionally dorsal roots. Its diagnosis requires neurological episodes separated by time and in different regions of the CNS white matter.

Optic neuritis is often present. Other eye signs include diplopia secondary to internuclear ophthalmoplegia. Life risk of developing MS after a single episode of optic neuritis in women is 50%.

Four patterns: (i) relapsing remitting course with recurrent episodes of neurological deficits ($\frac{2}{3}$ of cases); (ii) chronic progressive course with constant gradual deterioration; (iii) chronic stable course with fixed deficits but little progression; and (iv) incidental finding at autopsy.

Diagnosis is mostly on history supported by evidence of raised cerebrospinal fluid (CSF) IgG and oligoclonal bands in the presence of a normal protein level, and slowed or abnormal evoked responses. More than 90% of MRI scans are abnormal, with periventricular involvement the most common pattern. With gadolinium uptake it is likely that disease is active.

DIFFERENTIAL DIAGNOSIS OF MULTIPLE CENTRAL NERVOUS SYSTEM LESIONS WITH A RELAPSING REMITTING COURSE

1. Multiple sclerosis
2. Vascular disease (vasculitis (including SLE), cerebrovascular occlusive disease)
3. Sarcoidosis

THERAPY

Acute episodes may be treated with high-dose intravenous glucocorticoids. Progressive disease is sometimes treated with low-dose oral methotrexate. Subcutaneous interferon-β reduces the frequency and progression (shown on MRI) in relapsing remitting disease, which reduces disability from the disease.

PARKINSONISM

PATHOPHYSIOLOGY

Decreased availability of dopamine in the substantia nigra. In Parkinson's disease, there is cell death, which leads to the depletion.

Drugs which may block dopamine receptors include haloperidol, chlorpromazine, metoclopramide, prochlorperazine, alpha-methyldopa and reserpine.

CLINICAL CLUES

Tremor at rest
Rigidity
Hypokinesis
Impaired balance

TREATMENT

Standard treatment still involves carbidopa-levodopa (Sinemet), including sustained release form.
Dopamine agonists (bromocriptine, pergolide) are also of symptomatic benefit.
Selegiline (monoamine oxidase B inhibitor) is an adjunct to levodopa.

PARKINSON'S PLUS

This should be suspected if there is
1. No rest tremor
2. No response to levodopa/dopamine agonists
3. Added neurological signs.

Clinical entity	*Clinical clue*
Progressive supranuclear palsy	Parkinsonism plus conjugate gaze paresis especially downward gaze
Striatal-nigral degeneration	Parkinsonism plus hyper-reflexia
Olivopontocerebellar atrophy*	Parkinsonism plus poor coordination
Shy-Drager syndrome*	Parkinsonism plus hypotension and dysautonomia

HEADACHES

MIGRAINE

Episodic headaches and or cerebral disturbances where no structural abnormality can be found. Classic migraine (seen in about 30% of people with migraines) includes an aura (often visual), paraesthesiae or speech disturbances followed by a short self-limiting headache. It is more common in females and peaks during the reproductive years. Although cerebral blood flow is affected during an acute attack, it rarely causes permanent deficit.

TENSION

Headaches which may occur up to daily especially in stressful situations. They are characterised by a feeling of tightness in the frontal and temporal muscles.

CLUSTER

Relatively rare and predominantly seen in males. Historically, the pattern is of retro/periorbital headaches on an almost daily basis for weeks or months followed by months or years free from symptoms. Sometimes these become chronic rather than episodic.

DIFFERENTIAL DIAGNOSIS OF HEADACHES WITH AN IDENTIFIED CAUSE

- Temporal arteritis
- Acute glaucoma
- Structural problems (dental abscess, acute sinusitis, cervical spine damage)
- Benign intracranial hypertension and other causes of raised intracranial pressure
- Visual disorders

CEREBRAL HEMISPHERE LESIONS

Vascular lesions (thrombosis, embolism, haemorrhage) occur in specific vascular territories; primary or secondary compressive and infiltrative lesions tend to occur in the lobes of the brain.

---

*Also termed multiple systems atrophy.

CEREBROVASCULAR DISEASE

Table 8.11 *Symptoms and signs of transient ischaemic attacks (TIAs) in the carotid and vertebrobasilar territories*

Carotid arterial disease	Vertebrobasilar insufficiency (VBI)
Amaurosis fugax (visual loss in the eye on the same side as diseased carotid)	Dizziness (with vertigo and ataxia)
	Diplopia
Sensory and motor loss in a single limb or side (contralateral)	Dysarthria
	Dysphagia
Transient aphasia	'Demi-anaesthesia' (ipsilateral face, contralateral limb)
Carotid bruit (associated with stenosis >50% of diameter of lumen)	Quadriparesis (indicates basilar artery involvement)

Remember that transient loss of consciousness is very rarely associated with a TIA, and TIA symptoms are rarely 'positive' (rather there is loss of power, sensation etc.).

Differential diagnosis of a TIA includes migraine, tumour and epilepsy.

Table 8.12 *Intracerebral thrombosis or embolism: clinical features*

Middle cerebral artery	Posterior cerebral artery	Anterior cerebral artery
Main branch	*Main branch*	UMN leg; cortical sensory loss leg only; urinary incontinence.
Infarction middle third of hemisphere: UMN face, arm > leg; homonymous hemianopia; aphasia or non-dominant hemisphere signs (depending on side); cortical sensory loss.	Effects variable as anastomosis with middle cerebral artery; homonymous hemianopia (complete). *Perforating artery* Hemianaesthesia (loss of all modalities)	
Perforating artery Internal capsule infarction: UMN face; UMN arm > leg		

UMN = upper motor neurone lesion.

THERAPEUTIC PRINCIPLES IN CEREBROVASCULAR DISEASE

1. Stroke prevention in the setting of symptomatic carotid artery disease
   A greater than 70% carotid stenosis with ipsilateral signs or symptoms of ischaemia should be treated with endarterectomy.
2. Aneurysmal bleed causing subarachnoid haemorrhage
   Surgical clipping of the Circle of Willis aneurysm is the treatment of

choice. Antifibrinolytics reduce rebleeding but increase infarction (due to local vasospasm). For inoperable aneurysms other treatment options include embolisation and nimodipine. For inoperable non-saccular aneurysms, stereotactic radiotherapy can be an option.

3. Cerebral infarction and progressive stroke
   Anticoagulants are used with large vessel disease (carotid or basilar artery thrombosis) where the lesion is incomplete and CT scan has excluded a bleed, although there is no proof that this alters the course of the disease.

4. Atrial fibrillation (chronic or paroxysmal) and stroke prevention
   Anticoagulants reduce the risk of stroke by about eight times.

5. Intracerebral haematoma
   Surgical evacuation is of no value for lobar haematomas unaccompanied by raised intracranial pressure and is of no value for large haematomas causing transtentorial herniation; surgery may be of some value for cerebellar or lobar haematomas with signs of raised intracranial pressure. Steroids are of limited value.

6. Source of emboli
   It is important to consider the likely anatomical source of an embolus causing stroke. The carotid arteries should be imaged. If no source is found following transthoracic echocardiography, consideration should be given to emboli arising from the aorta; this is best imaged with a transoesophageal echocardiogram.

NEOPLASTIC DISEASE

In adults, cerebral tumours are usually supratentorial; a posterior fossa tumour in an adult is usually a metastasis (e.g. from lung, breast, kidney or melanoma).

Other features which may indicate cerebral neoplasia include:

1. Papilloedema.
2. False localising signs from raised intracranial pressure, e.g. VI nerve palsy (because of its long intracranial path).
3. Transtentorial herniation (appears only late in disease course).
4. A mass in one hemisphere may result in displacement of the uncus (medial temporal lobe) inferiorly through the temporal notch, causing compression of cranial nerve III with hemiparesis on the opposite side; consciousness is lost late.
5. A more centrally located mass may cause central herniation compressing the upper midbrain resulting in small, equal and reactive pupils and early coma.
6. Foramen magnum herniation ('coning') with a cerebellar mass.

LUMBAR PUNCTURE (LP) RESULTS

- A normal LP includes no polymorphonuclear cells but may include up to 4 lymphocytes/mL
- Xanthochromia: consider subarachnoid haemorrhage—often positive after 'sentinel' bleed when cerebral CT scan is normal.
- Raised protein: meningitis, multiple sclerosis, Guillain-Barré, malignancy.

Table 8.13 *Acute bacterial meningitis*

Organism	Gram stain	Age groups	Predisposing factors	Therapy	Alternatives
Streptococcus pneumoniae (pneumococcus)	Gram +ve coccus	Adults (50%) Children (15%)	Alcoholism CSF rhinorrhoea Lymphoma Myeloma Splenectomy	Penicillin*	Chloramphenicol Cefotaxime
Neisseria meningitidis	Gram −ve coccus	Adults (30%) Children (30%)	Crowding Terminal complement deficiencies	Penicillin*	As for pneumococcus
Haemophilus influenzae type b	Gram −ve bacillus	Adults (3%) Children (50%)	Hypogammaglobulinaemia Anatomical defects	Third-generation cephalosporin e.g. ceftriaxone	Ampicillin[†] and chloramphenicol
Escherichia coli	Gram −ve rod	Adults (rare) Neonates	Spontaneous bacteraemia	Third-generation cephalosporin (ceftazidime)	
Listeria[‡]	Gram −ve bacillus	Adults (rare)	Immunocompromised e.g. acute myeloid leukaemia	Penicillin Ampicillin	

*Ceftriaxone is usually commenced with penicillin until it is established that the organism is penicillin sensitive.
[†]Increasing ampicillin resistance occurring in children.
[‡]Resistant to all cephalosporins.

PROPHYLAXIS OF ACUTE BACTERIAL MENINGITIS

Haemophilus influenzae
Treat all household contacts and day-care centre children 4 years of age and under with rifampicin or trimethoprim-sulfamethoxazole.

Neisseria meningitidis
Treat intimate contacts only with rifampicin for 2 days.

DETERIORATION DURING ANTIBIOTIC THERAPY FOR MENINGITIS

If there is:

- recrudescence (of the same bacteria during therapy), consider whether the correct treatment was given;
- relapse (same bacteria 3–14 days after stopping therapy), consider a para-meningeal focus;
- recurrence with the same or new bacteria, consider whether there is a congenital or acquired dural defect.

Table 8.14 *Chronic meningitis*

Causes	Chronic neutrophilic meningitis	Chronic lymphocytic meningitis
Bacteria	Nocardia, Actinomyces, Brucella, TB	*Treponema pallidum* (acute), Leptospira, Lyme disease, TB
Virus		HIV
Fungi	Candida, Aspergillus, Blastomyces, Coccidioides	Candida, *Cryptococcus neoformans*, Coccidioides, *Histoplasma capsulatum*, *Blastomyces dermatitidis*
Parasites*		Toxoplasmosis
Non-infectious (rare)	SLE, intrathecal drugs, contents of craniopharyngioma or epidermoid tumour liberated into CSF	Lymphoma, sarcoidosis, multiple sclerosis, arteritis, Behçet's syndrome, non-steroidal anti-inflammatory drugs

*May cause eosinophilic meningitis, especially angiostrongyliasis.

'FAINTS AND FUNNY TURNS'

Lightheadedness, unsteadiness or transient loss of consciousness.

Table 8.15 *Some causes to consider*

Young adults	Elderly
Vasovagal episodes	Cardiac arrhythmias
Hypoglycaemia	Hypoglycaemia
Cardiac arrhythmias	Micturition syncope
Hyperventilation	Cough syncope
Epilepsy	Seizures
Hysteria	Postural hypotension including autonomic
Phaeochromocytoma (rare)	neuropathy
Micturition syncope	Hyperventilation
Orthostatic hypotension	

EPILEPSY

Epilepsy can be characterised as abnormal synchronisation or amplitude of neuronal discharge.

Lifetime risk 5% of having a single seizure.

Predisposing factors include:

- Structural brain lesions
- Alcohol
- Drug withdrawal
- Encephalopathy

Treat patients with multiple seizures and those with predisposing factors. Treating patients with a single fit with no obvious cause is generally not warranted.

Clinical presentation of disease	Subclassification	Drug therapy preferred
Partial seizures		
Associated with an aura and focal in nature when they begin	simple complex secondary generalised	carbamazepine valproic acid
Primary generalised		
Starts with loss of consciousness and includes convulsive, non-convulsive and myoclonic epilepsy		phenytoin primidone

Other second-line agents available include clonazepam, ethosuximide, lamotrigine, gabapentin, vigabatrin, topiramate and tiagabine.

Table 8.16 *Differentiating epilepsy from vasovagal syncope*

Timing	In favour of epilepsy	In favour of vasovagal syncope
Before episode	For primary generalised seizure, there is no warning	Often associated with weakness, sweating and fading vision
During episode	Generalised tonic clonic movement with loss of consciousness	Secondary tonic or myoclonic phase especially if patient prevented from falling. Patient appears pale and limp.
After episode	Post-ictal confusion common	Usually lucid within moments

DEMENTIA versus DELIRIUM

DELIRIUM

- Reversible
- Disturbed consciousness
- Changed cognition
- Develops over a short period of time
- Aetiological cause can be defined

COMMON CAUSES

- drugs, including withdrawal
- metabolic causes (hypoxia, uraemia, hypercalcaemia, hepatic failure, hyponatraemia, hypernatraemia)
- sepsis
- intracerebral disease etc.

It is important to remember that patients with delirium may be hypoactive especially in metabolic and encephalopathic settings and with intoxication.

Hyperactive delirium is best characterised by withdrawal syndromes.

Table 8.17 *Dementia versus delirium*

Feature	Dementia	Delirium
Onset	gradual	often rapid
Orientation	sometimes impaired	mostly impaired
Short-term memory	impaired	impaired
Long-term memory	often intact	often impaired
Aetiology	rarely identifiable	mostly identifiable
Sleep pattern	intact	disturbed
Clinical course	steady progression	fluctuation
Other neurological signs	minimal	overt signs often present
Hallucinations/perceptions	none/preserved	often/impaired

DEMENTIA

Dementia is characterised by multiple cognitive deficits that include short-term memory loss.

It is most commonly due to Alzheimer's disease, a diagnosis of exclusion. Pathophysiological changes include amyloid protein beta-A4 deposition, reduced parietotemporal perfusion and decreased acetylcholine in the nucleus basalis of Meynert.

Investigating these patients is undertaken with a view to excluding treatable causes of dementia. Tests may include:

1. TSH—hypothyroidism.
2. Biochemical screen—calcium (hypercalcaemia or hypocalcaemia); sodium (hyponatraemia); urinalysis, urea and creatinine (renal failure—dialysis dementia is not reversible); fasting blood sugar (hypoglycaemia or hyperglycaemia).
3. Serum B_{12} and folate.
4. Liver function tests—hepatic encephalopathy of subacute onset.
5. Full blood count and erythrocyte sedimentation rate—vasculitis.
6. VDRL—cerebrovascular syphilis.
7. Chest X-ray—lung cancer.
8. CT or MRI scan of brain—to exclude resectable tumour, subdural haematoma (headache and mental changes), or normal pressure hydrocephalus (altered mentation, abnormal gait and urinary incontinence). It can also define multiple infarcts.
9. 24-hour urine for lead and mercury.
10. Lumbar puncture—rule out chronic infection such as cryptococcal meningitis if there is a subacute onset.
11. HIV test.
12. Antinuclear antibody tests looking for systemic lupus erythematosus.

Always exclude drugs (e.g. sedatives, alcohol and thiamine deficiency in alcoholics, beta-blockers, digoxin) and depression.

URINARY INCONTINENCE

Table 8.18 Urinary incontinence

Type	Causes	Therapy
Detrusor instability (70%)*	Bladder irritation, e.g. cystitis, uterine prolapse. Neurological disease, e.g. dementia, normal pressure hydrocephalus.	Imipramine (anticholinergic action inhibits detrusor contractions) Bladder retraining
Overflow incontinence	Outflow obstruction, e.g. prostate Hypotonic bladder, e.g. drugs, autonomic neuropathy	Relieve obstruction Urinary catheter Bethanecol (cholinergic agonist increases detrusor contraction)

Table 8.18 *Continued*

Type	Causes	Therapy
Stress incontinence	Postmenopausal women who have decreased pelvic muscle support	Imipramine (anticholinergic and alpha-agonist effects increase sphincter tone) Topical oestrogen Repair urethrovesical angle surgically
Iatrogenic	Drugs e.g. diuretics	Alter therapy

*Causes urge incontinence.

POTENCY

Erection requires an intact parasympathetic reflex at S2 and S3, while ejaculation requires an intact sympathetic L1 root.

CAUSES OF LOST POTENCY

1. Spinal cord or cauda equina disease.
2. Autonomic neuropathy, e.g. diabetes mellitus.
3. Endocrine disease, e.g. hypogonadism.
4. Leriche syndrome and other vascular diseases.
5. Psychological states (very common).

COMA

This can be defined as at least 6 hours of failure to respond to noise or commands, move limbs in response to pain, or open the eyes either spontaneously or in response to pain.

CAUSES (MNEMONIC COMA)

C—CO_2 narcosis (respiratory failure—uncommon), carbon monoxide poisoning.

O—Overdose of drugs, e.g. opiates, tranquillisers, alcohol, salicylates, antidepressants (often taken together).

M—Metabolic, e.g. hypoglycaemia (this must never be missed), ketoacidosis, renal failure, hypothyroidism, hepatic coma, hypercalcaemia, adrenal failure, terminal cardiac failure, hypothermia.

A—'Apoplexy', e.g. head trauma, stroke, subdural or extradural haematoma, space-occupying lesions (tumour, abscess), meningitis, encephalitis, epilepsy, hypertensive crisis.

BRAIN DEATH

This results from total cessation of blood flow and global infarction of the brain.

DIAGNOSTIC TESTS WHILE ON ARTIFICIAL CARDIORESPIRATORY SUPPORT

Deeply comatosed patient with (on repeated testing over 24 hours)
1. Absent pupillary light reflexes (midbrain damage).
2. Absent corneal reflexes (pontine damage).
3. Absent vestibulo-ocular reflexes, i.e. Doll's eyes manoeuvres, ice water (caloric) stimulation (medullary damage).
4. Apnoea—demonstrated by removing the respirator while supplying oxygen: $PaCO_2$ rises 2 mmHg/min (0.027 kPa/min) in the brain dead; no respiratory movements should occur with a $PaCO_2$ >50 mmHg (6.67 kPa) (medullary damage).
5. Isoelectric EEG (widespread cortical damage).

Always exclude drug-induced coma and hypothermia.

If the pupils are *constricted*, beware of diagnosing brain death; on the other hand, spinal reflexes may be retained with brain death.

9

Endocrinology

INSULIN DEFICIENCY

CLINICAL CLUES

TYPE 1 DIABETES (INSULIN-DEPENDENT DIABETES MELLITUS)

- Acute/subacute onset, usually presenting with ketoacidosis
- Polyuria, polydipsia
- Dehydration, hypotension, tachycardia
- Ketone breath, Kussmaul respiration
- Mental confusion
- Bouts of ketoacidosis frequently associated with infection
- Glycosuria, ketonuria

TYPE 2 DIABETES (NON-INSULIN-DEPENDENT DIABETES MELLITUS)

- Chronic symptoms
- Polyuria, polydipsia
- Frequent infection (e.g. Candida balanitis/vulvitis, recurrent urinary tract infection)
- Fatigue
- Visual disturbance
- Vascular disease
- Glycosuria

Table 9.1 *Differential diagnosis in diabetic coma*

Type	Glucose (plasma)	Ketones (urine)*	Acidosis (increased anion gap)	Dehydration	Hyperventilation
Ketoacidosis	+++	+++	+++	+++	+++
Hyperosmolar non-ketotic	+++	—	—	+++	—
Hypoglycaemia	Low	—	—	—	—

Table 9.1 (*Continued*)

Type	Glucose (plasma)	Ketones (urine)*	Acidosis (increased anion gap)	Dehydration	Hyperventilation
Lactic acidosis	Low to ++	+	++++	+	+++
Alcoholic ketoacidosis[†] (non-diabetic)	Normal	+++	+++	++	++

+ = inceased.
*Nitroprusside test measures only acetoacetate.
[†]Alcoholics may also develop lactic acidosis and/or hypoglycaemia.

PATHOPHYSIOLOGY

TYPE 1 (insulin-dependent diabetes mellitus)

- Autoimmune damage to islet cells leads to a reduced capability to produce insulin.
- Certain HLA types more susceptible (DR3, DR4).
- Insulin lack relative to counter-regulatory hormones (e.g. glucagon) stimulates gluconeogenesis, lipolysis and ketogenesis, resulting in the syndrome of diabetic ketoacidosis.
- Hypoglycaemia unawareness is common in long-standing disease, due to an inability to release glucagon and/or adrenaline when hypoglycaemic. This may be, in part, due to autonomic neuropathy.
- Responsible for less than 15% of total cases of diabetes mellitus.

TYPE 2 (non-insulin-dependent diabetes mellitus)

- Usually results from a combination of reduced insulin secretion and impaired tissue response to the actions of insulin.
- More common in older, obese individuals.
- Residual levels of insulin prevent development of ketoacidosis, but hyperglycaemia and the resulting diuresis can cause a severe hyperosmolality with circulatory compromise. This condition carries a significant mortality.
- Hypoglycaemia unawareness may occur with long-standing disease.

DISEASE STATES

DIABETES MELLITUS

Diagnostic criteria

Fasting plasma glucose of 7.0 mmol/L (127 mg/dL) or more, or a random blood glucose level of 11.1 mmol/L (200 mg/dL) or more, on more than one occasion.

CAUSES

Primary
1. Type 1 or insulin-dependent diabetes.
2. Type 2 or non-insulin dependent diabetes.
3. Maturity-onset diabetes of the young (MODY). This syndrome is auto-somal dominant, and is due to mutations in the gene encoding for the enzyme glucokinase. The phenotype is for mild hyperglycaemia and resistance to ketosis.

Secondary
1. Counter-regulatory hormone excess, e.g. pregnancy, acromegaly, Cushing's syndrome, phaeochromocytoma, glucagonoma.
2. Drugs, e.g. corticosteroids, thiazide diuretics (secondary to hypo-kalaemia), phenytoin, HIV protease inhibitors, diazoxide (inhibits insulin secretion), streptozotocin.
3. Pancreatic disease—chronic pancreatitis, carcinoma, haemochromatosis.
4. Insulin resistance syndromes (rare).
    a) Lipoatrophic diabetes—generalised lipoatrophy, hepatomegaly, hirsutism, hyperpigmentation, hyperlipidaemia.
    b) Type A syndrome—usually young females with acanthosis nigricans and polycystic ovaries.
    c) Type B syndrome—acanthosis nigricans and autoimmune disease.

Table 9.2 *Features of Type 1 and Type 2 diabetes mellitus*

Characteristic	Type 1	Type 2
Prevalence	0.2 to 0.3% (equal sex predilection)	3–6% (commoner in women)
Age of onset	Usually <30 years	Usually >40 years
Genetics	HLA B8, B15, DR3, DR4 50% concordance in twins	No HLA association Nearly 100% concordance in twins
Islet cell antibodies	Acute disease (90%) at presentation	Nil
Anti-GAD antibodies	Yes	No
Insulin secretion	Absolute deficiency	Insulin resistance
Glucagon secretion	Increased	Increased
Obesity	Rare	Usual
Ketoacidosis	Prone	Not prone
Association with other autoimmune diseases	Occasionally	No

GAD = glutamic acid decarboxylase.

CHRONIC COMPLICATIONS OF DIABETES MELLITUS

A Microangiopathic sequelae
1. Retinopathy—present in 50% of Type 1 patients by 10–15 years, 80% by 20 years; in Type 2 diabetes 50% will be affected by 15 years.

a) Non-proliferative: dilated veins, microaneurysms, soft exudates, haemorrhages, hard exudates.
b) Proliferative: new vessels, vitreous haemorrhage, retinal detachment.
2. Neuropathy—present in approximately 30% of patients with diabetes of >10 years' duration.
a) Peripheral (may be painful).
b) Autonomic, e.g. diabetic diarrhoea, impotence, postural hypotension.
c) Dorsal column loss (diabetic pseudotabes).
d) Proximal myopathy (amyotrophy).
e) Mononeuritis (especially III cranial nerve with pupil sparing).
f) Tight diabetic control is helpful in preventing the development of neuropathy.
3. Nephropathy—present in 15% of IDDM patients after 15 years and 30–40% after 30 years. (See also page 169)
a) Glomerular sclerosis—diffuse, or less commonly nodular (Kimmelstiel-Wilson lesion).
b) Arteriolar disease.
c) Recurrent urinary tract infection.
d) Papillary necrosis.
e) Chronic renal failure.
f) Hyporeninaemic hypoaldosteronism (suspect if there is hyper-kalaemia out of proportion to the creatinine level).
g) Those at risk can be detected early by measuring microalbuminuria, with >30 mg/24 hours signifying the need for tight diabetic control to attempt to reverse the trend to overt nephropathy. Use of angiotensin converting enzyme inhibitors and tight control of hypertension at this stage may also improve prognosis.
h) Patients with diabetic nephropathy are at risk of rapid deterioration in renal function with the use of contrast dyes for diagnostic tests, particularly if underhydrated.

B Macroangiopathic sequelae
1. Coronary artery disease.
2. Cerebrovascular disease.
3. Peripheral vascular disease.

C Infections
1. Candidiasis.
2. Bacterial.
3. Rare but almost pathognomonic—malignant otitis externa due to *Pseudomonas aeruginosa*, rhinocerebral mucormycosis, emphysematous pyelonephritis and cholecystitis.

D Skin disease
1. Necrobiosis lipoidica diabeticorum.
2. Lipoatrophy, lipohypertrophy.

3. Pigmented scars.
4. Diabetic dermopathy ('shin spots').
5. Leg ulceration (neuropathy, vasculopathy).

E Other eye complications
1. Cataracts.
2. Glaucoma.
3. Transient lens changes due to hyperglycaemia resulting in blurred vision.

F Lipid abnormalities
 a) Type 1 diabetes
   In ketoacidotic states, very-low-density lipoprotein (VLDL) levels are often high and triglyceride levels may be very high.
 b) Type 2 diabetes
   If diabetic control is poor, VLDL, triglyceride and cholesterol levels may be elevated, and high-density lipoprotein levels low.

PREGNANCY AND DIABETES MELLITUS

1. Blood sugar levels are normally lower in pregnancy.
2. Renal threshold for glucose decreases, therefore glycosuria common.
3. Insulin requirements increase in the 2nd and 3rd trimester, due to the effects of human placental lactogen and human placental somatomammotrophin.
4. Insulin requirements dramatically decrease postpartum.
5. Gestational diabetes confers a greater risk of developing diabetes later in life.
6. Gestational diabetes increases the risk of fetal morbidity e.g. intrauterine death, macrosomia and neonatal hypoglycaemia and hypocalcaemia.
7. Tight glycaemic control during pregnancy improves fetal outcome.

CAUSES OF INSULIN RESISTANCE

1. Obesity (decreased receptor number): most common cause.
2. Insulin antibodies.
3. Insulin resistance syndromes.
4. Counter-regulatory hormone excess.
5. Other: haemochromatosis, lymphoma, injection into fibrotic areas, factitious.

MONITORING DIABETES MELLITUS

1. Haemoglobin A1c levels reflect control in the previous 8 to 12 weeks.
2. Levels decrease with haemolysis and pregnancy.
3. Fructosamine levels reflect diabetic control within the preceding 3 weeks. May be spuriously low in the presence of proteinuria.

THERAPY

1. Diet
   The ideal diabetic diet should consist of 50–60% complex carbohydrate,

15–20% protein, and the remainder fat (a low cholesterol content). Simple sugars should be avoided.
2. Exercise
   Regular exercise is essential to increase insulin sensitivity, assist weight loss and prevent cardiovascular disease.
3. Oral medication (Type 2 diabetes).

Table 9.3 Oral medications used in diabetes mellitus

Drug	Mechanism of action	Adverse effects
Oral sulfonylureas	Increase pancreatic insulin secretion	Hypoglycaemia, weight gain due to increased appetite, bone marrow suppression, cholestatic jaundice, skin rash
Individual agents		
Tolbutamide	Weak action, short duration	
Chlorpropamide	Moderate potency, very long duration of action	Unique effects include prolonged hypoglycaemia, hyponatraemia (SIADH), and a disulfiram-like effect when consumed with alcohol
Glibenclamide	Most potent agent in class	
2nd generation agents		
Glipizide	Potent, intermediate duration of action	
Biguanides	Inhibit gluconeogenesis and increase insulin receptor number and activity	
Metformin	Aids weight loss through appetite suppression	Lactic acidosis (very rare and in association with renal or hepatic disease); vitamin B_{12} malabsorption
Other		
Acarbose	Reduces glucose absorption	Flatulence
Troglitazone	↑ glucose disposal ↓ hepatic glucose output (no hypoglycaemia)	Hepatic failure Haematological problems

SIADH = syndrome of inappropriate secretion of antidiuretic hormone.

4. Insulin therapy

Table 9.4 *Insulins*

Insulin type	Examples	Onset (h)	Peak effect (h) (in diabetics)	Duration (h)
Rapidly acting	Actrapid, lispro*	0.25–1	2–4	5–8
Intermediate	NPH zinc suspension (Monotard), Protaphane, Humulin NPH	2–4	6–10	12–24
Long-acting	Ultralente	3–4	14–20	24–36

*Human insulin analogue with transposition of lysine and proline at 28′ and 29′. Very fast onset of action which better resembles a physiological response.

CAUSES OF DECREASING INSULIN REQUIREMENTS
IN A PREVIOUSLY STABLE DIABETIC

1. Decreased caloric intake
2. Increased exercise
3. Injection errors
4. Diabetic renal disease
5. Rarely: development of Addison's disease; panhypopituitarism; malabsorption; high levels of insulin antibodies; insulinoma (check C-peptide level)

HYPOGLYCAEMIA

DEFINITION

A blood glucose of <2.8 mmol/L (<50 mg/dL) in males and <2 mmol/L (<40 mg/dL) in females in the presence of consistent clinical symptoms.

CLINICAL CLUES

1. Adrenergic overactivity—diaphoresis, palpitations, tremor, pallor, anxiety, dilated pupils.
2. Nervous system glucose starvation—hunger, confusion, slurred speech, personality change, double vision, seizures, coma.

CAUSES

1. Postprandial or reactive hypoglycaemia
2. Fasting hypoglycaemia
   a) Hepatic disease—extensive liver pathology; hereditary enzyme deficiencies

b) Endocrine causes—insulinoma; insulin or oral hypoglycaemic excess;* hypopituitarism; cortisol deficiency
c) Extrapancreatic islet cell tumours—adenocarcinoma; adrenocortical carcinoma; mesenchymal tumours; hepatoma
d) Malnutrition
e) Alcoholism
f) Severe systemic illness
g) Pharmacological agents—β-blockers; salicylates; mushroom poisoning

INSULIN EXCESS

DISEASE STATES

INSULINOMA

- Rare tumours of pancreatic islet cells
- 80% have a single benign tumour
- 10% are multiple
- 10% are malignant
- 10% occur in the setting of multiple endocrine neoplasia Type I.

DIAGNOSIS

- 72 hour fast—symptoms of hypoglycaemia are accompanied by a progressive rise in the ratio of plasma insulin to glucose and C-peptide. The majority of patients will have a percentage of proinsulin >25%.
- Tumour localisation is the next step; this involves imaging of the pancreas with CT or MRI scanning, angiography, selective venous sampling of the pancreas, or intraoperative ultrasonography.

POSTPRANDIAL HYPOGLYCAEMIA

- Very rare
- Due to excessive insulin secretion relative to glucose levels
- Symptoms occur 1–5 hours after a meal
- Types:
  a) Idiopathic
  b) Hereditary childhood form
  c) Patients with impaired glucose tolerance who have a delayed insulin response
  d) 'Alimentary' hypoglycaemia, occurring in patients who have had surgical alteration to the upper gastrointestinal tract and have rapid

---

*Covert insulin use can be detected by absence of C-peptide, and sometimes circulating insulin antibodies. Covert sulfonylurea use can be picked up with a urinary drug screen.

delivery of large glucose loads into the small intestine, resulting in a surge of insulin secretion.

DIAGNOSIS

- 72 hour fast—symptoms should be accompanied by low blood glucose.

THYROID HORMONE EXCESS

CLINICAL CLUES

TYPICAL PRESENTATIONS

- Heat intolerance, excessive sweating
- Weight loss
- Dyspnoea (even without congestive cardiac failure)
- Increase in frequency of bowel movements
- Weak muscles
- Emotional lability
- Nervousness/difficulty sleeping
- Atrial fibrillation (especially in the elderly)
- Decreased menstrual flow

ATYPICAL PRESENTATIONS

- Unexplained atrial arrhythmias in the middle-aged
- Severe proximal myopathy with normal creatine phosphokinase levels
- Unmasking or deterioration of myasthenia gravis
- Hypokalaemic periodic paralysis especially in Asians
- Gynaecomastia
- Chronic diarrhoea

PATHOPHYSIOLOGY

- Low TSH is often the first laboratory abnormality in hyperthyroidism.
- Low TSH may also be seen with:
  a) administration of glucocorticoids, dopamine
  b) severe illness
  c) pituitary disease

HYPERTHYROIDISM

EXOGENOUS CAUSES—excess thyroid hormone ingestion.

PITUITARY CAUSES—(rare) autonomous TSH secretion due to a pituitary secreting adenoma. In this case TSH will be normal or high; T4 and T3 will be high.

THYROID CAUSES

AUTONOMOUS HORMONE PRODUCTION

1. Hot nodule
2. Toxic multinodular goitre
3. Struma ovarii (rare)

EXCESS STIMULATION OF THYROID

1. Immunoglobulins in Graves' disease

EXCESS RELEASE OF THYROID HORMONE

1. Painful subacute thyroiditis
2. Silent lymphocytic thyroiditis

IODINE LOAD—may cause hyperthyroidism in the setting of areas of autonomous function (hot nodule, toxic multinodular goitre)

SOURCES OF IODINE LOAD

1. Drugs—amiodarone, cough medicines
2. Radiocontrast material
3. Surgical exposure to povidone iodine

In the setting of previous iodine deficiency, iodine loading causing hyperthyroidism is called the Jod Basedow phenomenon.

DISEASE STATES

GOITRE (DIFFUSE)

1. Idiopathic
2. Puberty
3. Pregnancy
4. Graves' disease
5. Thyroiditis
   - Hashimoto's thyroiditis
   - Subacute thyroiditis (tender)
6. Iodine deficiency
7. Goitrogens, e.g. iodine, phenylbutazone, lithium

CAUSES OF A SOLITARY NODULE

5% of all people, rate increases with age. 20–50% of adults have thyroid nodules.

1. Benign
   a) Dominant nodule in multinodular goitre
   b) Adenoma or cyst
2. Malignant
   a) Carcinoma (primary)

GRAVES' DISEASE

- Thyroid stimulating antibodies (TSAB)—stimulate TSH receptors
- Increased frequency in HLA B8, DR3
- Pretibial myxoedema, exophthalmos, clubbing are immune-mediated, not thyroid-mediated, changes
- More common in women
- Diffuse goitre with diffuse radioactive iodine uptake (RAIU)

PAINFUL SUBACUTE THYROIDITIS

- HLA-B35 related
- Occurs after a viral illness
- Excess release of stored thyroid hormone
- Raised erythrocyte sedimentation rate (ESR), decreased RAIU
- Tender thyroid, clinical hyperthyroidism with fever, raised ESR lasting for months often followed by transient hypothyroidism then a return to euthyroid state

SILENT LYMPHOCYTIC THYROIDITIS

- Autoimmune
- Non-painful thyroid, normal to mildly raised ESR
- May occur several times in life
- RAIU absent in hyperthyroid phase
- 25% go on to persistent hypothyroidism
- Seen in   5% of unselected pregnancies
　　　　　 30% of pregnancies with diabetes
　　　　　 75% of pregnancies with pre-existing Hashimoto's thyroiditis

HASHIMOTO'S THYROIDITIS

- Chronic inflammatory disease of the thyroid with goitre
- May present as initial hyperthyroidism

PHARMACOLOGY

METHIMAZOLE OR CARBIMAZOLE

- Mechanism: decreases thyroid hormone synthesis by decreasing the incorporation of iodide into thyroglobulin
- Side effects: fever, rash, arthralgia, myalgia, leucopenia, agranulocytosis, hepatitis
- Indications: hyperthyroidism, thyrotoxic crisis

PROPYLTHIOURACIL

- Mechanism: decreases thyroid hormone synthesis, decreases peripheral conversion of T4 to T3
- Side effects: fever, rash, arthralgia, myalgia, leucopenia, agranulocytosis
- Indications: hyperthyroidism, thyrotoxic crisis

RAI (^{131}I)

- Mechanism: beta particle emitter preferentially taken up by the thyroid, hence major tissue destruction in the thyroid
- Side effects: occasional acute thyrotoxicosis (7–10 days after treatment), late hypothyroidism (>50% at 10 years)
- Indications: non-pregnant patients more than 30 years old. A large goitre is a relative contraindication.

THYROID HORMONE DEFICIENCY

CLINICAL CLUES

- Weight gain
- Constipation
- Cold intolerance
- Lethargy
- Depression
- Dementia
- Hoarse voice
- Menorrhagia

PATHOPHYSIOLOGY

- TSH is usually raised in primary hypothyroidism as the first laboratory abnormality. T3 drops after T4 and low T3 is therefore a sign of severe hypothyroidism.
- TSH may be raised in: (a) adrenal insufficiency; (b) recovery from severe illness.

CAUSES OF HYPOTHYROIDISM

1. Without a goitre
   - Primary
     a) Idiopathic atrophy
     b) Ablation (^{131}I, radiotherapy for Hodgkin's disease, or surgery)
     c) Thyroid agenesis
   - Secondary
     a) Pituitary disease
   - Tertiary
     a) Hypothalamic disease
2. With a goitre (failure of hormone synthesis)
   - Primary
     a) chronic thyroiditis (Hashimoto's)
     b) drugs (lithium, amiodarone, iodide)
     c) iodine deficiency
     d) inborn errors of metabolism

DISEASE STATES

HASHIMOTO'S THYROIDITIS

- Chronic inflammatory disease of the thyroid with goitre
- Common in middle-aged women
- Lymphocytic infiltration of the gland
- Raised serum antithyroglobulin antibodies, antithyroid peroxidase (anti-TPO) antibodies (positive in 95–98%), antimicrosomal antibodies (85%)
- Association with other autoimmune diseases
- Seen in areas of iodine deficiency
- Patients with Hashimoto's are more likely to develop postpartum thyroiditis and *vice versa*
- Frank hypothyroidism eventually seen in 80% of patients with Hashimoto's

SUBCLINICAL HYPOTHYROIDISM

20% of patients over 65 years have a raised TSH; of these 20%, 3–5% per year will go on to frank hypothyroidism.

PHARMACOLOGY

THYROXINE

- L-thyroxine has a long half-life, so once daily dosing is possible.
- Introduce slowly, especially in the elderly.
- More rapid metabolism with phenytoin, rifampicin, phenobarbitol, carbamazepine.
- Decreased absorption—cholestyramine, ferrous sulphate, sucralfate.

THYROID IN PREGNANCY

PHYSIOLOGICAL CHANGES

1. Small goitre (relative iodine deficiency).
2. Tachycardia and heat intolerance (increased basal metabolic rate).
3. Increased thyroid binding globulin (TBG).

To exclude hyperthyroidism, measure TSH.
Graves' disease may go into remission in the third trimester but may flare postpartum.
Radioactive iodine is absolutely contraindicated in pregnancy; antithyroid medications are used.

CORTISOL EXCESS (CUSHING'S SYNDROME)

CLINICAL CLUES

1. Cushingoid appearance—moon-shaped face, facial plethora, buffalo hump, supraclavicular fat pads, central obesity, striae, bruising, pigmentation

2. Acne, hirsutism (adrenal androgen excess)
3. Proximal myopathy
4. Osteoporosis, pathological fractures
5. Hypertension, oedema (aldosterone effect)
6. Symptoms/signs of diabetes mellitus
7. Symptoms/signs of pituitary tumour (in Cushing's *disease*)
8. Mental changes (depression, psychosis)
9. Hyperpigmentation if excess ACTH present

PATHOPHYSIOLOGY

CAUSES OF CUSHING'S SYNDROME

1. Excess administration of endogenous steroid or ACTH
2. Adrenal hyperplasia
   a) Secondary to pituitary ACTH production (Cushing's disease) from a microadenoma or macroadenoma (70% of cases).
   b) Secondary to an ACTH-producing tumour (20% of cases), e.g. small cell carcinoma of the lung (note, these people do not usually appear Cushingoid, but have hypokalaemia and virilisation).
3. Adrenal tumour (10% of cases)
   a) Adenoma
   b) Carcinoma (also causes virilisation)
4. CRH-producing tumour, e.g. bronchial carcinoid, pancreatic cancer, thymus tumour.

SIGNS SUGGESTIVE OF THE UNDERLYING AETIOLOGY

1. Adrenal carcinoma
- Palpable abdominal mass
- Virilisation
- Gynaecomastia

2. Ectopic ACTH
- Cushingoid features absent
- Prominent oedema and hypertension
- Myopathy
- Hyperpigmentation
- Cachexia

DISEASE STATES

CUSHING'S SYNDROME

SCREENING TESTS

1. *Overnight dexamethasone suppression test*: 1 mg of cortisol at midnight results in suppression of plasma cortisol to <140 nmol/L (<5 mg/dL) in normal people. Patients with Cushing's syndrome usually have values >280 nmol/L (>10 mg/dL). These levels can also be found in obesity, alcoholism, depression, those taking the oral contraceptive pill, and those on

medications that hasten the metabolism of dexamethasone, e.g. phenytoin and barbiturates.
2. *24-hour urinary free cortisol* is elevated in the vast majority of those with
Cushing's syndrome. It can also be elevated in obesity, alcoholism and
depression, and after trauma and surgery.

Table 9.5 *Cause and diagnosis of Cushing's syndrome*

Cause	Clinical features	Laboratory abnormalities
Cushing's disease	Predominantly affects young and middle-aged women Gradual onset of illness	ACTH levels normal or mildly increased. *Low-dose* dexamethasone suppression test* fails to suppress. *High-dose* dexamethasone suppression test† suppresses in 70%. 50% have pituitary tumours on CT or MRI. May need petrosal sinus ACTH levels sampled. Polycythaemia, neutrophil leucocytosis. Hyperglycaemia.
Ectopic ACTH-producing tumours	Mainly older men. Tumour types: lung carcinoma, thymoma, phaeochromocytoma, medullary carcinoma of the thyroid, carcinoma of the pancreas. Rapid onset of illness. Cushingoid features absent. Weakness, hypertension, oedema, hyperpigmentation	Elevated ACTH, >twice normal. *High-dose* dexamethasone suppression test fails to suppress. Urinary 17-ketosteroids, 17-ketogenic steroids, and 17-hydroxysteroids are grossly elevated. Hypokalaemic alkalosis.
Iatrogenic Cushing's syndrome	Most common cause of the syndrome	
Adrenal adenoma	Usually a typical clinical picture of cortisol excess (as in Cushing's disease, but without the	Very low ACTH. *High-dose* dexamethasone suppression test fails to suppress. Urinary 17-ketosteroids normal; urinary 17-ketogenic steroids, and

Table 9.5 Continued

Cause	Clinical features	Laboratory abnormalities
	pigmentation of ACTH excess).	17-hydroxysteroids are mildly increased. Adrenal mass on abdominal CT scan. ↑ DHEA.
Adrenal carcinoma	Adrenal carcinoma tends to cause a mixture of clinical effects of cortisol, androgen, and mineralocorticoid excess; therefore virilisation, hypertension and oedema occur in addition to Cushingoid features.	Very low ACTH. High-dose dexamethasone suppression test fails to suppress. Urinary 17-ketosteroids markedly increased; urinary 17-ketogenic steroids, and 17-hydroxysteroids are mildly increased. Adrenal mass on abdominal CT scan. ↑↑ plasma DHEA.

*Low-dose dexamethasone suppression test is performed by giving oral dexamethasone 0.5 mg every 6 hours for 2 days.
†High-dose dexamethasone suppression test is performed by giving 2 mg oral dexamethasone every 6 hours for 2 days.
DHEA = dehydroepiandrosterone.

TREATMENT

- Cushing's disease: trans-sphenoidal surgery to remove the adenoma. Metyrapone, ketoconazole, aminoglutethamide, stereotactic radiotherapy.
- Ectopic ACTH: if curative treatment of the primary tumour is not possible, adrenal blockade is attempted using aminoglutethamide, o,p'-DDD (mitotane) or ketoconazole. Bilateral adrenalectomy is a last resort.
- Adrenal adenoma: surgical excision.
- Adrenal carcinoma: surgical excision, with pharmacological adrenal blockade if residual disease is present.

CORTISOL DEFICIENCY

CLINICAL CLUES

- Fatigue
- Syncope

- Hypotension—postural and/or resting, shock
- Hyperpigmentation
- Vitiligo (20 times more common than in the general population)
- Cortisol deficiency from causes other than autoimmune adrenal disease (e.g. sudden withdrawal of long-term iatrogenic prednisolone, or hypopituitarism) is not accompanied by pigmentation or vitiligo.

PATHOPHYSIOLOGY

CAUSES

CHRONIC

1. Primary
   - Autoimmune adrenal disease (>80% of all cases)
   - Infection—tuberculosis, histoplasmosis
   - Demyelinating disease (Schilder's disease)
   - Metastatic malignancy
   - Lymphoma
   - Medication—following heparin therapy (bilateral adrenal haemorrhage), aminoglutethamide, ketoconazole
   - Congenital adrenal hyperplasia or hypoplasia
2. Secondary
   - Pituitary or hypothalamic disease

ACUTE

- Meningococcal septicaemia
- Bilateral adrenalectomy
- Any stress in a patient with chronic hypoadrenalism or abrupt cessation of prolonged high-dose steroid therapy

DIAGNOSIS OF ADRENOCORTICAL FAILURE

1. *Short Synacthen test:* 0.25 mg of synthetic ACTH (Synacthen) is given intramuscularly or intravenously. A normal response is a rise in plasma cortisol by >200 nmol/L (>7 mg/dL) and a peak of >500 nmol/L (>18 mg/dL). A normal response excludes primary adrenocortical failure but does not exclude hypothalamic-pituitary disease.
2. *Insulin hypoglycaemia testing:* Induction of hypoglycaemia by administration of insulin results in a plasma cortisol of >500 nmol/L (>18 mg/dL) if the hypothalamic-pituitary-adrenal axis is intact, but fails to distinguish adrenal from hypothalamic-pituitary disease.
3. The *ACTH level* is critical in distinguishing adrenal from hypothalamic-pituitary disease. Levels >44 pmol/L (>200 pg/mL) are seen in Addison's disease.

DISEASE STATES

AUTOIMMUNE ADDISON'S DISEASE

UNIQUE CLINICAL FEATURES

- Associated autoimmune disorders such as vitiligo, autoimmune thyroid disease, pernicious anaemia, Type 1 diabetes mellitus and hypoparathyroidism are common.

LABORATORY ABNORMALITIES

- Anti-adrenal antibodies (70%)
- Anti-thyroid antibodies (80%)
- Hyponatraemia, hyperkalaemia, hyperchloraemic acidosis, elevated urea
- Lymphocytosis and eosinophilia may be present

TREATMENT OF ADRENOCORTICAL FAILURE

1. Chronic
- Hydrocortisone or prednisolone in replacement doses.
- Mineralocorticoid replacement therapy, in the form of fludrocortisone, is often only necessary in cases of primary adrenal failure.
2. Acute
- For minor illnesses or surgery, triple the dose of the usual replacement glucocorticoid.
- For severe illness or major surgery, give intravenous hydrocortisone 100 mg every 6 hours.
- For adrenal crisis, give intensive fluid resuscitation, and intravenous hydrocortisone 100 mg every 6 hours.

PHAEOCHROMOCYTOMA

CLINICAL CLUES

- Headache
- Diaphoresis
- Palpitations
- Anxiety
- Pallor
- Heat intolerance
- Weight loss
- Hypertension: in >90%
- Postural hypotension may occur secondary to volume depletion
- Family history of multiple endocrine neoplasia syndrome (IIA or IIB)

PATHOPHYSIOLOGY

- Chromaffin tumours, usually located in the adrenal gland, but potentially in sites in the abdomen, or rarely the chest or neck.
- Small percentage are malignant.
- Generally secrete adrenaline and noradrenaline.

DIAGNOSIS

- 24 hour urine collection should reveal elevated levels of catecholamines and their metabolites metanephrine and vanillylmandelic acid.
- CT scanning or MRI will localise the tumour in the majority of cases. In special cases where localisation is problematic, radiolabelled I-metaiodobenzylguanidine may be of value.

TREATMENT

- Definitive surgery.
- Alpha-adrenergic blockade with phenoxybenzamine is the mainstay of medical treatment in the perioperative period.

ALDOSTERONE EXCESS (CONN'S SYNDROME)

CLINICAL CLUES

Hypertension, persistent hypokalaemia, weakness and polyuria in the absence of oedema and diuretic use should raise the possibility of Conn's syndrome.

PATHOPHYSIOLOGY

Aldosterone alone is raised and renin release is decreased. (If renin is raised, it suggests secondary hyperaldosteronism seen in 'malignant' hypertension.) This leads to hypokalaemia, metabolic alkalosis and hypernatraemia. High urinary potassium is maintained. Aldosterone is not suppressed with intravenous normal saline loading, fludrocortisone or angiotensin converting enzyme inhibitors.

DISEASE STATES

Primary excess—females-more commonly adrenal adenoma.
males-more commonly diffuse adrenal hyperplasia.
CT will distinguish between these two entities.

ALDOSTERONE DEFICIT

CLINICAL CLUES

Incidental finding of hyperkalaemia.

PATHOPHYSIOLOGY

Inability to increase aldosterone during salt restriction.
Low plasma renin—hyporeninaemic hypoaldosteronism
Especially seen in adult diabetics with mild renal impairment. Aldosterone

probably fails to rise after renin fails to rise in response to salt restriction and volume depletion.

Normal/high plasma renin—normoreninaemic hypoaldosteronism
Severe illness (adrenal necrosis, diminished mineralocorticoid response to ACTH).
Inherent (corticosterone methyloxidase defect).
Heparin.

PHARMACOLOGY

Fludrocortisone—0.05–0.15 mg/24 hours. Higher doses required for hyporeninaemic hypoaldosteronism.
In hypertensive patients with mild renal impairment ± cardiac failure, frusemide may be used alone in this setting or in combination with fludrocortisone.

PROLACTIN EXCESS

CLINICAL CLUES

* Women   amenorrhoea
             galactorrhoea
             loss of libido
             infertility
* Men   hypogonadism (decreased LHRH release in the hypothalamus)

PATHOPHYSIOLOGY

High blood levels but normal state
* pregnancy/early post-partum period, sleep, stress
Drugs
* dopamine antagonists—metoclopramide, phenothiazines/thioxanthenes, butyrophenones
* dopamine depletion—methyldopa, reserpine
* others—oestrogens, opiates
Disease states
* Pituitary tumours—prolactinomas
* Pituitary adenomas causing pituitary stalk compression
* Hypothalamic disease—craniopharyngioma, sarcoidosis, stalk section, empty sella syndrome
* Other causes—chronic renal failure (decreased clearance), cirrhosis

PITUITARY TUMOURS

* Prolactinoma—size of adenoma correlates with the output of prolactin. Prolactin >150 µg/L consistent with an adenoma in the non-pregnant state.

- Microadenomas more common in women, causing hyperprolactinaemia and hypogonadism. Usually successfully treated medically with bromocriptine. Return to normal levels of serum prolactin occurs in up to 30% of patients not treated.
- Macroadenomas more common in men, can cause other pituitary hormone deficiency by their compression of normal tissue. Although shrinkage is seen with bromocriptine, surgery or ablative radiotherapy need consideration in non-responders.

PHARMACOLOGY

Bromocriptine and cabergoline, dopamine agonists, causes a rapid return to normal serum levels of prolactin once therapeutic levels are achieved.

Nausea, vomiting, fatigue and postural hypotension are common as treatment is initiated.

PROLACTIN INSUFFICIENCY

This is very rare and is due to either panhypopituitarism or specific damage to lactotrophs—infarction of the hypertrophied lactotrophs postpartum (Sheehan's syndrome), autoimmune lymphocytic hypophysitis (late in pregnancy) or postpartum infarction in diabetic patients.

GROWTH HORMONE EXCESS

ACROMEGALY

CLINICAL CLUES

- Increasing shoe or hat size
- Headache
- Diaphoresis
- Heat intolerance
- Visual field defect
- Symptoms of diabetes mellitus, glycosuria
- Hypertension
- Goitre
- Coarsening of facial features
- Oiliness of skin
- Carpal tunnel syndrome
- Skin tags

SIGNS OF ACTIVE DISEASE

- Headache, increasing ring or hat size
- Increasing number of skin tags (molluscum fibrosum)
- Excessive sweating
- Presence of diabetes mellitus
- Increasing visual field loss
- Enlarging goitre
- Hypertension

PATHOPHYSIOLOGY

- Growth hormone (GH) excess is due to overproduction of the hormone by a pituitary tumour in all but the very rare situation of an ectopic GH-producing tumour, e.g. lung or pancreatic cancer, or hypothalamic GHRH producing tumour.
- GH excess after puberty results in acromegaly. Prior to puberty, GH excess causes pituitary gigantism.

DIAGNOSIS

- An oral glucose tolerance test is required for diagnosis. GH is measured 60 to 120 minutes after the glucose load, and normally should suppress to <1 µg/L (<1 ng/mL). In acromegaly, this fails to happen.
- If results are equivocal, a thyrotrophin-releasing hormone (TRH) test can be performed. In acromegaly, a paradoxical rise in GH levels will follow TRH administration in 80% of cases.
- Insulin-like growth factor-1 (IGF-1 or somatomedin-C) levels are elevated in active disease.
- Biochemical confirmation of the disorder should be followed by CT or MRI scanning of the pituitary fossa to localise the pituitary tumour. Map the visual fields.

TREATMENT

- Trans-sphenoidal surgery.
- Radiotherapy.
- Pharmacotherapy—bromocriptine or somatostatin analogues.

PANHYPOPITUITARISM

CLINICAL PRESENTATION

Presentation will depend on whether all or some pituitary hormones are affected. See each of the hormones separately.

Table 9.6 *Anterior pituitary hormones*

Hormone	Hypothalamic regulatory hormone	
	Stimulatory	**Inhibitory**
Growth hormone (GH)	Growth hormone-releasing hormone (GHRH)	Somatostatin
Prolactin	—	Dopamine
Follicle stimulating hormone (FSH) and luteinising hormone (LH)	Gonadotrophin-releasing hormone (GnRH)	—
Thyrotrophin (TSH)	Thyrotrophin-releasing hormone (TRH)	—
Corticotrophin (ACTH), and B lipotrophin (B-LPH) and B endorphin (B-END)	Corticotrophin-releasing hormone (CRH)	

CAUSES

PITUITARY DAMAGE

1. Pituitary adenoma
2. Pituitary surgery
3. Pituitary radiation
4. Closed head trauma
5. Infarction in the postpartum period (Sheehan's syndrome)
6. Lymphocytic hypophysitis—autoimmune pituitary destruction (more common in women with diabetes mellitus in the postpartum period or late stages of pregnancy)

STALK DAMAGE

1. Sarcoidosis
2. Metastatic carcinoma
3. Midline germ cell tumours
4. Histiocytosis
5. Craniopharyngiomas

SYSTEMIC 'FUNCTIONAL' HYPOPITUITARISM

1. Anorexia nervosa
2. Systemic illness
3. Severe stress

REPLACEMENT THERAPY

1. *ACTH deficiency:* especially in response to stress—basal levels may be maintained in a 'well' person—cortisone acetate 25 mg mane, 12.5 mg nocte; or hydrocortisone 20 mg mane, 8 mg nocte. Always ensure adequate glucocorticoid replacement before commencing thyroid replacement.
2. TSH deficiency: thyroxine 2–3 µg/kg/day using lean body mass or

levothyroxine 0.05–0.15 mg/day. Monitor free T4 in this situation rather than TSH.
3. Vasopressin: desmopressin 0.05–0.1 mL intranasally twice daily.
4. LH/FSH deficiency: females—daily combined oral contraceptive pill or hormone replacement therapy.
males—oral, implantable or intramuscular testosterone.
5. Growth hormone: optimum dosage yet to be determined.

VASOPRESSIN DEFICIENCY

Vasopressin (antidiuretic hormone) usually acts by concentrating urine.
Failure of release—central diabetes insipidus (DI).
Failure of renal response to vasopressin—nephrogenic diabetes insipidus.
In central DI, exogenous administration of vasopressin will reverse the pattern of hypotonic polyuria. In nephrogenic DI, there will be no change because the abnormality is in the kidney's inability to respond to vasopressin.

CLINICAL CLUES

1. Polydypsia
2. Polyuria
   In mild DI urine concentration of 290–600 mmol/kg.
   In severe DI urine concentration less than 290 mmol/kg.
3. Mild elevation of the serum sodium can be an early subtle clue.

Polydipsia and polyuria are closely matched, so in normal circumstances relative euvolaemia is maintained. A mismatch can occur following anaesthesia or after disabling trauma, which is when patients are at greatest risk of severe dehydration.

DIAGNOSIS

1. Exclude other causes of polyuria
2. Confirm diabetes insipidus
   a) Screening—plasma osmolality high, urine osmolality low (suggesting either central or nephrogenic DI). N.B. plasma osmolality may be normal if a high fluid intake has been maintained.
   b) Antidiuretic hormone (ADH) given if plasma osmolality high—in central DI urine volume decreases and urine osmolality rises (>600 mOsm/L over 6 hours).
   c) Water deprivation test if plasma osmolality is normal—in DI urine volume does *not* fall and urine osmolality does *not* rise >600 mOsm/L (ADH is given then to differentiate central from nephrogenic DI). N.B. in primary polydipsia (excessive water intake) the water deprivation test causes a fall in urine volume and a rise in urine osmolality, but this may take days.

In central DI, exclude pituitary space-occupying lesions.

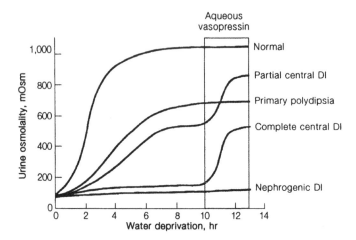

Figure 9.1 *Patterns of changes in urine osmolality in response to prolonged water deprivation. DI denotes diabetes insipidus.* Reproduced, with permission, from Wyngaarden JB, Smith LH, editors. Cecil's Textbook of Medicine, 18th ed. Philadelphia: WB Saunders, 1988.

CAUSES

1. Idiopathic
2. Head trauma
3. Primary brain tumour—preoperatively
4. After excision of primary brain tumour
5. After hypophysectomy

TREATMENT

- Desmopressin intranasally every 12 hours.
- Non-hormonal agents include chlorpropamide, clofibrate and carbamazepine.

VASOPRESSIN EXCESS

CLINICAL CLUES

- Mild—lethargy, nausea, vomiting, anorexia
- Severe—body weight increase; cerebral oedema with signs of central nervous system irritation may be prominent

- Hyponatraemia
- Serum osmolality <275 mmol/kg
- Urine osmolality inappropriately high
- Urinary sodium >20 mmol/L
- Low serum uric acid level

PATHOPHYSIOLOGY

'PHYSIOLOGICAL' EXCESS

1. Follows sodium retention to maintain plasma osmolality—e.g. cardiac failure
2. Hypotension in patients with adrenal insufficiency

'PATHOLOGICAL' EXCESS

Syndrome of inappropriate excretion of antidiuretic hormone—SIADH (see page 155)

SEX HORMONE EXCESS

MALES

Increased oestrogen
- Obesity (increased conversion of androgens to oestradiol and oestrone)
- Increased plasma precursors (liver and adrenal disease)
- Increased testicular production (tumours or testosterone resistance)

Gynaecomastia is the most common feature of oestrogen excess in males.

HIRSUTISM

Hirsutism is excessive hairiness in women, while virilisation is the appearance of male secondary sexual characteristics (clitoromegaly, frontal hair recession, male body habitus, and deepening of the voice due to androgen excess).

CAUSES

1. Constitutional
2. Ovarian disease
   a) Idiopathic
   b) Polycystic ovaries
   c) Tumour
3. Adrenal disease
   a) Congenital adrenal hyperplasia (21 and 11-hydroxylase deficiency)
   b) Cushing's syndrome
   c) Virilising adrenal tumours

4. Drugs
   a) Androgens, glucocorticoids
   b) Minoxidil, phenytoin, diazoxide, streptomycin
5. Other
   a) Acromegaly
   b) Porphyria cutanea tarda

Table 9.7 *Congenital adrenal hyperplasia*

Enzyme deficiency	Virilised	Salt wasting	Hypertension
21-hydroxylase	+	±	–
11-hydroxylase	+	–	+ (renin decreased)
17-hydroxylase*	–	–	+ (renin decreased)

*Female phenotype.

SEX HORMONE DEFICIENCY

MALE

CLINICAL CLUES

- Decreased libido
- Decreased potency

PATHOPHYSIOLOGY

Testosterone is made by the cells of Leydig under the control of pituitary luteinising hormone (LH)—peripherally it can be converted to dihydrotestosterone or oestrogen. Follicle stimulating hormone (FSH) may further slightly increase testosterone secretion.

Seminiferous tubules are more directly under the control of FSH and so are needed for spermatogenesis together with androgens.

DISEASE STATES

- Testicular disease (primary)—hypergonadotrophic hypogonadism (high LH, FSH)
- Klinefelter's syndrome (XXY karyotype), gonadal dysgenesis, androgen resistance, testicular enzyme defects, castration, trauma, orchitis
- Secondary hypogonadotrophic hypogonadism (normal/low LH, FSH)
- Pituitary or hypothalamic disease

THERAPEUTICS

- Testosterone (oral or implantable)
- 100–200 mg testosterone ethanoate intramuscularly 1–2 weekly, or dermal patches.

FEMALE

CLINICAL CLUES

- Secondary amenorrhoea
- Pregnancy/menopause are the commonest causes

PATHOPHYSIOLOGY

LH and FSH are glycoproteins produced by gonadotrophs in 10% of the anterior pituitary. FSH acts on the granulosa cells in the ovary—responsible for oestradiol production.
LH works on ovarian theca cells.
Prolactin production inhibits LHRH release, so prolactinomas can cause secondary amenorrhoea.

DISEASE STATES

- Hypothalamic disease—obesity, anorexia nervosa, extreme exercise, cessation of oral contraceptive pill
- Pituitary disease—prolactinoma, Sheehan's syndrome
- Thyroid disease—hyperthyroidism or hypothyroidism
- Adrenal disease—adrenal hyperplasia
- Ovarian disease—polycystic ovaries, hypergonadotrophic ovarian failure (resistance to LH, FSH)
- Uterine disease—endometrial atrophy
- Systemic disease—chronic renal failure

THERAPEUTICS

In premenopausal women, this can be treated with a combined oestrogen/progesterone oral contraceptive pill or hormone replacement therapy.

MINERALOCORTICOID DEFICIENCY

CAUSES

1. Mineralocorticoid and glucocorticoid deficiency (plasma renin is high)
   a) Congenital 21-hydroxylase deficiency (rare)
   b) Analdosteronism (rare)
2. Isolated mineralocorticoid deficiency
   a) With low plasma renin
      i) Hyporeninaemic hypoaldosteronism
   b) With normal or high plasma renin
      i) Normoreninaemic hypoaldosteronism
      ii) Heparin

Table 9.8   Steroids

Type	Equivalent anti-inflammatory doses (mg)	Mineralocorticoid potency	Biological half-life (hours)
Hydrocortisone	20	1.0	8 to 12
Cortisone	25	0.8	8 to 12
Prednisolone	5	0.8	12 to 36
Dexamethasone	0.75	0	24 to 48

ORAL CONTRACEPTIVE PILL

SIDE EFFECTS

OESTROGEN RELATED

1. Oedema, weight gain
2. Nausea, vomiting
3. Headaches, migraine
4. Hypertension
5. Depression,* lethargy, irritability
6. Breast tenderness*
7. Mucorrhoea
8. Venous stasis in the legs, deep venous thrombosis
9. Hepatic adenoma, hepatic nodular hyperplasia, peliosis hepatis, Budd-Chiari syndrome

PROGESTERONE RELATED

1. Hypomenorrhoea
2. Decreased libido
3. Dry vagina, monilial vaginitis
4. Depression

PRO-ANDROGENIC EFFECTS

1. Acne, hirsutism, alopecia
2. Chloasma, galactorrhoea

METABOLIC EFFECTS

1. Abnormal carbohydrate tolerance
2 Increased cholesterol, triglycerides
3. Increased plasma proteins

---

*also related to progesterone.

CONTRAINDICATIONS TO PRESCRIBING ORAL CONTRACEPTIVES

ABSOLUTE

1. History of thromboembolic disease
2. History of cerebrovascular disease
3. Oestrogen dependent tumour (breast, uterus)
4. History of cholestatic jaundice in pregnancy
5. Undiagnosed vaginal bleeding

RELATIVE

1. Hypertension
2. Family history of cerebrovascular disease
3. Hyperlipidaemia
4. Epilepsy
5. Diabetes mellitus
6. Migraine
7. Heavy smoker
8. >40 years of age
9. Cardiac disease

GYNAECOMASTIA

CAUSES OF PATHOLOGICAL GYNAECOMASTIA

INCREASED OESTROGEN-LIKE PRODUCTION

1. Leydig cell tumour (oestrogen)
2. Adrenal carcinoma (oestrogen)
3. Ectopic human chorionic gonadotrophin (HCG), e.g. lung carcinoma, testicular tumours
4. Liver disease (?increased conversion of oestrogen from androgen)
5. Thyrotoxicosis (increased conversion of oestrogen from androgen)
6. Starvation

DECREASED ANDROGEN PRODUCTION (HYPOGONADAL STATES)

1. Klinefelter's syndrome (47XXY karyotype)
2. Secondary testicular failure: orchitis, castration, trauma, torsion, tumour, myotonic dystrophy

TESTICULAR FEMINISATION SYNDROME

DRUGS

1. Oestrogen receptor binders: oestrogen, digoxin, marijuana
2. Antiandrogens: spironolactone, cimetidine, methyldopa

PARATHYROID GLAND

HYPERCALCAEMIA

CLINICAL CLUES

1. Anorexia, nausea, vomiting
2. Constipation
3. Polyuria, polydipsia
4. Hypotonia, hyporeflexia
5. Lethargy, confusion, depression, weakness
6. Coma
7. Renal colic due to nephrolithiasis
8. Chronic renal failure secondary to nephrocalcinosis
9. Pancreatitis (rarely)

PATHOPHYSIOLOGY

ACTIONS OF PARATHYROID HORMONE (PTH)

1. Causes enhanced action of osteoclasts on bone, resulting in mobilisation of calcium and phosphate.
2. This can only occur in the presence of activated vitamin D (calcitriol).
3. PTH stimulates calcium resorption in the distal tubules, and enhances phosphate excretion.
4. PTH stimulates conversion of vitamin D to the active form in the proximal tubule. Vitamin D then causes increased absorption of calcium and phosphate from the intestine.
5. PTH is released from the parathyroid gland in response to low serum calcium.

CAUSES OF HYPERCALCAEMIA

1. Primary or tertiary hyperparathyroidism
2. Malignancy—PTH-related peptide(PTHrP)-dependent, or bony metastases
3. Drugs—thiazides, lithium
4. Exogenous vitamin D excess, or excessive production of vitamin D metabolites—sarcoidosis, some T cell lymphomas
5. Thyrotoxicosis, hypothyroidism
6. Addison's disease
7. Phaeochromocytoma
8. Acromegaly
9. Multiple myeloma
10. Prolonged immobilisation with Paget's disease
11. MEN I or II
12. Familial benign hypercalcaemia
13. Familial hypercalcaemic hypocalciuria—an asymptomatic autosomal dominant condition with an increased PTH
14. Milk-alkali syndrome

HYPERPARATHYROIDISM

CLINICAL CLUES

- Often asymptomatic and found on random blood test
- Symptoms and signs of hypercalcaemia (see above)
- Bone disease—osteopenia, osteitis fibrosa cystica

PATHOPHYSIOLOGY

1. Primary—adenoma (80%), hyperplasia, carcinoma. Adenoma can rarely be ectopic in other organs, e.g. thymus, thyroid. May occur in association with MEN I or IIA.
2. Secondary—following chronic renal failure.
3. Tertiary—autonomous hyperparathyroidism following secondary hyper-parathyroidism.

DIAGNOSIS

- Hypercalcaemia
- Hypophosphataemia
- Serum chloride may be increased and bicarbonate decreased
- PTH level is elevated despite hypercalcaemia

TREATMENT

- Surgical adenomectomy or subtotal parathyroidectomy

HYPOCALCAEMIA

CLINICAL CLUES

1. Tetany, muscle spasms (Trousseau's sign)
2. Seizures
3. Cardiac arrhythmias
4. Lethargy
5. Abdominal pain, nausea, vomiting

PATHOPHYSIOLOGY

CAUSES OF HYPOCALCAEMIA

With high serum phosphate
1. Hypoparathyroidism
2. Pseudohypoparathyroidism
3. Chronic renal failure

With low or normal serum phosphate
1. Malabsorption (vitamin D deficiency)
2. Hypophosphataemic rickets
3. Magnesium deficiency, e.g. in alcoholics
4. Acute pancreatitis

HYPOPARATHYROIDISM

Hypoparathyroidism presents with tetany due to hypocalcaemia. Causes include:
1. Postoperative (thyroidectomy, parathyroidectomy)
2. Hereditary, e.g. Di-George syndrome, autoimmune polyglandular deficiency
3. Infiltrative disease, e.g. haemochromatosis

PSEUDOHYPOPARATHYROIDISM

Pseudohypoparathyroidism may present with tetany. It is an inherited disorder characterised by end-organ resistance to the action of PTH.
1. Type IA is due to reduced activity of the stimulatory guanyl nucleotide-binding protein that is linked to adenylate cyclase. There are characteristic skeletal deformities (short fourth or fifth digit, short stature, round face, short neck) and mental retardation.
2. Type IB is probably the result of a PTH receptor defect.
3. Type II is due to a post-receptor defect.

PSEUDO-PSEUDOHYPOPARATHYROIDISM

Presents with *normal* calcium levels but characteristic skeletal deformities; there is also reduced activity of the stimulatory guanyl nucleotide-binding protein.

BONE DISEASE

OSTEOPOROSIS

This is defined as a decreased bone mass per unit volume, with a normal mineral content. Patients often present with back pain, fractures (especially T12) and spinal deformity.

CAUSES
1. Idiopathic in postmenopausal females and the elderly
2. Steroid excess—Cushing's syndrome
3. Thyrotoxicosis
4. Hyperparathyroidism
5. Hypogonadism
6. Alcoholism
7. Drugs—chronic heparin administration, cyclosporin A
8. Malignancy
9. Immobilisation

10. Genetic disorders of collagen synthesis—Ehlers-Danlos syndrome, homocystinuria, osteogenesis imperfecta
11. Malnutrition, coeliac disease

DIAGNOSIS

1. Bone densitometry
2. Identify the cause

TREATMENT

1. Hormone replacement (in oestrogen-deficient women and androgen-deficient men)
2. Bisphosphonates
3. Vitamin D and calcium supplementation

OSTEOMALACIA

Rickets is defined as a defective mineralisation of bone and the growth plate in children, while osteomalacia is defective mineralisation of the adult skeleton.

CLINICAL CLUES

- Bone pain
- Proximal muscle weakness
- X-rays show decreased bone density. Looser's zones (radiolucent bands) in the femoral neck, pelvis, outer scapula, upper fibula and metatarsals may be seen

PATHOPHYSIOLOGY

Causes
- Vitamin D deficiency (poor diet, malabsorption, chronic renal failure, phenytoin)
- Renal tubular acidosis
- Phosphate depletion (antacids, vitamin D resistant rickets due to decreased tubular phosphate reabsorption)
- Fanconi syndrome

DIAGNOSIS

- Vitamin D deficiency states—low or normal calcium, high PTH
- Non-vitamin D-dependent osteomalacia—normal calcium and PTH (Table 9.9)
- Radiographic changes

TREATMENT

- Vitamin D replacement
- Calcium supplementation
- Oral phosphate supplements if hypophosphataemic

Table 9.9 *Calcium metabolism and bone*

Disease	Calcium	Phosphate	25-OH vitamin D	PTH	Alkaline phosphatase (bone)
Osteoporosis	N	N	N	N	N
Osteomalacia or rickets due to malabsorption or dietary lack	Low-N	Low-N	Decreased	Increased-N	Increased
Osteomalacia with renal bone disease	Variable	N-increased	Variable	Increased-N	Increased
Familial hypophosphataemic rickets	N	Decreased	N	N	Increased
Primary hyperparathyroidism	Increased	Decreased-N	N	Increased	Increased-N
Paget's disease	N	N	N	N	Increased

N = normal.

PAGET'S DISEASE

CLINICAL CLUES

- Predominantly a disease of older individuals
- Bone pain, deformity, fracture
- Skull enlargement
- Erythema and warmth of overlying skin
- Transformation to osteogenic sarcoma
- High-output cardiac failure
- Angioid streaks in optic fundus
- Nerve entrapment syndromes
- Hypercalcaemia with immobilisation

PATHOPHYSIOLOGY

- Cause unknown
- Disorganised bone remodelling gives rise to weakened bone, pain and deformity
- May be monostotic or affect multiple bones

DIAGNOSIS

- Raised serum alkaline phosphatase
- Characteristic radiographic changes
- Increased uptake on bone scan in affected areas

TREATMENT

- Calcitonin
- Bisphosphonates

SHORT STATURE

CAUSES

1. Normal variant
2. Disease (mnemonic—IS NICCE)
   I— Intrauterine growth retardation, e.g. maternal alcoholism.
   S— Skeletal disease, e.g. achondroplasia, rickets.
   N—Nutritional, e.g. malabsorption, starvation.
   I— Iatrogenic growth retardation, e.g. glucocorticoids, spinal irradiation.
   C—Chromosomal, e.g. Turner's syndrome.
   C—Chronic disease e.g. cyanotic congenital heart disease, cystic fibrosis, chronic liver or renal impairment.
   E—Endocrine e.g. hypothyroidism, growth hormone deficiency, Cushing's syndrome (in childhood), congenital adrenal hyperplasia (tall children but short adults), precocious puberty.

MULTIPLE ENDOCRINE NEOPLASIA (MEN)

MEN I

- Autosomal dominant
- Abnormal gene is located on chromosome 11
- Primary hyperparathyroidism is almost invariable
- Islet cell neoplasia, with tumours potentially secreting a variety of hormones including pancreatic polypeptide, gastrin, insulin, vasoactive intestinal polypeptide, glucagon and somatostatin
- Approximately 15% of patients also have pituitary tumours, most commonly prolactinoma
- Carcinoid tumour, thyroid and adrenal adenomas, and lipomas may also occur in these patients

MEN II

- Autosomal dominant
- Abnormal gene is located on chromosome 10

MEN IIA

- Medullary carcinoma of the thyroid
- Phaeochromocytoma
- Hyperparathyroidism

MEN IIB

- As per type IIA but hyperparathyroidism does not occur
- The medullary carcinoma of the thyroid develops earlier in life
- Mucosal neuromas, intestinal ganglioneuromatosis, and marfanoid features occur

AUTOIMMUNE CLUSTER

1. Autoimmune thyroid disease, hypoparathyroidism
2. Addison's disease, vitiligo
3. Pernicious anaemia
4. Diabetes mellitus, mucocutaneous candidiasis
5. Primary ovarian failure
6. Coeliac disease, dermatitis herpetiformis

10

Haematology

CLINICAL CLUES

LYMPHADENOPATHY

CAUSES

Generalised
1. Lymphoma, leukaemia (chronic lymphocytic and acute lymphoblastic leukaemia particularly).
2. Infections: viral (e.g. Epstein-Barr virus, cytomegalovirus (CMV), rubella, HIV); bacterial (e.g. TB, brucellosis, syphilis); protozoal (e.g. toxoplasmosis).
3. Autoimmune diseases, e.g. rheumatoid arthritis, systemic lupus erythematosus (SLE).
4. Infiltrations, e.g. sarcoidosis.
5. Drugs, e.g. phenytoin (pseudolymphoma).

Localised
1. Local acute or chronic infection, e.g. TB, cervical adenopathy.
2. Metastases (often hard, fixed and non-tender) from carcinoma or other solid tumours.
3. Lymphoma (often rubbery, mobile and firm), especially Hodgkin's disease.

N.B. Epitrochlear lymphadenopathy occurs in non-Hodgkin's lymphoma and uncommonly in chronic lymphocytic leukaemia, intravenous drug abuse, infectious mononucleosis and sarcoidosis.

Virchow's node (enlarged left supraclavicular fossa node) is found most often with a gastrointestinal malignancy.

SPLENOMEGALY

Splenomegaly refers to splenic enlargement. Hypersplenism refers to sequestration in the spleen of red cells, white cells and platelets.

CAUSES

Massive
1. Chronic myeloid leukaemia.
2. Myelofibrosis.

3. Malaria, kala azar.
4. Primary lymphoma of the spleen.

Moderate

Above causes plus

1. Portal hypertension.
2. Lymphoma.
3. Leukaemia (acute or chronic).
4. Thalassaemia.
5. Storage diseases, e.g. Gaucher's disease.

Mild

Above causes plus

1. Other myeloproliferative diseases—polycythaemia rubra vera, essential thrombocythaemia.
2. Haemolytic anaemia.
3. Infections—viral (e.g. infectious mononucleosis, hepatitis), bacterial (e.g. infective endocarditis).
4. Autoimmune diseases, e.g. rheumatoid arthritis, SLE, polyarteritis nodosa.
5. Infiltrations, e.g. amyloidosis, sarcoidosis.

GENERALISED LYMPHADENOPATHY AND SPLENOMEGALY

CAUSES

1. Infections.
2. Haematological malignancies (lymphoma, chronic lymphocytic leukaemia, acute lymphoblastic leukaemia).
3. Inflammatory and immunological diseases.

FEVER, LYMPHADENOPATHY AND/OR SPLENOMEGALY

CAUSES

1. Mononucleosis-like syndromes—Epstein-Barr virus, CMV, toxoplasmosis, HIV.
2. Infective endocarditis
3. Salmonella infection, syphilis, TB.
4. Lymphoma.
5. Sarcoidosis.

HEPATOSPLENOMEGALY

CAUSES

1. Chronic liver disease with portal hypertension.
2. Haematological disease, e.g. myeloproliferative disease, lymphoma, leukaemia.
3. Infection, e.g. acute viral hepatitis, Epstein-Barr virus, CMV, HIV.

4. Infiltrations, e.g. amyloidosis, sarcoidosis.
5. Autoimmune disease, e.g. SLE.
6. Acromegaly.

SPLENOMEGALY AND JAUNDICE

1. Chronic liver disease and portal hypertension.
2. Epstein-Barr virus/CMV/HIV infection with haemolytic anaemia.
3. Infective endocarditis with haemolysis.
4. SLE/chronic lymphoblastic leukaemia/non-Hodgkin's lymphoma with warm IgG haemolytic anaemia.
5. Cold haemolytic anaemia (primary or secondary to non-Hodgkin's lymphoma).
6. Paroxysmal nocturnal haemoglobinuria (PNH).
7. Hereditary spherocytosis.
8. Budd Chiari (hepatic vein thrombosis) with PNH, myeloproliferative disorders.

SPLENIC ATROPHY OR ABSENCE

CAUSES

1. Splenectomy.
2. Coeliac disease.
3. Multiple splenic infarcts (autosplenectomy), e.g. sickle cell disease.
4. Congenital absence.

The post-splenectomy blood film may show Howell-Jolly bodies, target cells and crenated cells; there may also be thrombocytosis or leucocytosis.

Splenic atrophy results in increased susceptibility to infections with encapsulated organisms including:

1. *Streptococcus pneumoniae*
2. *Neisseria meningitidis*
3. *Haemophilus influenzae*

and non-encapsulated organisms including:

1. *Babesia* (a protozoa that causes acute febrile haemolytic anaemia)
2. Malaria.

Staphylococcus aureus and *Escherichia coli* may also be implicated in some infections in the presence of asplenism.

LABORATORY CLUES

ERYTHROCYTE SEDIMENTATION RATE (ESR)

FACTORS THAT RESULT IN ESR RISING

1. Hyperfibrinogenaemia
2. Hyperglobulinaemia
3. Lipaemia

Internal Medicine

Causes of an esr >100 mm/h

1. Multiple myeloma, paraproteinaemia
2. SLE, rheumatoid arthritis
3. Temporal arteritis and polymyalgia rheumatica
4. Carcinoma (e.g. renal), chronic infection, pulmonary infarction, drug fever

A low ESR (<3mm/h) occurs in polycythaemia rubra vera, hypofibrinogenaemia and severe hypogammaglobulinaemia.

Table 10.1 Red cell changes and disease

Change	Description	Causes
Autoagglutination	Red cells joined together in clumps	Cold agglutinin disease (cold IgM antibody)
Anisocytosis	Variation in size	Megaloblastic anaemia, thalassaemia, iron deficiency anaemia
Basophilic stippling	Stippling seen in the cytoplasm of the cells	Ribosomal aggregates: lead poisoning; chronic renal failure; thalassaemia
Burr cells	Irregularly shaped cells	Chronic renal failure
Heinz bodies	Crystal violet stains to demonstrate precipitated haemoglobin	Denatured globulin: haemolysis after oxidant stress ± G-6-PD deficiency
Howell-Jolly bodies	Nuclear remnants in cells	Post-splenectomy; B_{12} and folate deficiencies
Leucoerythro-blastic picture	Immature myeloid cells and nucleated red cells in peripheral film	Infiltration of marrow by malignant cells or fibrosis
Nucleated red cells	Nuclei still clearly seen	Marrow infiltrative disease (e.g. fibrosis, tumour), haemolysis (excess demand); severe anoxia
Poikilocytes	Irregularly shaped cells	Iron deficiency and many primary marrow disorders
Round macrocytes	Excess membrane cholesterol	Alcohol; cirrhosis; reticulocytosis; marrow infiltration; myelodysplastic syndrome: hypothyroidism
Rouleaux	Red cells joined together in lines	Red cell loses -ve charge: any cause of an elevated ESR
Schistocytes	Red cell fragments	Splenectomy; DIC; TTP; cardiac haemolysis
Sickle cells	Elongated crescent shaped cells	Sickle cell disease; heterozygous sickle thalassaemia

Table 10.1 Continued

Change	Description	Causes
Siderocytes	Iron granules in a perinuclear ring	Alcohol; haemolysis
Spherocytes	Small densely staining spherical cells	Decreased surface/volume ratio; hereditary spherocytosis; warm antibody autoimmune haemolytic anaemia; haemolytic transfusion reactions; microangiopathic haemolysis
Spur cells	Bizarre shaped red blood cells with thorn-like projections	Decreased surface/volume ratio and increased membrane cholesterol; liver disease (advanced)
Target cells	Central staining in the red cell	Increased surface/volume ratio decreases osmotic fragility: liver disease; splenectomy; haemoglobinopathy
Tear drop cells	Tear drop shaped cells	Extramedullary haematopoiesis; myelofibrosis

DIC = disseminated intravascular coagulation, TTP = thrombotic thrombocytopenic purpura, G-6-PD = glucose 6 phosphate dehydrogenase.

ALL CELL LINES

DECREASED CELL LINES: PANCYTOPENIA

CLINICAL CLUES

May be asymptomatic.
Leucopenia mostly characterised by recurrent bacterial infections or bacterial infections that respond poorly to appropriate antibiotics. The infection often presents with masked symptoms and signs, e.g. minimal pyuria in urinary tract infection, reduced erythema/swelling in cellulitis.

Table 10.2 Pancytopenia

Mechanisms		Clinical setting
Decreased production	Decreased number of normal myeloid cells at all stages of production	Bone marrow aplasia Myelofibrosis Myelodysplasia Acute leukaemias Metastatic infiltration of bone marrow HIV infection Severe systemic sepsis Paroxysmal nocturnal haemoglobinuria

Table 10.2 *Continued*

Mechanisms	Clinical setting
Normal numbers of marrow cells with impaired maturation of cells	Infection e.g.HIV, disseminated *Mycobacterium avium complex* B$_{12}$/folate deficiency Autoimmune Drug effect
Increased destruction/ sequestration	Splenomegaly Autoimmune Sepsis HIV infection Drug effect Felty's syndrome

BONE MARROW APLASIA
(also known as aplastic anaemia)

CLINICAL CLUES

Most patients present with symptoms of anaemia (lethargy, dyspnoea, tachycardia), sepsis (especially bacterial sepsis in the face of prolonged neutropenia) or evidence of a tendency to bleed (from thrombocytopenia).

CAUSES

1. Idiopathic
2. Drugs
   a) Dose-related, e.g. antineoplastic drugs, ionising radiation
   b) Idiosyncratic, e.g. chloramphenicol, indomethacin, phenylbutazone, phenytoin, sulfonamides, gold salts
3. Other exogenous causes—benzene
4. Viruses
   a) hepatitis B, C
   b) haemorrhagic fever viruses (e.g. dengue)
5. SLE (IgG-mediated stem cell damage)
6. Oestrogens
7. Fanconi syndrome
8. Immune-mediated stem cell damage (antibodies and cytokines)

N.B. exclude PNH as a cause of apparent marrow failure.

LABORATORY CLUES

Severe aplasia: absolute neutrophil count <500/μL (very severe <200/μL)
                  absolute reticulocyte count <20000/μL
                  platelet count <20000/μL
                  marrow biopsy cellularity <25%

Blood film: normal appearing platelets, red and white cells on peripheral blood film.

Bone marrow biopsy: in aplasia, 0–25% of the normal number of cells in the marrow.

Causes of a dry bone marrow tap:

- technical difficulties
- bone marrow fatty, empty or markedly hypocellular (e.g. acute leukaemia)
- irradiated marrow
- marrow fibrosis

TREATMENT OF MARROW APLASIA

Supportive
- Red cell transfusion for symptomatic anaemia.
  If marrow transplant is considered, avoid transfusion from close relatives to reduce risk of sensitisation and subsequent graft rejection.
- Platelet transfusion for symptomatic thrombocytopenia (bleeding).
- Antibiotics for bacterial infections.

Disease modifying
- Antithymocyte globulin: 5–10 day course, maximum benefit at 2–3 months—mechanism unknown.
- Immunosuppressive agents e.g. steroids. cyclophosphamide, cyclosporin.
- Bone marrow transplantation: success rate highest in those <20 years with matched sibling donors transplanted before receiving 20 units of packed cells.

CELL LINE PROLIFERATION—MYELOPROLIFERATIVE DISEASES

PATHOPHYSIOLOGY

A stem cell disorder characterised by effective, ordered overproduction of one or more cell lines. Most are due to monoclonal disorders. All can be associated with marrow fibrosis which may disappear with bone marrow transplantation.

1. Polycythaemia rubra vera.
2. Myeloid metaplasia with myelofibrosis (characterised by bone marrow fibrosis with splenomegaly).
3. Chronic myeloid leukaemia.
4. Essential thrombocythaemia: characterised by sustained elevation of the platelet count without any primary cause, megakaryocytic hyperplasia in the bone marrow (>95%) and splenomegaly (40%).

All have the potential for acute leukaemic transformation (>30% blasts). Other marrow cell lines are usually depressed with leukaemic transformation. The risk of transformation increases in patients previously treated with alkylating agents.

CLINICAL CLUES

- Incidental finding on routine blood tests
- Splenomegaly
- Fevers, night sweats, weight loss
- Coagulation disturbances (both arterial and venous occlusion may occur).
  In polycythaemia rubra vera, haematocrit of >50% increases the likelihood of thrombosis. Thrombotic problems are rarely seen in secondary polycythaemia.

TREATMENT

Symptomatic treatment, if the underlying cause cannot be treated, is by phlebotomy and judicious use of cytotoxic agents. Hydroxyurea is helpful, and in older patients radioactive phosphorus may be used. Busulfan, widely used in the past, probably increased the rate of leukaemic transformation.

RED CELLS

POLYCYTHAEMIA (ERYTHROCYTOSIS)

This is an elevated haemoglobin concentration and can result from either an increased red cell mass (which may be primary or secondary) or a decreased plasma volume.

CAUSES

Consider the diagnosis in the setting of raised haemoglobin concentration and raised haematocrit.

Absolute polycythaemia (red cell mass increased)
1. *Polycythaemia rubra vera*

Diagnostic criteria:

Category I
- Increased red cell mass
- PaO_2 normal
- Splenomegaly

Category II
- Platelets >400000/mm^3
- White cell count >12000/mm^3 in the absence of infection or fever
- Neutrophil alkaline phosphatase score elevated >100
- Serum B_{12} elevated

Diagnosis = all category I; or 2 of category I plus any 2 of category II.

2. *Secondary polycythaemia*
- Increased erythropoietin secretion:

  Renal disease: polycystic kidneys, hydronephrosis, tumour
  Malignancy: hepatoma, haemangioblastoma
  Uterine fibroma
  Endocrine: virilising syndromes, Cushing's syndrome, phaeochromocytoma

- Hypoxic states (erythropoeitin secondarily increased):
  Smokers' polycythaemia, chronic lung disease, sleep apnoea, cyanotic congenital heart disease, high altitude

Relative polycythaemia (decreased plasma volume)
1. Dehydration
2. Stress polycythaemia

Polycythaemia rubra vera

Treatment
Phlebotomy to keep haematocrit below 46%. Hydroxyurea can be used. Busulfan and radioactive phosphorus are reserved for patients >65 years because of the leukaemic risk.

DECREASED OR ABNORMAL RED CELLS: ANAEMIA

Chronic anaemia is often well tolerated with few symptoms.

Mechanisms

Blood loss, cell breakdown, sequestration—normal or high reticulocyte count. Underproduction—low reticulocyte count (<20000/μL)*

Hypochromic microcytic anaemia

Causes
1. Iron deficiency
   a) Blood loss—chronic (gastrointestinal tract usually; rarely genitourinary tract)
   b) Decreased absorption—postgastrectomy, small bowel disease
   c) Increased requirements—heavy menstrual loss, pregnancy, hookworm infection
   d) Poor diet (very rarely the primary cause)
   Often associated with a thrombocytosis.
   Laboratory clues
   - total iron binding capacity increases
   - transferrin saturation with iron falls
   - serum ferritin (reflecting body iron stores) falls (but this is also an acute phase reactant so may be normal in some cases of iron deficiency)
2. Thalassaemia
3. Sideroblastic anaemia
   Sideroblasts are red cell precursors containing non-haem iron granules.
   a) Congenital. X-linked or autosomal recessive—may or may not respond to pyridoxine.

---

*Bone marrow biopsy may be of use but is rarely of benefit if reticulocyte count is normal or raised.

b) Acquired. Myelodysplastic syndrome (usually in the elderly; rarely responds to pyridoxine).
c) Secondary. Myeloproliferative disease: lymphoma; myeloma; carcinoma; connective tissue disease; alcohol; drugs (anti-tuberculous drugs, chloramphenicol, cytotoxics).
4. Chronic systemic illness.

If iron deficiency anaemia is unresponsive to iron supplementation, consider:
a) Non-compliance
b) Blood loss continuing (reticulocytosis persists)
c) Malabsorption
d) Incorrect diagnosis (thalassaemia; sideroblastic anaemia/myelodysplastic syndrome; chronic illness).

Macrocytic anaemia

Causes
Megaloblastic bone marrow, oval macrocytes, hypersegmented neutrophils on peripheral blood film.
1. Vitamin B_{12} (cobalamin) deficiency
   a) Malabsorption
      • Lack of intrinsic factor (e.g. pernicious anaemia, gastrectomy).
      • B_{12} malabsorption: ileal disease or >60cm resection, small bowel bacterial overgrowth (which may produce folate), fish tapeworm
      • Pancreatic disease
   b) Drugs, e.g. phenytoin, colchicine, neomycin
   c) Diet (rare—seen in true vegans).
2. Folate deficiency
   a) Most commonly inadequate diet, especially in alcoholics
   b) Malabsorption: coeliac disease, tropical sprue
   c) Increased demand
      • Pregnancy
      • Increased cell turnover: myeloproliferative disease; malignancy; chronic haemolysis; chronic inflammation—psoriasis, rheumatoid arthritis
   d) Drugs
      • Dihydrofolate reductase inhibitors, e.g. methotrexate, trimethoprim
      • Decreased absorption, e.g. phenytoin, cholestyramine, sulfasalazine
      • Anti-retroviral agents e.g. zidovudine
Normoblastic bone marrow (round macrocytes on the blood film)
1. Alcohol
2. Cirrhosis
3. Reticulocytosis, e.g. haemolysis, haemorrhage
4. Hypothyroidism
5. Marrow infiltration especially with malignant cells
6. Myelodysplastic syndrome
7. Myeloproliferative disease

NORMOCYTIC NORMOCHROMIC ANAEMIA

Causes
1. Bone marrow failure
   a) Bone marrow aplasia (also known as aplastic anaemia)
   b) Ineffective haematopoiesis (normal or increased bone marrow cellularity)
      i) Myelodysplastic syndrome
      ii) Paroxysmal nocturnal haemoglobinuria
   c) Bone marrow infiltration (leucoerythroblastic blood film)
      i) Leukaemia, lymphoma, carcinoma, myeloma, granuloma, myelofibrosis
2. Chronic systemic disease (bone marrow iron stores normal or increased) —anaemia of chronic disease
   a) Chronic inflammation, e.g. infection (abscess, TB), connective tissue disease, malignancy
   b) Endocrine deficiencies, e.g. hypothyroidism, hypopituitarism, Addison's disease, hypogonadism
   c) Liver disease
   d) Chronic renal failure
   e) Malnutrition
3. Haemolysis—see below
4. Acute marrow toxins, e.g. alcohol (may simply suppress normal erythropoiesis), isoniàzid, lead

Erythropoietin
Low in chronic renal failure—anaemia in this setting responds well to exogenous erythropoietin if there are normal iron and folate stores. In the setting of high aluminium levels, response to erythropoietin is blunted.

HAEMOLYTIC ANAEMIA

Classification
Intracorpuscular defects (problems of the red cell wall or contents)
1. Congenital
   a) Membrane defect, e.g. hereditary spherocytosis, elliptocytosis
   b) Haemoglobin defect, e.g. sickle cell disease, thalassaemia
   c) Enzyme defect, e.g. G-6-PD, pyruvate kinase deficiency
2. Acquired
   a) Paroxysmal nocturnal haemoglobinuria

Extracorpuscular defects (problems related mainly to plasma or vessel walls)
1. Immune
   a) Autoimmune
   b) Haemolytic disease of the newborn, incompatible blood transfusion
2. Non-immune
   a) Mechanical trauma, drugs, hypersplenism

Diagnosis of haemolysis
Clinically, acute haemolysis may present with fever, chills, back pain, acute renal failure and shock.

Internal Medicine

1. *Confirm haemolysis is present*
   a) Increased reticulocyte count (also occurs with blood loss and partially treated anaemia)
   b) Reduced haptoglobin level
   c) Release of red cell components—increased unconjugated bilirubin, lactate dehydrogenase (LDH)
   d) Bone marrow—erythroid hyperplasia
2. *Determine if there is an underlying red cell change*
   a) On history
      i) Onset at an early age or a family history—intrinsic red cell defect
      ii) Ethnicity: African Americans, Mediterranean background—G-6-PD deficiency.
      African Americans—sickle cell disease.
      People of southern Mediterranean descent—thalassaemia
   b) In the laboratory
      i) On blood film—target cells (thalassaemia, sickle cell disease), spherocytes (hereditary spherocytosis, immune haemolysis), fragments (microangiopathic haemolysis)
      ii) Direct Coombs' test—see below
      iii) Haemoglobin electrophoresis (at pH 8.6 and 6.8) for thalassaemia
      iv) G-6-PD and pyruvate kinase screening tests.
      v) Ham's test—see below
3. *Determine if there is free haemoglobin in the blood (intravascular haemolysis)*
   a) Decreased haptoglobin—binds to haemoglobin freed into the plasma
   b) High methaemalbumin—free haem bound to albumin
   c) Haemoglobinuria—haemoglobin free in plasma filtered through the glomerulus and passed directly into urine
   d) Urine haemosiderin—sloughed iron-rich renal tubular cells from haemoglobin dimers which have been filtered and reabsorbed. Found for up to weeks after intravascular haemolysis
   Causes of intravascular haemolysis (mnemonic MCP)
   M—Microangiopathic haemolytic anaemia (irregularly fragmented red cells; may be helmet cells on the blood film, seen in up to 25% of disseminated intravascular coagulation (DIC))
   M—March haemoglobinuria
   C—Chronic cold agglutinin disease
   C—Cardiac (valvular) disease
   P—Paroxysmal nocturnal haemoglobinuria
   P—Paroxysmal cold haemoglobinuria
4. *If not, is there extravascular haemolysis?*
   a) Idiopathic
   b) Splenomegaly or occasionally liver disease. The spleen normally destroys senescent red blood cells. Destruction of red cells can be accelerated with any cause of splenomegaly or as an immune-mediated phenomenon.
   c) Red cell antibodies against erythrocyte surface antigens.

i) alloantibodies—pregnancy, blood transfusion
ii) warm (IgG) antibodies—chronic lymphocytic leukaemia, non-Hodgkin's lymphoma, SLE, alpha methyldopa, penicillin, quinidine
iii) cold (IgM) antibodies (<15°C)—*M. pneumoniae*, Epstein-Barr virus, lymphoma

Laboratory clues
Blood film may show erythrocyte clumping (autoagglutination).
Coombs' test assesses the presence of IgG and complement on the cell surface and is positive in extravascular immune-mediated haemolysis.

Treatment
Remove or treat underlying cause if possible.
May respond to high-dose steroids.

Clinical settings
1. DIC, thrombotic thrombocytopenic purpura (TTP), haemolytic uraemic syndrome. These patients are also thrombocytopenic.
2. Prosthetic heart valves or fibrin deposition on heart valves (cardiac haemolysis).
3. Malignant hypertension, toxaemia of pregnancy.
4. Vasculitis, e.g. Wegener's granulomatosis.
5. Malignancy.

MYELODYSPLASIA

Pathophysiology
- Ineffective and disordered blood cell generation
- Defect in the maturation of one or more cell lines
- Seen most often in the elderly
- Varying degrees of (usually macrocytic) anaemia, leucopenia and thrombocytopenia

Current FAB (French-American-British) classification
- Refractory anaemia (RA)
- RA with ringed sideroblasts (RARS)
- RA with excess blasts (RAEB) 5–20% blasts
- RAEB in transformation (RAEB-t) 21–30% blasts
- Chronic myelomonocytic leukaemia (CMML)

Clinical clues
Two groups of patients:
- those with a stable cell maturation defect
- those with evolving acute non-lymphoblastic leukaemia (ANLL) from RAEB and RAEB-t

RARS have a better prognosis than RAEB or RAEB-t.

Marrow: normal or hypercellular for most patients

10–15% hypocellular or aplastic marrow

10–15% have moderate to severe fibrosis and decreased cellularity.

Often become transfusion dependent—iron overload is therefore one of the long-term sequelae.

Death commonly caused by severe sepsis in the face of sustained neutropenia.

Platelet transfusions should be avoided in the chronic setting if possible.

Worsening prognosis is associated with increasing blasts on bone marrow biopsy, marrow fibrosis, marrow hypoplasia, clusters of immature precursor cells, increasing numbers of circulating blasts in the peripheral blood, suppression of other cell lines and increasing age.

Treatment
- Stimulating factors (granulocyte macrophage colony stimulating factor (GM-CSF), granulocyte colony stimulating factor (G-CSF) and erythropoietin) are of little benefit.
- Intensive chemotherapy has little benefit on survival in the aged.
- Myeloablative therapy followed by allogeneic bone marrow transplantation has a role in patients under 50 years of age.

HEREDITARY SPHEROCYTOSIS

Clinical clues

Autosomal dominant

1. Anaemia (with reticulocytosis, spherocytosis and an increased mean corpuscular haemoglobin concentration (MCHC)).
2. Splenomegaly (and a good response to splenectomy).
3. Jaundice (due to haemolysis (high unconjugated bilirubin) or pigment stone obstruction of the biliary tree).
4. Aplastic crises, leg ulcers, spinal cord lesions.

Diagnosis
1. Spherocytosis on the blood film with negative Coombs' test.
2. Increased osmotic fragility (increased lysis in the presence of low osmotic fragility).
3. Family studies.

Treatment

Splenectomy for symptomatic patients stops haemolysis.

SICKLE CELL ANAEMIA

Pathophysiology

HbS has valine substituted for glutamic acid at the sixth position of the beta globin chain; the haemoglobin affected has an abnormal response to deoxygenation, acidosis, and increased 2,3 DPG.

- Heterozygous—sickle cell trait: benign condition (unless also heterozygous for another haem abnormality such as β thalassaemia).
- Homozygous—sickle cell anaemia.

Occlusion of microvasculature by sickled cells presents with painful crises, aseptic necrosis of bone, renal failure or retinal haemorrhages.

Clinical clues
Features of acute crises
1. Microcirculatory occlusion by sickled cells (misshapen, rigid cells) causing:
   a) Joint pain and swelling (especially knees, elbows)
   b) Abdominal pain
   c) Nervous system haemorrhage including retinal haemorrhages
   d) Renal failure
   e) Aseptic necrosis of bone
   f) Lung disease (pulmonary infarction).
2. Infection is the most common cause of death:
   a) *Streptococcus pneumoniae* (pneumonia, peritonitis, bacteraemia)—prophylactic antibiotics should be given from 4 months of age
   b) *Salmonella* (bacteraemia, osteomyelitis)
   c) *Haemophilus influenzae* (meningitis)
   d) *Mycoplasma pneumoniae* (pneumonitis)
   e) *Escherichia coli* (bacteraemia).

Diagnosis
The diagnosis should be considered in any African American or African patient with haemolytic anaemia, even in the presence of adult onset disease without sickle cells on blood film. A history of painful crises or arthropathy is helpful. Blood films reveal normochromic, normocytic anaemia with characteristic sickled cells. Haemoglobin electrophoresis shows excess haemoglobin F (2–20%).

Treatment
- Bone marrow transplantation is the only cure for sickle cell disease.
- Supportive measures in a crisis—oxygen, hydration, analgesia.
- Strokes, especially in the young, should be treated with an aggressive exchange transfusion regimen. Bone marrow transplantation should be considered if an HLA-identical donor can be found.
- Erythropoeitin and hydroxyurea increase haemoglobin F production which is relatively protective against sickling.

Paroxysmal nocturnal haemoglobinuria (pnh)

Pathophysiology
The principal defect is the loss of cell surface proteins normally attached to the cell membrane by phosphatidyl inositol (PI). The defect is in the PIG-A gene.

In this disease, there is increased sensitivity to complement-mediated lysis. This is a stem cell disease although most of the syndrome is associated with red cells. There are cell membrane deficiencies which normally inhibit complement activation and cell lysis.

Internal Medicine

Clinical clues
1. Haemoglobinuria, especially at night (as more acidotic at night).
2. Pancytopenia.
3. Venous thrombosis (limbs, portal, brain—50% deaths).

Precipitants: infection, dehydration, surgery, acidosis.
50% of patients have low-grade intravascular haemolysis.
50% of patients have a prothrombotic tendency.

Laboratory tests
- Urinary haemosiderin—indicates recent intravascular haemolysis.
- Sucrose haemolysis test—lysis of red cells in a solution of decreased ionic strength.
- Ham's test—lysis of red cells under acidic conditions.
- Neutrophil alkaline phosphatase score low.
- Immunophenotyping for PI-linked proteins.

Treatment
- Folate/iron supplements.
- Prednisolone treatment may be life-saving.
- Warfarin can be used to treat thromboembolic events.
- Transfusion in patients who are symptomatically anaemic.
- Severe marrow aplasia/hypoplasia—allogeneic bone marrow transplantation.

THALASSAEMIA

Pathophysiology
Normal: 4 alpha globin genes (chromosome 16)
              2 beta globin genes (chromosome 11)

Alpha thalassaemia
- Common in Asians and Africans
- diagnose with southern blot or with polymerase chain reaction.
  1 alpha-globin gene deletion—carrier state
  2 alpha-globin gene deletions—no symptoms through to mild anaemia, microcytosis
  3 alpha-globin gene deletions—haemoglobin H disease
  4 alpha-globin gene deletions—death *in utero* (hydrops fetalis)

Beta thalassaemia
- diagnose with haemoglobin electrophoresis.

Inactivation of one or both of the beta-globin genes.

Clinical clues
Most problems are due to anaemia either because of reduced haemoglobin synthesis or haemolysis in haemoglobin H disease.

Treatment
Alpha-thalassaemia: haemoglobin H disease is usually a well tolerated microcytic anaemia. HbH cells (which contain precipitated haemoglobin) confirm the diagnosis.

Beta-thalassaemia is classified by clinical course:
- thalassaemia trait (asymptomatic)
- thalassaemia intermedia (not transfusion dependent)
- thalassaemia major (transfusion dependent).

Supportive treatment for beta-thalassaemia major—blood transfusion (with desferrioxamine cover to avoid iron overload)—is often complicated by alloimmunisation to minor red cell antigens in the long term.

Disease modifying treatment—bone marrow transplantation.

OTHER HAEMOGLOBIN VARIANTS

Haemoglobin E up to 30% in some South East Asian countries—unstable beta globin chain which in homozygotes produces microcytosis and mild haemolytic anaemia. Also diagnosed by haemoglobin electrophoresis.

ENZYME RELATED RED CELL DISEASE

Glucose-6-phosphate dehydrogenase (G-6-PD) deficiency: seen almost always in males. Oxidation of haemoglobin by fava beans, sulfonamides, primaquine or infection causes intravascular haemolysis. Mild to moderate G-6-PD deficiency is seen in Africans, with clinically more severe disease seen in people of Mediterranean descent.

Pyruvate kinase deficiency—autosomal recessive. Haemolysis seen, with splenectomy reversing the process.

WHITE CELLS

Neutrophil alkaline phosphatase (NAP) score

Low NAP score
1. Chronic myeloid (granulocytic) leukaemia.
2. Paroxysmal nocturnal haemoglobinuria (PNH).
3. Infectious mononucleosis.
4. Hypophosphatasia.

High NAP score
1. Polycythaemia rubra vera.
2. Myeloid metaplasia, leukaemoid reactions, leucocytosis.
3. Pregnancy, pyogenic infections (reactive leucocytosis).

Table 10.3 *Differential diagnosis of an elevated white cell count*

Feature	Chronic myeloid leukaemia	Leukaemoid reaction	Myelofibrosis with myeloid metaplasia
White cells	May be >100000 with myelocyte and neutrophil peaks	Rarely >100000, mostly neutrophils	Typically <100000 with early myeloid forms
Red cells	Occasional nucleated cells	Normal	Nucleated and tear drop cells

Table 10.3 *Continued*

Feature	Chronic myeloid leukaemia	Leukaemoid reaction	Myelofibrosis with myeloid metaplasia
NAP score	Low (<20)	High	Normal or high
Bone marrow	Panhypercellular	Myeloid hyperplasia	'Dry tap', fibrosis
Philadelphia chromosome	Seen in 95% of cases	Absent	Absent

ACUTE LEUKAEMIA

RISK FACTORS

1. Radiation.
2. Chemicals—benzene, alkylating agents.
3. Chromosomal abnormalities—Down, Turner's, Klinefelter's, Bloom's syndromes; Fanconi's anaemia.
4. Immunodeficiencies—ataxia telangiectasia, X-linked agammaglobulin-aemia.
5. Chronic bone marrow disorders—myeloproliferative disorders, bone marrow aplasia, myeloma, paroxysmal nocturnal haemoglobinuria.

Table 10.4 *Features of acute leukaemia*

Feature	Acute non-lymphoblastic leukaemia	Acute lymphoblastic leukaemia
FAB classification	M1—AML without differentiation M2—AML with differentiation (myeloblasts, promyelocytes) M3—Acute promyelocytic leukaemia, associated with DIC, all-trans-retinoic acid may be of benefit M4—Acute myelomonocytic leukaemia, marrow eosinophilia M5—Acute monocytic leukaemia, associated with hypokalaemia M6—Erythroleukaemia M7—Acute megakaryoblastic leukaemia. Down syndrome associated	L1—small lymphoblastic (20%) L2—large pleomorphic (80%) L3—undifferentiated. Rare. Often associated with massive tumour lysis*

Table 10.4 *Continued*

Feature	Acute non-lymphoblastic leukaemia	Acute lymphoblastic leukaemia
Proportion of acute leukaemias in adults	80–90%[†]	10–20%[†]
Clinical presentation	Symptomatic hyperleucocytosis more common	Bone pain, arthralgia, central nervous system involvement, organomegaly and lymphadenopathy more common
Light microscopy, immuno-peroxidase stains of bone marrow	Large irregular cells. Multiple nucleoli. 50% have Auer rods. Myeloperoxidase positive	Small regular lymphocytes. One prominent nucleolus T cell (20%), B cell (5%) Common acute lymphoblastic leukaemia antigen (50%)
Treatment	Induction, consolidation chemotherapy	Induction, consolidation, cranial irradiation and maintenance
	Any central nervous system signs should be investigated and if due to leukaemia treated with intrathecal chemotherapy	
Role of bone marrow transplantation	Used in first remission with 60% long-term survival	Used in *second* remission with 20–40% long-term survival[‡]
Prognostic factors	Younger patients with leukaemia arising *de novo* do better than if a secondary leukaemia due to pre-existing haematological problems such as myelodysplasia	Best prognosis in females 3–9 yrs old with white cell counts of less than 10×10^9/L. L1 subtype also has a better prognosis

AML = acute myeloid leukaemia. DIC = disseminated intravascular coagulopathy.
[*]Hyperuricaemia, hyperphosphataemia, hyperkalaemia and hypocalcaemia. Treated with hydration, allopurinol, urine alkalinisation and calcium.
[†]Up to 20% of acute leukaemias in adults have cell surface markers of both myeloid and lymphoid cell lines (biphenotypic) which carries a much worse prognosis.
[‡]Bone marrow transplantation and chemotherapy have similar outcome with first remission treatment.

CHRONIC LYMPHOCYTIC LEUKAEMIA (CLL) AND OTHER CHRONIC LYMPHOID HAEMATOLOGICAL DISORDERS

CLASSIFICATION

1. CLL
99% B cell, usually in elderly males. An incidental finding of lymphocytosis (>15000/mL peripherally; >40% bone marrow) is the presentation of 25%; may present with lymphadenopathy, anaemia, Coombs' positive autoimmune haemolysis (10%), bleeding (low platelets), hypogammaglobulinaemia (50%) or monoclonal gammopathy (10%).

Modified Rai classification of staging with median survival

Staging		Median survival
0:	lymphocytosis	10 years
I/II:	0 and lymphadenopathy and/ or hepatosplenomegaly	7 years
III/IV:	I/II and anaemia or thrombocytopenia	1.5 years

Other poor prognostic factors include: doubling of lymphocyte count in less than 12 months; and diffuse bone marrow involvement.

Often associated with hypogammaglobulinaemia.

Treatment
• Chlorambucil ± prednisolone
• Fludarabine (nucleoside analogue derived from cytosine arabinoside).

2. Hairy cell leukaemia
Mononuclear cells with prominent cytoplasmic projections (hairs) are characteristic. Usually occurs in men older than 40 and is associated with splenomegaly, bone marrow infiltration, pancytopenia and infections. Death most frequently from sepsis from atypical organisms (mycobacteria, legionella, nocardia).

Treatment
• Alpha interferon—10% complete response, 90% partial response.
• New agents such as 2' deoxycoformycin (DCF) has a 55% complete response rate.
• 2-chlorodeoxyadenosine (2-CDA) 80% complete response (febrile neutropenia the most common toxicity).

3. Sézary syndrome
Abnormal T cells associated with erythroderma, pruritus and lymphadenopathy.

4. Prolymphocytic leukaemia
80% B cells, usually elderly patients; associated with infections and splenomegaly. It is rare with >55% nucleated cells as prolymphocytes.

Clinically, patients have high white cell counts (>100 000/mL), massive splenomegaly and minimal lymphadenopathy. Very poor prognosis.

5. Large granular lymphoproliferative disorder (T-gamma lymphocytosis syndrome)
Often a benign proliferative disorder. Patients present with splenomegaly, anaemia or neutropenia. More than 30% of patients have rheumatoid arthritis.

CHRONIC MYELOID LEUKAEMIA (CML)

CLINICAL CLUES

1. CML—Philadelphia chromosome diagnostic: splenomegaly (90%), anaemia, bleeding, hepatomegaly (40%), blood film shows increased neutrophils, metamyelocytes, myelocytes and promyelocytes; bone marrow shows less than 20% blasts unless a blast crisis is imminent.
2. Atypical CML—Philadelphia chromosome negative by standard cytogenetics has a poorer prognosis.
3. Chronic myelomonocytic—elderly usually.
4. Chronic neutrophilia—very rare.
5. Eosinophilia—rare.

Leucostasis due to high white cell counts manifest primarily as diffuse interstitial pulmonary infiltrates or neurological deficits.

BLAST CRISIS

After the first year of diagnosis, 20% of patients with CML have an acute blastic transformation per year. Clinical features suggesting transformation to a blast crisis may include:
1. Weight loss
2. New, unexplained fever
3. Rapidly increasing spleen size
4. Cutaneous infiltrates
5. Lytic bone lesions
6. Resistance to previously effective chemotherapy.

Laboratory features suggesting transformation to a blast crisis may include:
1. Progressive anaemia, basophilia or thrombocytosis
2. Thrombocytopenia
3. Hypercalcaemia
4. Progressive myelofibrosis
5. Increasing blasts peripherally and in the bone marrow (>30%)
6. NAP score becomes normal or increased
7. Cytogenic clonal evolution.

Median survival is 2–4 months if transformation is to myeloblastic leukaemia, but 6–12 months with transformation to lymphoblastic leukaemia.

CML: Hydroxyurea is used to control the white cell count. Alpha interferon induces normalisation of cytogenetics in about 25% of patients. Allogeneic bone marrow transplantation is associated with 60% long term disease free survival if done in the chronic phase of disease.

For any of the myeloproliferative conditions, splenectomy can be of benefit in selected patients for severe symptomatic anaemia or thrombocytopenia secondary to hypersplenism.

LYMPHOMA

STAGING OF DISEASE

To determine extent of disease and prognosis.
Given that Hodgkin's disease tends to spread to contiguous nodes, staging is of more importance than for non-Hodgkin's lymphoma, which tends to be more widespread at presentation.

I   Disease confined to a single node region, or a single extralymphatic site (Ie).
II Disease confined to 2 or more lymph node regions on the *same* side of the diaphragm.
III Disease confined to lymph node regions on *both* sides of the diaphragm, with localised involvement of the spleen (IIIs), other extra-lymphatic organ or site (IIIe), or both.
IV Diffuse disease of one or more extralymphatic organs (with or without lymph node disease).

For any stage
A: no symptoms.
B: fever, weight loss (>10% of body weight), and night sweats.
Pruritus may also be an important prognostic indicator.

NON-HODGKIN'S LYMPHOMA (NHL)

There is no ideal single clinicopathological classification for NHL.

Table 10.5   *Classification of non-Hodgkin's lymphoma*

Rappaport	International Working Formulation
Considers architecture of lymph node (low power microscopy) and cytology of cells (high power microscopy)	Combination of current knowledge which incorporates immunohistochemical and cytogenetic observations

I. Favourable prognosis group
  1. Diffuse lymphocytic, well differentiated
	I. Low-grade lymphoma
	
	  1. Small lymphocytic cell

Table 10.5 Continued

Rappaport	International Working Formulation
2. Nodular lymphocytic, poorly differentiated	2. Follicular, mixed cleaved cell
3. Nodular mixed	3. Follicular, mixed small cleaved and large cell
II. Intermediate prognosis group	II. Intermediate grade lymphoma
1. Nodular histiocytic	1. Follicular large cell
2. Diffuse lymphocytic, poorly differentiated	2. Diffuse small cleaved cell
3. Diffuse mixed	3. Diffuse mixed small cleaved cell
4. Diffuse histiocytic	4. Diffuse large cell
III. Unfavourable prognosis group	III. High grade lymphoma
1. Diffuse histiocytic	1. Large cell immunoblastic
2. Lymphoblastic convoluted/non-convoluted	2. Lymphoblastic cell
3. Diffuse undifferentiated	3. Small non-cleaved cell (Burkitt and non-Burkitt)

Clinical clues

Painless lymphadenopathy which is more than 1 cm in size and persists for more than 6 weeks without an obvious infective cause should be investigated. The differential diagnosis should include bacterial, viral and parasitic infections.

Symptoms tend to be associated with where the lymphadenopathy is: e.g. mediastinal lymphadenopathy may lead to a dry cough or stridor.

Treatment

High-grade lymphomas are aggressive with a very poor prognosis if untreated. They are sensitive to cytotoxic chemotherapy.

By contrast, low-grade lymphomas are often indolent and relatively less responsive to chemotherapy.

Bone marrow transplantation is an option in younger patients with otherwise unresponsive disease.

NEUTROPENIA

Mild: 1000–1500 neutrophils/mL
Moderate: 500–1000 neutrophils/mL
Severe: <500 neutrophils/mL

Tolerated better in the chronic state with high cell turnover.

Internal Medicine

- Cyclic neutropenia—intermittent low neutrophil counts for 3–10 days every 21–28 days with oral ulcers, pharyngitis and lymphadenitis during the period with a low count.
- Drugs—cytotoxic agents, chloramphenicol, phenytoin, phenothiazines, but consider any drug as a potential cause.
- Autoimmune disorders—SLE, rheumatoid arthritis (this plus neutropenia and splenomegaly constitutes Felty's syndrome).
- Infections—viral: influenza, hepatitis, HIV; bacterial: typhoid, brucellosis, tuberculosis, rickettsia, staphylococcus.

TREAT

- Withdraw offending drug.
- Treat underlying autoimmune disease.
- Growth factors such as granulocyte macrophage colony stimulating factors (GM-CSF) can shorten the duration of chemotherapy-induced neutropenia.

PLATELETS

OVERPRODUCTION — THROMBOCYTOSIS

Causes of thrombocythaemia
Platelets >400 000

1. Following haemorrhage or surgery
2. Postsplenectomy
3. Iron deficiency
4. Chronic inflammatory diseases (ulcerative colitis, vasculitis, rheumatoid arthritis)
5. Malignancy
6. Chronic infection (tuberculosis, osteomyelitis)

Platelets >800 000

1. Myeloproliferative disease
2. Recent splenectomy or malignancy occasionally

Essential thrombocytosis (a diagnosis of exclusion)

Treatment
Platelet counts should be suppressed if symptomatic—central nervous system thromboembolic disease or digital ischaemia. Thrombocythaemia can be treated with either alpha interferon or hydroxyurea.

UNDERPRODUCTION/DESTRUCTION OF PLATELETS — THROMBOCYTOPENIA

Causes
1. Immune-mediated decreased survival
   a) Immune thrombocytopenic purpura (ITP)—acute (10%) or chronic (90%) in adults.

b) Evan's syndrome—consists of ITP and autoimmune haemolytic anaemia.
c) SLE.
d) Drugs, e.g. quinine, quinidine, thiazides, sulfonamides, methyldopa, heparin, penicillins, gold.
2. Increased consumption/ destruction
   a) DIC, thrombotic thrombocytopenic purpura, haemolytic uraemic syndrome.
   b) Infection, e.g. meningococcal septicaemia.
   c) Mechanical heart valves
   d) Drugs—heparin (more common than a true immune-mediated heparin-induced thrombocytopenia)
3. Decreased production
   a) Pancytopenia due to marrow aplasia, myelofibrosis or marrow infiltration.
   b) Drugs (cytotoxic chemotherapy, alcohol, thiazide diuretics).
   c) Infections.
   d) Toxins.
   e) Megaloblastic anaemia (ineffective thrombopoiesis).
4. Sequestration—hypersplenism, passive congestion in the liver.
5. Dilution (e.g. massive transfusion) or loss (e.g. massive bleeding).
6. Factitious—secondary to autoanalysers not detecting platelet clumps from blood samples collected in EDTA tubes.

Treatment
Consider transfusion of platelets when there is
- no evidence of platelet destruction *and*
- uncontrolled bleeding. The risk of spontaneous bleeding (especially intracranial) increases as the platelet count drops below 20 000/mL.

IMMUNE THROMBOCYTOPENIC PURPURA (ITP)

Autoantibodies directed against platelets (platelet transfusion therefore rarely indicated unless there is active bleeding)

Causes
- Idiopathic
- HIV related
- SLE, other autoimmune disease
- Drugs (see 1(d) above)

Treatment
- Glucocorticoids.
- If recurrent, splenectomy.
- If refractory, immunoglobulins or immunosuppression with cyclophosphamide, azathioprine or vincristine. Danazol sometimes helps in ITP refractory to other treatments.

BLEEDING DISORDERS

Table 10.6 Clinical clues on history

Symptom (clue)	Suggests
Recurrent bleeding from the time of childhood, family history of bleeding problems	Inherited coagulation problem or platelet abnormality
History of deep spontaneous bleeding (haematomas or haemarthroses) or delayed bleeding after trauma	Coagulation factor deficiency
Cutaneous/mucosal bleeding, arterial thrombosis	Platelet or vascular endothelial defect

INVESTIGATING BLEEDING PROBLEMS

- Prothrombin time (PT) (or international normalised ratio (INR)) reflects the extrinsic or tissue factor dependent pathway.
- Activated partial thromboplastin time (APTT) reflects the intrinsic coagulation pathway.
- Thrombin time (TT) reflects rate of conversion of fibrinogen to fibrin.
- Bleeding time—of use only when specifically testing for von Willebrand's disease or qualitative platelet abnormalities.

Causes of 'normal' laboratory studies but clinically significant bleeding
- Dysfibrinogenaemia—prolonged thrombin time.
- Mild clotting factor deficiency.
- Plasminogen activator inhibitor deficiency.
- Factor XIII (fibrin stabilising factor) deficiency (delayed bleeding, impaired wound healing).

QUALITATIVE PLATELET DEFECTS

1. Congenital.

Table 10.7 *Congenital qualitative platelet defects*

Characteristic	Glanzmann's thrombasthenia	Bernard-Soulier syndrome
Inheritance	Autosomal recessive	Autosomal recessive
Mechanisms	Platelet fibrinogen receptor (glycoprotein IIb and IIIa) deficiency	Platelet vWF receptor (glycoprotein Ib) deficiency
Platelets	Normal number and morphology	Decreased number and giant forms
Aggregation with ADP	No	Normal
Aggregation with ristocetin	Yes	No
Bleeding time	Prolonged	Prolonged (markedly)

vWF = von Willebrand factor. ADP = adenosine diphosphate.

2. Acquired
   a) Drugs, e.g. aspirin, NSAIDs.
   b) Myeloproliferative disease.
   c) Chronic renal failure.
   d) Paraproteinaemia.

COAGULATION DISORDERS

Table 10.8 *Haemophilia*

Characteristic	Haemophilia A	Haemophilia B
Deficiency	Factor VIII	Factor IX
Incidence	1:10000	1:40000
Inheritance	X-linked mutations of genes (male disease)	
Clinical presentation	Clinically similar with bleeding including haemarthroses and haematomas	
Treatment	Mild disease—desmopressin Severe disease—factor VIII concentrate*	Factor IX concentrate

*Up to 15% of patients treated with Factor VIII will eventually develop anti factor VIII IgG.

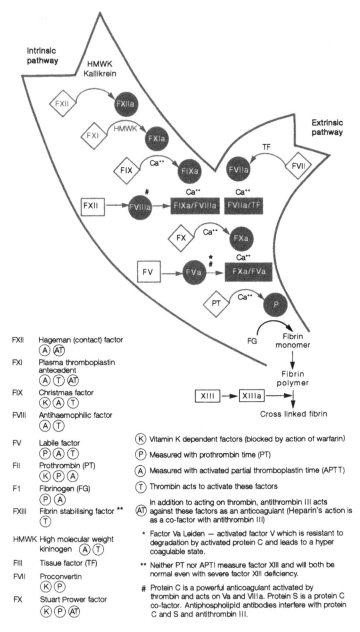

FXII Hageman (contact) factor
       Ⓐ Ⓐ̄ᴛ

FXI   Plasma thromboplastin
       antecedent
       Ⓐ Ⓣ Ⓐ̄ᴛ

FIX   Christmas factor
       Ⓚ Ⓐ Ⓣ

FVIII Antihaemophilic factor
       Ⓐ Ⓣ

FV   Labile factor
       Ⓟ Ⓐ Ⓣ

FII   Prothrombin (PT)
       Ⓚ Ⓟ Ⓐ

F1   Fibrinogen (FG)
       Ⓟ Ⓐ

FXIII Fibrin stabilising factor **
       Ⓣ

HMWK High molecular weight
       kininogen Ⓐ Ⓣ

FIII   Tissue factor (TF)

FVII   Proconvertin
       Ⓚ Ⓟ

FX   Stuart Prower factor
       Ⓚ Ⓟ Ⓐ̄ᴛ

Ⓚ Vitamin K dependent factors (blocked by action of warfarin)

Ⓟ Measured with prothrombin time (PT)

Ⓐ Measured with activated partial thromboplastin time (APTT)

Ⓣ Thrombin acts to activate these factors

Ⓐ̄ᴛ In addition to acting on thrombin, antithrombin III acts against these factors as an anticoagulant (Heparin's action is as a co-factor with antithrombin III)

* Factor Va Leiden — activated factor V which is resistant to degradation by activated protein C and leads to a hyper coagulable state.

** Neither PT nor APTI measure factor XIII and will both be normal even with severe factor XIII deficiency.

Protein C is a powerful anticoagulant activated by thrombin and acts on Va and VIIIa. Protein S is a protein C co-factor. Antiphospholipid antibodies interfere with protein C and S and antithrombin III.

Figure 10.1 *The coagulation cascade.*

270

VON WILLEBRAND'S DISEASE

Up to 1% of the adult population.
von Willebrand factor (vWF) mediates platelet adhesion to the subendothelial matrix.

Table 10.9 von Willebrand's disease

Characteristic	Type I	Type IIa	Type IIb	Type III
Inheritance	Autosomal dominant	Varied	Varied	Autosomal recessive
Clinical presentation	Superficial cutaneous and mucosal bleeding	Mild/moderate bleeding	Mild/moderate bleeding	Severe bleeding
Laboratory findings	Prolonged bleeding time, prolonged aPTT, vWF 20–50% of normal	vWF level normal, ristocetin cofactor very low (unable to form large vWF multimers needed for clot formation)	Normal ristocetin and vWF levels but increased platelet aggregation in response to ristocetin	Absent vWF
Percentage of von Willebrand disease	70%	15%	15%	Very rare
Mechanism	Quantitative deficiency	Qualitative deficiency	Qualitative deficiency	Quantitative deficiency
Treatment	Desmopressin (DDAVP) (releases vWF from storage in endothelial cells), cryoprecipitate		Cryoprecipitate or purified factor VIII (which contains vWF)	

Table 10.10 Haemophilia A contrasted with von Willebrand's disease Type 1

Characteristic	Haemophilia A	von Willebrand's disease (Type I)
Inheritance	Sex linked recessive	Autosomal dominant (incomplete penetrance usually)
Factor VIII coagulant*	Decreased	Decreased
Ristocetin cofactor activity	Normal	Decreased
Bleeding time	Normal	Prolonged
Clinical bleeds	Haemarthroses Haematomas	Epistaxis Mucocutaneous bleeding

Table 10.10 Continued

Characteristic	Haemophilia A	von Willebrand's disease (Type I)
PT (INR)	Normal	Normal
APTT	Prolonged	Prolonged
Therapy	Cryoprecipitate Factor VIII concentrates	Cryoprecipitate DDAVP

*Necessary for coagulation; measured by a clotting assay: <1% severe disease; >10% mild disease.
PT = prothrombin time.
APTT = activated partial thromboplastin time.
DDAVP = 1-desamino-8-D-arginine vasopressin.
INR = international normalised ratio.

Table 10.11 Major blood products available for promoting coagulation

Type	Contents	Indications
Cryoprecipitate	Factor VIII C, vWF; Factor XIII; Fibrinogen	Haemophilia A* von Willebrand's disease Factor XIII deficiency Hypofibrinogenaemia
Cryosupinate	Factors II, VII, IX, X	Correct prothrombin time (viral infection risk)
Fresh frozen plasma	All coagulation factors (fluid phase) and plasma proteins	Use if others not appropriate

*Not first-line therapy.

REPLACEMENT THERAPY FOR HAEMOPHILIA A

Factor VIII

1 unit coagulation factor = amount in 1 mL of plasma.

Total VIII coagulant is 2500 units (i.e. 2.5 L plasma); $t^{1/2}$ VIII is 12 hours.

Therefore, to increase factor VIII by 100%, approximately 2500 units every 12 hours are needed.

1 bag of cryoprecipitate contains 150 units, factor VIII concentrate contains 300 units.

In bleeding episodes, 30% to 50% levels of VIII are needed; before surgery 50% to 60% levels of VIII are required.

Units to be given = (desired factor concentration % minus initial factor concentration %) × plasma volume X weight (kg).

N.B. Plasma volume = 41 mL/kg if the haematocrit is normal.

Add 30% to the calculated dose to account for extravascular distribution.

DISSEMINATED INTRAVASCULAR COAGULATION (DIC)

Laboratory abnormalities in DIC:

1. Increased fibrin degradation products (FDPs), prothrombin time (PT), activated partial thromboplastin time with kaolin (APTT) and thrombin time.
2. Decreased platelets, fibrinogen and factors V and VIII.
3. Mild microangiopathic haemolytic anaemia.
4. Clinically may result in thrombosis or bleeding.

CAUSES (mnemonic HOT MISS)

H—Hepatic: liver failure.
O—Obstetric: amniotic fluid embolus, eclampsia.
T— Trauma or surgery, or tissue necrosis.
M—Malignancy: mucin secreting carcinoma, prostatic carcinoma, acute promyelocytic leukaemia.
I— Immune: anaphylaxis, incompatible blood transfusion.
S— Sepsis.
S— Shock, from any cause.

Trousseau's syndrome—chronic low grade DIC in the setting of cancer.

THROMBOTIC THROMBOCYTOPENIC PURPURA (TTP)

This syndrome, which may rarely follow taking the contraceptive pill or infection, is classically characterised by a pentad:

1. Microangiopathic haemolytic anaemia.
2. Thrombocytopenia (normal coagulation profiles, unlike DIC).
3. Fluctuating neurological symptoms and signs.
4. Renal disease with proteinuria, haematuria and casts.
5. Fever.

Widespread platelet thrombi in small arterioles and capillaries occur secondary to an unknown insult to vascular endothelium.

Plasmapheresis and plasma exchange using fresh frozen plasma is the treatment. If this fails, glucocorticoids can be used. Platelet transfusions are contraindicated because they exacerbate platelet thrombus formation.

HAEMOLYTIC URAEMIC SYNDROME

This condition usually affects children and results in vascular and glomerular lesions like TTP. It is thought to be due to verotoxin-producing enteropathic *Shigella* or *Escherichia coli*.

Treatment options are the same as for TTP.

DISEASES PREDISPOSING TO THROMBOSIS

These account for less than 10% of deep venous thromboses without apparent predisposing factors.

1. Factor V Leiden—a point mutation on factor V which makes activated factor V (Va) relatively resistant to activated protein C.

2. Antithrombin III deficiency.
   a) This may be autosomal dominant or secondary to the contraceptive pill, pregnancy, heparin therapy, or after surgery.
   b) Symptomatic patients need anticoagulation for life.
3. Protein C deficiency.
   a) Autosomal dominant.
   b) In homozygotes, warfarin may induce skin necrosis.
4. Protein S deficiency.
5. Myeloproliferative disorders.
6. Cancer, peripartum, oral contraceptive pill, postoperative, prolonged immobilisation.
7. Tissue plasminogen activator (tPA) deficiency.

Factor V Leiden is responsible for primary and recurrent thromboembolism, including venous thrombosis during pregnancy, with the use of the oral contraceptive pill and in the presence of other anticoagulant abnormalities. It is carried by approximately 4% of Caucasians and is much lower in other population groups. For those with this abnormality, the risk of thromboembolism is 7 times higher than the population in general.

Testing for proteins C and S and for antithrombin III should be done after the acute thrombotic episode has resolved and while the patient is not on anticoagulant therapy. All three are inherited as autosomal dominant traits.

ANTIPHOSPHOLIPID ANTIBODY SYNDROME

See Immunology (page 317)

Table 10.12 *Interactions with warfarin: mechanisms*

Increased sensitivity	Increased resistance
1. Vitamin K deficiency, e.g. malabsorption, antibiotics, clofibrate	1. Increase in Vitamin K
2. Albumin binding displacement, e.g. phenylbutazone, indomethacin, phenytoin, oestrogen, oral hypoglycaemics	2. Reduced drug absorption, e.g. cholestyramine, malabsorption
3. Synergism with warfarin, e.g. anabolic steroids	3. Increased metabolism of warfarin e.g. barbiturates, carbamazepine, rifampicin
4. Blocking warfarin metabolism, e.g. phenytoin, chloramphenicol, cimetidine, tricyclic antidepressants, erythromycin	4. Hereditary warfarin resistance
5. Mechanism unknown, e.g. quinidine, phenothiazines, amiodarone	

MIXED CRYOGLOBULINAEMIA

CLINICAL FEATURES

1. Purpura, cold urticaria, Raynaud's phenomenon.
2. Polyarthralgia.
3. Peripheral neuropathy.
4. Immune complex nephritis.
5. Hepatosplenomegaly, lymphadenopathy.

LABORATORY FINDINGS

Cold precipitins, raised ESR, diffuse hypergammaglobulinaemia, positive rheumatoid factor, no monoclonal band on EPG.

Diagnosis is made by incubating serum at 0–4°C.

MONOCLONAL GAMMOPATHIES

Electrophoretograms (EPG) and immunoelectrophoretograms (IEPG)

B lymphocytes produce immunoglobulins. There are 5 heavy chain isotypes of immunoglobulin (M, G, A, D, E) and 2 light chain variations (kappa and lambda). Electrophoretograms analyse the components of proteins in serum or urine quantitatively, and in monoclonal gammopathies usually have a spike in the gamma region.

Immunoelectrophoretograms confirm the monoclonal nature of such a spike qualitatively by defining the light and heavy chains involved.

MULTIPLE MYELOMA

This is a disseminated disease of plasma cells that typically affects the elderly and is more common in males.

A better prognosis is associated with minimal tumour burden (low level of monoclonal component, normal serum calcium, normal haemoglobin concentration), normal renal function and low levels of $\beta2$ microglobulin and C reactive protein.

CLINICAL FEATURES

1. Anaemia (marrow infiltration or secondary to renal failure).
2. Purpura (marrow infiltration or thrombocytopenia).
3. Infections.
4. Bone tenderness, pathological fractures of osteolytic bone lesions, hypercalcaemia.
5. Skin disease, e.g. hypertrichosis, erythema annulare, yellow skin, secondary amyloid deposits.
6. Renal failure
   a) Acute—due to hypercalcaemia, hyperuricaemia, dehydration, hyperviscosity, contrast studies, nephrotoxic antibodies.
   b) Chronic—due to above causes, nephrotoxic light chains, casts causing tubular obstruction, pyelonephritis, amyloid, plasma cell infiltration.

Internal Medicine

1. EPG of serum and urine, and an IEPG—monoclonal globulin peak is found in 97% of cases.
2. Bone marrow—plasma cells >20%.
3. Bone destruction—lytic lesions, fractures and osteoporosis.

TREATMENT

Anti-tumour effects

Melphalan and prednisolone are still the standard treatment.

There may be a role for alpha interferon in the setting of light chain disease (as evidenced by urinary Bence Jones protein), IgA disease or in the setting of maintenance after induction therapy.

Autologous bone marrow transplantation may be of benefit in young patients with myeloma.

Supportive therapy

- Erythropoietin may improve the anaemia in myeloma.
- Bisphosphonates have demonstrated benefit in reducing bone pain, reducing the number and delaying the onset of fractures and episodes of hypercalcaemia.

DIFFERENTIAL DIAGNOSIS

1. Benign monoclonal gammopathy.
2. Waldenstrom's macroglobulinaemia (monoclonal IgM peak on the EPG, splenomegaly and anaemia, hyperviscosity common, treated with alkylating agents).
3. Localised myeloma (plasmacytoma).

OTHER MONOCLONAL GAMMOPATHIES

Monoclonal gammopathy of undetermined significance (MGUS)

- M component <3 g/dL.
- <5% plasma cells in bone marrow.
- Up to 2% of the population over 50 years of age.
- 17% risk of developing lymphoproliferative disease at 10 years, 33% at 20 years.

POEMS

Acronym for

- **P**olyneuropathy—demyelinating sensorimotor neuropathy.
- **O**rganomegaly—splenomegaly, hepatomegaly and lymphadenopathy.
- **E**ndocrinopathy—amenorrhoea, impotence and gynaecomastia in men, diabetes, hyperprolactinaemia.
- **M**onoclonal gammopathy—osteosclerotic myeloma or IgG or IgA M proteins with lambda light chains.
- **S**kin changes—hyperpigmentation, thickening of the dermis, hyperhydrosis, hirsutism.

AMYLOIDOSIS

Primary
1. Fibrils are composed of monoclonal immunoglobulin light chains (AL protein)

Secondary
2. Chronic inflammatory disease: composed largely of amyloid associated (AA) protein—an acute-phase reactant protein.
3. Heredofamilial amyloid where the proteins are variants of prealbumin (AF protein).
4. Senile cardiac and senile brain (AS protein) derived from variant pre-albumin.

Simplest and most useful diagnostic test: subcutaneous abdominal fat-pad biopsy (sensitivity ~90%). If not diagnostic, biopsy of involved organ or rectal biopsy.
   Presentations include

- nephrotic syndrome.
- congestive cardiac failure (worst prognosis).
- carpal tunnel syndrome.
- malabsorption.
- infiltrative peripheral neuropathy.

   Thrombin time may be prolonged.
   Occasional acquired factor X deficiency.

Table 10.13   Blood transfusion reactions

Transfusion reaction	Clinical features	Management
Fever	Fever, urticaria (white cell antibody sensitisation usually)	Pretreat with antihistamines and/or steroids
Allergy	Fever, urticaria, anaphylaxis (donor plasma protein sensitisation usually)	Use buffy-coat-poor blood Antihistamines and/or steroids Use washed or frozen red cells
Major haemolysis (blood incompatibility)	Shock, fever, back pain, intravascular haemolysis (acute renal failure, DIC)	Stop transfusion (send blood and a fresh sample of patient's blood to laboratory) Hydrate, maintain high urine flow, support blood pressure

Miscellaneous complications: infection (hepatitis B, hepatits C, HIV, syphilis, malaria), circulatory overload, hyperkalaemia, elevated citrate (increasing bleeding), haemosiderosis, air embolus.

Red blood cells do not express HLA antigens, but platelets and white cells do. Leucocyte depletion filters can eliminate febrile reactions to transfusions contaminated with leucocytes. Pruritic reactions are usually due to IgG or IgE allergic response to donor plasma proteins.

With platelet transfusions, the more times a transfusion is given, the more likely there will be alloimmunisation to donor white cells. Patients likely to need recurrent blood product support should therefore be covered with third-generation leucocyte filters when blood is being given.

BONE MARROW TRANSPLANTATION

Two major types
1. Allogeneic—for stem cell abnormalities needing transplantation (e.g chronic myeloid leukaemia), this replaces the patient's stem cells with normal cells from an HLA matched donor.
2. Autologous—where stem cells are intact, the patient's own marrow can be used. For example, the marrow suppressing effect of high-dose chemotherapy can be tolerated with the use of autologous stem cell transplantation.

Table 10.14 *Types of bone marrow transplantation*

Feature	Allogeneic	Autologous
Initial damage	Damaged stem cell lines	Intact stem cell lines
Current age limitations	<55 years of age	Can be used in older patients
Complications	Risk of graft-versus-host disease. Seen in 50% of such transplants	
Matching process	Major histocompatibility loci matching—6 major loci matched. With more than one unmatched locus, the risk of graft-versus-host becomes unacceptable	'Pre-matched'

Early complications (less than 4 months)
- Related to marrow-ablative chemotherapy and radiotherapy conditioning.
- Acute graft-versus-host disease: rash, diarrhoea and abnormal liver function tests. Rates lessened with immunosuppression with methotrexate or cyclosporin.
- CMV infection presenting as pneumonitis: treat with intravenous ganciclovir.

Acute mortality between 5 and 20%.

Late complications (>6 months after transplant)
- Infections: herpes viruses (reactivation of varicella zoster, CMV or herpes simplex), *P. carinii*, encapsulated organisms (patients need reimmunising after bone marrow transplantation).
- Skin: scleroderma like syndrome.

Colony stimulating factors
- Granulocyte-macrophage/granulocyte colony stimulating factors (GMCSF/GCSF)
- Administration of colony stimulating factors can reduce severity and duration of
  - chemotherapy-induced neutropenia
  - idiopathic bone marrow aplasia
  - idiopathic neutropenia
  - cyclic neutropenia.

11

Oncology and Palliative Medicine

Our current understanding of cancer is that the disease is caused by abnormally functioning genes. In the vast majority of cases, genetic damage is acquired rather than inherited. Such damage may take the form of mutation, rearrangement, translocation, deletion or amplification. Genetic damage may arise directly by exposure to certain carcinogens (such as ionising radiation or tobacco). More commonly, changes in DNA arise because of the complexity of the human organism, and the need to replicate and repair DNA constantly throughout life. Thus common epithelial malignancies are diseases of ageing mediated by environmental influences.

DEFINING CHARACTERISTICS OF MALIGNANT CELLS

It is important to remember that cancers arising in different sites may behave in a different manner and may respond to different treatments. Nevertheless, certain generalisations can be made.

Clonality—cancers are derived from a single cell line.

Autonomy—cancers are not responsive to normal physiological control mechanisms in the cell cycle.

Anaplasia—cancer cells differ from normal cells in appearance.

Invasion/metastases—most cancer cells have the ability to grow at sites other than the primary site by direct invasion, or by spread via blood or lymph. Different cancer types have different propensities to metastasise.

Table 11.1 Most common cancers

Male	Female	All
Incidence (in order of occurrence)		
Prostate	Breast	Prostate
Lung	Colon/rectum	Breast
Melanoma*	Melanoma*	Lung
Colon/rectum	Lung	Melanoma*
Lymphomas	CUP*	Colon/rectum

Table 11.1 Continued

Male	Female	All
Deaths (in order of occurrence)		
Lung	Breast	Lung
Prostate	Colon/rectum	Colon/rectum
Colon/rectum	Lung	CUP†
CUP*	CUP*	Breast
Stomach	Pancreas	Prostate

*in Australia. †CUP = cancer with unknown primary.

CANCER WITH UNKNOWN PRIMARY (CUP)

By definition, this is metastatic cancer at presentation where the primary site of cancer is not known after history, physical examination and baseline tests such as full blood count, urea and electrolytes, liver function tests, urine analysis and chest X-ray.

Adequate tissue biopsy is required to exclude treatable metastatic cancers such as lymphoma, breast, prostate and germ cell primaries which can be diagnosed with a combination of histopathology and electron microscopy.

Exhaustively searching for the primary site of disease with scans and endoscopic procedures is unlikely to discover a primary site and will not change the clinical approach to such patients.

Peak incidence is at about 60 years of age, with a slight male preponderance.

Treatment should be symptomatic unless patients are in one of the treatable subgroups.

POTENTIALLY TREATABLE SUBGROUPS OF CUP

Females with isolated axillary lymphadenopathy should be treated as breast cancer, even with a normal mammogram and negative oestrogen/progesterone receptor status on biopsy.

Females with peritoneal carcinomatosis, which often behaves like ovarian cancer, should be offered treatment with platinum-based chemotherapy.

Males with an elevated prostate specific antigen (PSA) and blastic bone lesions should be treated as though they have metastatic prostate cancer.

Squamous cell carcinoma in lymph nodes of the upper $^2/_3$ of the head and neck without an obvious primary should be treated aggressively, as 5-year survival may be as high as 30% in this subgroup.

Males who fit the classification of midline germ cell tumour—age <50 years, mediastinal or retroperitoneal tumours (which may not stain for alphafetoprotein (AFP) or beta-chorionic gonadotrophin (BHCG)) may respond to platinum-based chemotherapy like germ cell tumours, with many longterm survivors. Patients with neuroendocrine histology and CUP may also respond well to platinum-based chemotherapy.

BREAST CANCER

RISK FACTORS

- Long unopposed oestrogen stimulation of breast tissue (early menarche, late menopause).
- Late first pregnancy, nulliparity.
- Hormone replacement therapy/oral contraceptive pill use have a very small increased risk counterbalanced by benefits.
- Family history of breast cancer.

Lifetime risk (with the increasing age of the population) is 1 in 9 of being diagnosed with breast cancer; 1 in 33 lifetime risk of dying from it. Women sometimes have a long interval between initial diagnosis and the diagnosis of metastatic disease.

PATHOLOGY

Ductal cancer tends to be localised and palpable, and accounts for more than 80% of breast cancers.

Infiltrating lobular cancer tends to be multicentric, may be bilateral with impalpable disease, and accounts for 10% of breast cancer histology.

More than 50% of breast cancers are oestrogen receptor positive, and the majority of these will respond to endocrine manipulation.

SCREENING

Finding early breast cancers can change the course of disease as smaller breast cancers are more likely to be curable. Randomised trials demonstrate a reduction in breast cancer related death of 20–30% with the use of screening mammography. The effect appears to be greater in women aged 50–69 than in women aged 40–49 years. There is increasing evidence of the need to screen women in the 40–49 age group.

Table 11.2 *Staging and treatment options for breast cancer*

Stage	Characteristics	Treatment options
Stage 1	<2 cm primary, no lymph node involvement.	Mastectomy or lumpectomy* plus radiation therapy. Consider systemic chemotherapy.
Stage 2	<5 cm primary ± lymph node involvement.	Excision of primary and adjuvant chemotherapy/hormone therapy. Radiotherapy if the breast is preserved. *Axillary clearance.
Stage 3	>5 cm ± chest wall involvement, nodal involvement.	Usually incurable. Local control of tumour is important with either radiotherapy or surgery. Chemotherapy or hormone therapy also used.

Table 11.2 Continued

Stage	Characteristics	Treatment options
Stage 4	Distant metastatic disease	Generally hormone therapy in postmenopausal women; chemotherapy in premenopausal women.

*Axillary clearance is a staging tool, not something which will itself add to cure rates. Radiotherapy improves the rate of local control and should be offered to all women who have breast conserving surgery.

Breast-conserving surgery should be offered to women except in the setting of multifocal breast disease or where the tumour is large (especially in relation to the rest of the breast tissue).

More recent staging advances include the number of capillaries as an index of the likelihood of metastases and amplification of oncogene HER-2/neu.

THERAPEUTICS

ENDOCRINE THERAPY

Ovarian ablation in premenopausal women and tamoxifen in both premenopausal and postmenopausal women have been shown to reduce the risk of relapse and improve overall survival in hormone receptor positive cancers.

Ovarian ablation can be achieved surgically with radiation or with the use of LHRH analogues such as goserelin. Ovarian ablation is effective in both early and advanced disease.

Tamoxifen is effective in both early and advanced disease. It has an antioestrogenic effect in breast cancer tissue, but some pro-oestrogenic effects in other tissues. There is evidence that tamoxifen reduces age-related bone loss, and may reduce the risk of heart disease. It is also associated with an increased risk of endometrial cancer. There is also a very small risk of thromboembolism.

Other endocrine agents used include progestins and aromatase inhibitors. Aromatase inhibitors inhibit the conversion of androstenedione to oestrone in adipose tissue. They are therefore effective in postmenopausal women. Aminoglutethimide is widely used. Newer and more effective agents include anastrozole and letrozole.

Withdrawal of long-term endocrine therapy at times may act as a therapeutic tool in the setting of endocrine-sensitive cancers such as breast cancer.

CHEMOTHERAPY FOR BREAST CANCER

For women with very small (i.e. <1 cm) tumours and no involved nodes, the benefits of chemotherapy are negligible.

Generally, node-positive women should be offered some kind of endocrine therapy if the tumour is endocrine receptor positive. Combination chemotherapy reduces the risk of relapse and improves overall survival in all women with invasive breast cancer.

Active drugs include:

- taxanes, e.g. docetaxel, paclitaxel
- anthracyclines, e.g. doxorubicin, epirubicin
- alkylating agents, e.g. cyclophosphamide
- antimetabolites, e.g. 5-fluorouracil, methotrexate, capecitabine.

Combinations of chemotherapy are more active than single agents. Commonly used combinations include:

- CMF (cyclophosphamide, methotrexate, 5-fluorouracil)
- AC (Adriamycin (doxorubicin), cyclophosphamide).

METASTATIC CANCER

Metastatic disease can sometimes be detected years or even decades after the initial presentation with breast cancer. The most frequent sites of metastatic disease include bone, liver, lung and brain. Measures that can improve quality of life and prolong survival include endocrine therapies and systemic chemotherapy. Radiotherapy is useful for local disease.

PROSTATIC CANCER

This is the most common malignancy diagnosed in males, but most do not die from the cancer. As the primary site of disease is often asymptomatic, metastatic disease is a common presentation. The natural history of prostate cancer is undefined as the rate at autopsies is higher than the clinical incidence, especially in older males.

STAGING

A—incidental finding at transurethral resection.
B—palpable nodule involving one lobe of the prostate (B2 is more diffuse involvement).
C—periprostatic tissue (C2 involves the seminal vesicles).
D—metastatic disease including regional lymph nodes.

THERAPEUTICS

Stage A–C—surgery and/or radical radiotherapy is the treatment of choice.
Stage D—hormone manipulation when symptomatic.

Despite the availability of blood tests for prostate specific antigen (PSA), the overall benefits of screening for prostate cancer have not been proven, hence the management of cancers diagnosed incidentally (by raised PSA or at surgery for prostatic hypertrophy) remains highly controversial. While disease at this stage can be cured with radical surgery, the side effects (urinary incontinence and impotence) are significant and common. In older men (>70 years), a reasonable policy may be to watch, as clinically significant disease may take more than 10 years to develop. In younger men, surgery is often recommended.

Luteinising hormone-releasing hormone (LHRH) agonist—goserelin—by monthly subcutaneous depot injection effectively down-regulates LHRH receptor to cause a chemical castration.

Anti-androgens—flutamide—block androgen receptors on tumour cells and are used ideally in combination with medical or surgical castration ('total androgen blockade'). The timing of total androgen blockade (at the time of diagnosis or when symptoms manifest) remains controversial.

Recent studies have demonstrated some benefit from the use of cyclophosphamide and prednisolone in the setting of advanced prostatic cancer.

Strontium[89] is useful for the treatment of diffuse bone pain from metastatic prostate cancer. A single injection can be given every three months. Side effects include transient cytopenia in about 10% of patients and more severe or prolonged cytopenia in about 1% of patients.

PRINCIPLES OF CHEMOTHERAPY

Chemotherapy is a compromise between toxicity to malignant cells and toxicity to normal cells. Mechanisms of action are broadly categorised but most chemotherapy has more than one mechanism of action.

The interval and dose of chemotherapy are generally defined by the amount of myelosuppression caused. When the bone marrow has recovered, further chemotherapy can be given.

With each dose of chemotherapy, a fixed percentage of cells is killed (log kill) rather than an absolute number of cells.

CELL CYCLE SPECIFIC DRUGS

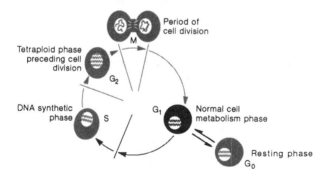

Figure 11.1 *A diagrammatic representation of the events during the cell cycle. M is the period mitosis—approximately one hour from prophase to cell division. G_1 reflects normal cell metabolism prior to DNA synthesis and usually constitutes more than half the total cell generation time. Cells not actively undergoing replication are described as G_0; here they may remain indefinitely or be recruited back into the cycle. The DNA synthetic (S) phase is generally 6 to 24 hours.*

Internal Medicine

S-PHASE SPECIFIC

Cytosine arabinoside
5-Fluorouracil
6-Mercaptopurine
Methotrexate

M-PHASE SPECIFIC

Vinblastine/vincristine

G2-PHASE SPECIFIC

Bleomycin

PREDOMINANTLY CYCLE SPECIFIC AND *NON*-PHASE-DEPENDENT DRUGS

Busulfan
Chlorambucil
Cyclophosphamide

NOT CYCLE SPECIFIC (lethal to non-dividing cells in G_0-phase)

Melphalan
Nitrogen mustard
Daunorubicin/doxorubicin
Cisplatinum
Procarbazine
Nitrosoureas (carmustine (BCNU), lomustine (CCNU))

Table 11.3 Cancer chemotherapy

Drug class and examples	Acute toxicity	Major delayed toxicity	Comment
Alkylating agents			
Cyclophosphamide	Nausea, vomiting, type I hypersensitivity	Bone marrow depression, cardiac arrhythmias and failure, haemorrhagic cystitis, bladder cancer, reversible alopecia, SIADH, pulmonary infiltration.	Activated in the liver. An important part of breast cancer treatment.
Chlorambucil	Minimal nausea	Bone marrow depression, hepatic toxicity, myelodysplasia or leukaemia.	Does not cause alopecia. Useful especially for low grade lymphoma.

Table 11.3 *Continued*

Drug class and examples	Acute toxicity	Major delayed toxicity	Comment
Antimetabolites			
Methotrexate	Minimal nausea, vomiting	Bone marrow depression, mucositis, cirrhosis, acute tubular necrosis (large doses), pulmonary interstitial disease.	Monitor liver enzyme levels. Diuretics, probenecid may interfere with renal excretion. Sulfonamides, phenytoin may displace drug from albumin. The presence of ascites or pleural effusions greatly increases toxicity due to prolongation of exposure—for this folinic acid rescue should be prescribed.
Mercaptopurine (6MP) and azathioprine	Nausea, vomiting, diarrhoea	Bone marrow depression, cholestasis, mucositis, pancreatitis.	Azathioprine converted to 6MP (must decrease dose with allopurinol).
5-Fluorouracil (5FU)	Minimal nausea, diarrhoea	Bone marrow depression, mucositis.	Mainstay of colorectal cancer treatment (adjuvant or advanced).
Cytosine arabinoside	Nausea, vomiting, diarrhoea	Bone marrow depression.	
Antibiotics			
Bleomycin	Minimal nausea and vomiting, fever common.	Pulmonary fibrosis, rash.	Check lung function before beginning therapy. Not myelosuppressive.
Daunorubicin; doxorubicin (Adriamycin)	Nausea, vomiting, red urine	Dose-related cardiomyopathy, bone marrow depression, hyperbilirubinaemia, stomatitis, alopecia.	Cardiac toxicity from sugar moiety—check left ventricular function before therapy.
Epirubicin			Less cardiac toxicity than doxorubicin.

Table 11.3 Continued

Drug class and examples	Acute toxicity	Major delayed toxicity	Comment
Vinca alkaloids			
Vinblastine	Mild nausea and vomiting	Bone marrow depression, SIADH.	
Vincristine	Mild nausea and vomiting	Peripheral and autonomic neuropathy, SIADH.	Not myelosuppressive
Vinorelbine	Mild nausea and pain at injection site	Myelosuppression.	Role in several cancers e.g. breast, lung.
Taxanes			
Paclitaxel	Mild nausea, hypersensitivity reactions	Myelosuppression, peripheral neuropathy.	Taxanes require steroid prophylaxis because of potential hypersensitivity reactions.
Docetaxel	Mild nausea	Myelosuppression.	
Miscellaneous			
Carboplatin	Mild nausea	More myelosuppression than cisplatin.	Minimal renal and neurotoxicity compared to cisplatin.
Cisplatin	Severe nausea, vomiting	Acute tubular necrosis (reversible), ototoxicity (mild), bone marrow depression (mild), neuropathy.	Check creatinine clearance before therapy. Adequate prehydration greatly reduces renal toxicity.
Procarbazine	Nausea, vomiting, Disulfiram-like effect	Bone marrow depression, stomatitis, alters mental state.	Inhibits monoamine oxidase.
Dacarbazine (DTIC)	Severe nausea, vomiting, flu-like syndrome	Bone marrow depression.	Activated in the liver.
Gemcitabine		Fatigue and myelosuppression.	New agent with potential role in pancreatic and non-small cell lung cancer.
L-asparaginase	Nausea, vomiting, fever, anaphylaxis	Decreased clotting factors, abnormal liver function, altered mental state, acute haemorrhagic pancreatitis.	

SIADH = syndrome of inappropriate secretion of antidiuretic hormone.

TOXICITY OF CYTOTOXIC CHEMOTHERAPY

Assume all cytotoxics cause
- nausea and vomiting
- bone marrow suppression
- alopecia

Taxanes and anthracyclines almost invariably cause alopecia. When used as single agents, 5-fluorouracil, vinorelbine and carboplatin cause little hair loss.

CYTOTOXICS THAT ARE RELATIVELY NON-MYELOSUPPRESSIVE

1. Vincristine
2. Bleomycin
3. Cisplatin
4. Streptozotocin

Note that most cytotoxics that are myelosuppressive cause a nadir at 10 to 14 days after treatment, but stem-cell poisons (e.g. busulfan, melphalan, procarbazine) cause severe myelosuppression with a delayed nadir 6 to 8 weeks after therapy.

CYTOTOXICS THAT REQUIRE DOSE REDUCTION IN RENAL DISEASE

1. Increased toxicity systemically occurs with methotrexate, cyclophosphamide, bleomycin and BCNU.
2. Increased renal damage occurs with high-dose methotrexate, cisplatin, carboplatin, mithramycin, BCNU and streptozotocin.

CYTOTOXICS THAT CAUSE PROLONGED AZOOSPERMIA

1. Chlorambucil
2. Cyclophosphamide
3. Cisplatin

CYTOTOXICS THAT CAUSE OVARIAN FAILURE

Most combinations of cytotoxic chemotherapy will induce ovarian failure. Women in their 40s generally don't regain ovarian function.

1. Cyclophosphamide
2. Chlorambucil
3. Nitrogen mustard
4. Mitomycin C
5. Procarbazine

DRUGS WHICH TEND TO INCREASE THE RATE OF SECOND CANCERS

Since part of the mechanism of action of cytotoxic chemotherapy is to damage DNA, there is a small risk of second cancers. Most of these are haematological malignancies.

Table 11.4 *Second cancers after chemotherapy*

Drug	Second cancer	Time interval between treatment of first cancer and appearance of second cancer
Chlorambucil, melphalan cyclophosphamide, busulfan, lomustine	Acute myeloid leukaemia (AML) types M1 and M2	From 2–10 years. 2–5% incidence
Etoposide, teniposide, ?anthracyclines	AML (M4, M5)	2–3 years
Cyclophosphamide	Bladder cancer	Years

SUCCESSFULLY TREATED PRIMARY CANCERS WITH INCREASED RISK OF
SECONDARY CANCERS

- Hodgkin's (AML and solid tumours)
- Non-Hodgkin's lymphoma
- Testicular cancer
- Breast cancer
- Radiation may induce leukaemia (non-lymphocytic), myeloma, breast cancer, small cell lung cancer, sarcoma; low-dose thyroid irradiation may cause thyroid carcinoma.

OTHER DRUGS

Bisphosphonates act to decrease osteoclastic activity. They are of proven benefit in patients with metastatic breast cancer to bone and myeloma patients in reducing the rate of significant bone fractures and increasing time to the onset of bone pain. There is evidence of these drugs improving prognosis independent of their effect on bone in breast cancer.

PRINCIPLES OF RADIOTHERAPY

The main mechanism for cell death as a result of radiotherapy is damage to DNA. Malignant cells are far less able to repair damage, so there is a differential effect sparing normal cells. There may also be a contribution from apoptosis (programmed cell death), release of cytokines and switching on of signal transduction pathways. Although at times cells are not killed with radiotherapy, they may be rendered unable to replicate.

Various sources of radiotherapy are available. These include gamma rays from cobalt 60 decay, photons generated as X-rays or electrons in a linear accelerator and more recently neutrons and protons in a cyclotron. The dose of therapy is measured in Grays (Gy). One Gy equals one joule of energy per kilogram of tissue.

FRACTIONATION

Cells are most sensitive to ionising radiation immediately before mitosis. Multiple exposures to radiotherapy increase the likelihood of finding the cell in this particular part of the cycle. Fractionation also serves to limit the damage to normal tissues.

RADIATION EFFECTS

All normal tissues have a dose beyond which recovery will not occur after exposure to radiation. This defines the maximum dose of radiotherapy.

SHORT TERM

1. Dry and moist desquamation.
2. Epilation.
3. Mucosal damage—gastrointestinal tract, respiratory tract and bladder.
4. Acute organ damage/failure with high-dose radiotherapy involving the lung, brain, kidney and large volumes of bone marrow.

LONG TERM

1. Skin—fragile skin.
2. Second malignancies.
3. Damage to mucosal surfaces (late proctitis or cystitis, dry mouth).
4. Scarring (small volume bladder).

TREATMENT RESPONSIVENESS

ENDOCRINE RESPONSIVE

1. Breast cancer (anti-oestrogen)
2. Endometrial cancer (progesterone)
3. Prostate cancer (androgen blockade)
4. Thyroid cancer (thyroxine which suppresses TSH)
5. Carcinoid (somatostatin)

POTENTIALLY CURABLE FOLLOWING CHEMOTHERAPY

1. Germ cell tumours (mainly testicular cancer)
2. Hodgkin's disease
3. Non-Hodgkin's lymphoma (certain subtypes)
4. Acute leukaemias
5. Wilm's tumour
6. Ewing's sarcoma and rhabdomyosarcoma (embryonal)

TUMOURS VERY SENSITIVE TO CHEMOTHERAPY

1. Small cell lung cancer
2. Non-Hodgkin's lymphoma
3. Ovarian cancer

POTENTIALLY CURABLE FOLLOWING RADIOTHERAPY

1. Seminoma
2. Hodgkin's disease (early stage)
3. Head and neck, or laryngeal cancers (early stage)
4. Cervical carcinoma (early stage)
5. Prostate (early stage)
6. Bladder (early stage)

Note that colorectal carcinoma, pancreatic adenocarcinoma, renal cell carcinoma, melanoma and mesothelioma are relatively resistant to cytotoxics and radiation.

Note also that rarely neuroblastoma, melanoma, Kaposi's sarcoma or renal cell carcinoma can undergo spontaneous regression.

THE NEUTROPENIC PATIENT

Patients undergoing cytotoxic chemotherapy are expected to have a fall in their white cells with most cytotoxic drugs 10–14 days after their administration. (In some patients, this is an important index that the dose of chemotherapy has been sufficient.)

If patients are unwell or febrile with this, it should be assumed they are neutropenic until proven otherwise. This is a medical emergency for, if untreated, overwhelming sepsis can intervene within a very short time.

Patients may have:

- fevers (>38.0°C), chills, rigors
- a flu-like illness
- malaise without fever or signs of sepsis.

The likelihood of sepsis increases with the length of time the absolute neutrophil count is less than 1000.

Patients are at higher risk of bacteraemia/septicaemia if they have evidence of mucosal damage—mouth ulcers or diarrhoea, advancing age or other co-morbidities.

Blood cultures are often negative even in the presence of overwhelming sepsis.

In the febrile neutropenic cancer patient, an empirical antibacterial regimen should be started expeditiously. The regimen should have a broad spectrum of activity (that includes activity against *Pseudomonas aeruginosa*), the ability to achieve high serum bactericidal levels, and be effective in the absence of neutrophils (e.g. aminoglycoside plus an antipseudomonal lactam e.g. Timentin, piperacillin, ceftazidime). If no infection is documented yet fever and neutropenia are still present on Day 7, consider adding an antifungal drug. In the setting of central line access, have a low threshold for considering vancomycin.

TUMOURS METASTATIC TO BONE

Bones most commonly involved (in order of frequency)

1. Vertebrae
2. Proximal femur

3. Pelvis
4. Ribs
5. Sternum
6. Proximal humerus

Tumours that most frequently metastasise to bone

1. Prostate (osteoblastic)
2. Breast (osteolytic and osteoblastic)
3. Lung
4. Thyroid, kidney, bladder
5. Hodgkin's disease (osteoblastic)

OSTEOBLASTIC METASTASES

1. No hypercalciuria
2. Serum calcium normal or decreased
3. Serum alkaline phosphatase greatly elevated

OSTEOLYTIC METASTASES

1. Hypercalciuria
2. Hypercalcaemia
3. Serum alkaline phosphatase normal or elevated

TUMOUR MARKERS IN SERUM

These markers predominantly have a role in following the course of disease. Almost all these markers can also be raised in non-malignant conditions.

1. Carcinoembryonic antigen (CEA)
Causes of an elevated level
- Colonic cancer (higher levels if the tumour is more differentiated or is extensive, or has spread to the liver).
- Lung or breast cancer; seminoma.
- Cigarette smokers.
- Cirrhosis, inflammatory bowel disease, rectal polyps, pancreatitis.
- Advanced age.

CEA is of no value in the preoperative diagnosis of colonic cancer or as a prognostic indicator. CEA is of value in the follow-up of resected colonic cancer; a consistently rising titre suggests metastatic disease and further diagnostic evaluation is indicated.

2. Alpha fetoprotein
Causes of an elevated level
- Hepatocellular cancer—very high titres (>500 ng/mL), or a rising titre are strongly suggestive, but >10% of patients do not have an elevated level.
- Hepatic regeneration including cirrhosis, and alcoholic or viral hepatitis.
- Cancer of the stomach, colon or pancreas, or lung.
- Teratocarcinoma or embryonal cell carcinoma (testis, ovary, extragonadal).

- Pregnancy.
- Ataxia telangiectasia.
- Normal variant.

3. CA-19-9[1]
Causes of an elevated level
- Pancreatic carcinoma (80% with advanced, well-differentiated cancer have an elevated level).
- Other gastrointestinal cancers: colon, stomach, bile duct.
- Other solid tumours e.g. breast.
- Acute or chronic pancreatitis.
- Chronic liver disease.
- Cholestasis (any benign or malignant cause).

4. HCG (human chorionic gonadotrophin)
- Non-seminomatous germ cell tumours (50%), pure seminoma (10%)
- Choriocarcinoma (nearly 100%).
- Solid tumours e.g. lung, colon, stomach, pancreas.

5. Prostate specific antigen
- Prostatic carcinoma.

6. CA 125
- Raised in ovarian cancer or peritoneal inflammation. Not a screening test, but useful to follow disease.

7. CA 15/3
- Raised in a range of solid tumours including breast cancer, but of limited clinical use.

8. Electrophoretogram (EPG) and immunoelectrophoretogram (IEPG)
- B cell malignancy.

SCREENING PROGRAMS

See Chapter 1.

FAMILIAL CANCERS

Cancers seem to be mediated in two distinct ways. The onset of a cancer may require both mechanisms to be activated. Tumour suppressor genes inhibit cell growth and may be related to programmed cell death (apoptosis). Oncogenes can cause malignant transformations by increasing growth factors or growth factor receptors.

One of the most thoroughly characterised cancer genes is the BRCA 1 gene. The familial cluster of cancers includes breast cancer, ovarian cancer and colonic cancer. The likelihood of this being the underlying cause of breast cancer is high in women who are diagnosed under the age of 40 years.

---

[1]Patients who cannot synthesise Lewis blood group antigens (~5% of the population) do not produce CA-19-9 antigen.

Table 11.5 *Frequently occurring familial cancers and their gene defects*

Cancer	Mode of inheritance	Gene implicated
Retinoblastoma	Autosomal dominant	Rb-1
Familial polyposis coli (FPC)	Autosomal dominant	5q21 adenomatous polyposis coli gene (APC) as well as other demonstrated mutations. This appears to be an oncogene.
Li-Fraumeni (sarcomas, breast, bone, brain, lung, laryngeal, leukaemia and adrenal cortex neoplasias in childhood and adults)	Autosomal dominant	p53 mutation (p53 is normally a tumour suppressor gene but is also involved in cell cycle regulation and apoptosis).
Breast cancer		17q21 breast cancer related gene (BRCA 1)

Table 11.6 *Carcinogens*

Occupational exposure	Cancer associated with exposure
Arsenic	Lung, liver, skin
Asbestos	Mesothelioma, lung (especially with smoking)
Benzene	Acute myeloid leukaemia
Chromium	Lung
Nickel	Lung, nasal sinuses
Ionising radiation	Most organ systems
Polycyclic hydrocarbons	Lung, skin
Vinyl chloride	Liver primary
Other exposures	
Tobacco	Lung, mouth, pharynx, larynx, oesophagus, pancreas, kidney, bladder, cervix
Viruses	
Human immunodeficiency virus (HIV)	Non Hodgkin's lymphoma
Human herpes virus 8 (HHV8)	Kaposi's sarcoma
Hepatitis B, hepatitis C	Hepatoma
Epstein-Barr virus (EBV)	Nasopharyngeal carcinoma, Burkitt's lymphoma
Drugs	See Table 11.4

Table 11.7 *Immunocytochemistry stains*

Tumour histology		Component detectable by immunostaining
Lymphoma		Leucocyte common antigen
Carcinoma		Cytokeratin
Specific carcinomas:	prostate	Prostate specific antigen
	follicular thyroid	Thyroglobulin
	medullary thyroid	Calcitonin
	neuroendocrine	Neurone-specific enolase, chromogranin
Germ cell		Beta subunit chorionic gonadotrophin, alpha-fetoprotein
Melanoma		s100, vimentin, HMB 45 antigen
Specific sarcomas:	rhabdomyosarcoma	Desmin
	angiosarcoma	Factor VIII antigen

PARANEOPLASTIC SYNDROMES

1. Anorexia, weight loss, fever
2. Endocrine
   a) Hypercalcaemia secondary to parathyroid hormone-related peptide, especially squamous cell
   b) Hyponatraemia due to the syndrome of inappropriate secretion of anti-diuretic hormone
   c) Ectopic ACTH production in oat cell carcinoma
   d) Carcinoid syndrome from small cell carcinoma
   e) Gynaecomastia due to gonadotrophin production
   f) Hypoglycaemia due to secretion of insulin-like peptide from squamous cell carcinoma or mesothelioma
   g) Hypercalcitoninaemia which is asymptomatic
3. Neuromuscular
   a) Eaton-Lambert syndrome
   b) Peripheral neuropathy
   c) Subacute cerebellar degeneration
   d) Polymyositis
   e) Cortical degeneration
4. Connective tissue and bone
   a) Acanthosis nigricans
   b) Clubbing
   c) Hypertrophic pulmonary osteoarthropathy (not small cell carcinoma or mesothelioma)
   d) Scleroderma (alveolar cell, adenocarcinoma)

5. Haematological
   a) Anaemia
   b) Leukoerythroblastosis
   c) Disseminated intravascular coagulation
   d) Migrating venous thrombophlebitis
6. Nephrotic syndrome due to membranous glomerulonephritis
7. Opportunistic infections

ADVANCED CANCERS

Advanced cancers manifest most of their effects systemically rather than locally where the cancer is growing. Patients with uncontrolled advanced cancer most frequently complain of:

- anorexia
- weight loss/cachexia
- lethargy

Progression of disease is often best monitored in these circumstances with level of function. Scales include Eastern Cooperative Oncology Group (ECOG) and Karnofsky Scale. Worsening functional status is one of the most reproducible measures of prognosis.

These symptoms can be seen in other life-limiting illnesses such as end-stage cardiac failure or advanced AIDS. In all, these changes seem to be mediated by the cytokine cascade. There are no data to support aggressive nutritional support in these circumstances in terms of prolonging survival, improving level of function or improving patient-defined quality of life.

PRINCIPLES OF PALLIATION

Palliation is aimed at maximising quality of life and level of function in the setting of a life-limiting illness. Patients with incurable cancer, end-stage organ failure, neurodegenerative disease and AIDS can all benefit from a palliative approach.

Quality of life is an entirely subjective concept—it will vary from person to person and also from time to time for the same person. A careful history will help elicit the facts needed to best address issues of quality of life.

All the life-limiting illnesses mentioned share similar end-stage physical characteristics of anorexia, weight loss and lethargy.

Facing a life-limiting illness is a time of huge change in a person's life. Clearly addressing the psychosocial, physical, emotional and spiritual issues at such a time can be helpful. An interdisciplinary approach to such issues is most likely to be helpful.

RATIONAL PRESCRIBING OF OPIOIDS

Opioids are safe and effective analgesics in the setting of chronic pain due to cancer. More than 85% of patients with advanced cancer will experience pain at some stage during their disease. Defining and treating the underlying cause of the pain is the best treatment. If the cause cannot be treated, then regular analgesia should be commenced for predictable pain.

Internal Medicine

Opioids available include morphine (oral solution, subcutaneous bolus or infusion, slow or sustained release preparations) and fentanyl (transdermal patch). Codeine and dextropropoxyphene have less predictable metabolism. Methadone has a role, but the half-life increases with duration of use and is therefore unpredictable.

In the setting of chronic malignant pain, regular morphine should be instituted. Between doses a breakthrough dose of one-half the four-hourly dose can be given. The total use over the past 24 hours can usually define the likely needs for the next 24 hours. If not, the dose should be adjusted on a percentage basis. Patients will rarely notice an increment in dose of less than 25%. For immediate release oral morphine solution and subcutaneous bolus doses, the dose should be adjusted to provide four hours of pain relief rather than adjusting the dose interval.

For slow or sustained release preparations, stabilise the patient on an immediate release solution first and then change to the same dose per 24 hours. Continue to use immediate release solution at a dose of $\frac{1}{6}$ to $\frac{1}{12}$ of the total daily dose as breakthrough.

12

Immunology and Allergy

CLASSIFICATION OF IMMUNE-MEDIATED REACTIONS

I ALLERGIC (IgE-MEDIATED)

IgE binds to sensitised cells (e.g. mast cells, eosinophils) releasing vasoactive substances on re-contact with antigen, e.g. anaphylaxis.

II CYTOTOXIC OR TISSUE-SPECIFIC ANTIBODY (IgG OR IgM-mediated)

Antibody reacts with antigen bound to the cell surface, e.g. Goodpasture's syndrome, blood transfusion reactions, post-streptococcal glomerulonephritis.

III CIRCULATING IMMUNE COMPLEXES (ARTHUS REACTION)

Free antigen and antibody combine and precipitate with complement fixation, e.g. SLE, serum sickness.

IV DELAYED HYPERSENSITIVITY (CELL MEDIATED)

Sensitised lymphocytes react with deposited antigen releasing lymphokines and monokines, e.g. tuberculosis, rheumatoid arthritis, Wegener's granulomatosis.

V ANTI-RECEPTOR ANTIBODIES

e.g. Graves' disease, myasthenia gravis.

HUMAN LEUCOCYTE ANTIGEN (HLA) SYSTEM

- Is controlled by several gene loci on the short arm of chromosome 6.
- The antigens these genes encode are transmembrane glycoproteins.
- There are 3 classes of genes:

Class I genes comprise HLA-A, HLA-B and HLA-C genes, and encode Class I antigens which are expressed on all nucleated cells, platelets, and some erythrocytes. They are not found on spermatozoa or placental trophoblasts.

Class II genes comprise HLA-DP, HLA-DQ and HLA-DR, which encode Class II antigens which are expressed on B lymphocytes, activated T lymphocytes, monocytes and epidermal cells.

Class III genes encode for some complement components and tumour necrosis factor.

HLA inheritance—a child has a 50% chance of inheriting HLA A or B from one parent, while siblings have a 25% chance of being identical for all four HLA A and B alleles.

COMPLEMENT SYSTEM

The complement system is designed to provide effector functions for humoral immunity; for example, as the final step in the elimination of bacteria.

──────────────────────────────────▶

Figure 12.1 *Components of the complement system.*
Overview of complement activation pathways. *The classical pathway is initiated by C1 binding to antigen-antibody complexes, and the alternative pathway is initiated by C3b binding to various activating surfaces, such as microbial cell walls. The C3b involved in alternative pathway initiation may be generated in several ways, including spontaneously, by the classical pathway, or by the alternative pathway itself (see text). Both pathways converge and lead to the formation of the membrane attack complex. In this and subsequent figures, bars over the letter designations of complement components indicate enzymatically active forms and dashed lines indicate proteolytic activities of various components.*
From Abbas et al. Cellular and molecular immunology. Philadelphia: WB Saunders, 1994. Reproduced with permission.

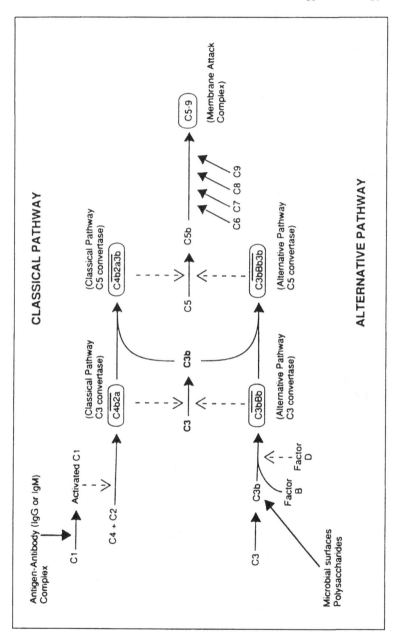

CLASSICAL PATHWAY

Antigen-Antibody (IgG or IgM) Complex

C1 → Activated C1

C4 + C2 → C4b2a (Classical Pathway C3 convertase)

C3 → C4b2a3b (Classical Pathway C5 convertase)

C3b

C5 → C5b

C6 C7 C8 C9 → C5-9 (Membrane Attack Complex)

ALTERNATIVE PATHWAY

C3 → C3b

Factor B, Factor D

C3bBb (Alternative Pathway C3 convertase)

C3bBb3b (Alternative Pathway C5 convertase)

Microbial surfaces Polysaccharides

ALLERGIC DISEASE

ANAPHYLAXIS

CLINICAL FEATURES

- Rash—erythema or urticaria
- Angio-oedema, especially face, oral cavity and upper airway
- Bronchospasm
- Abdominal pain, diarrhoea, vomiting
- Cardiovascular—hypotension, arrhythmia, shock

PATHOPHYSIOLOGY

- IgE (anaphylactic) or non-IgE (anaphylactoid) dependent mast cell degranulation
- Massive release of preformed vasoactive mediators
  histamine
  tryptase
  chymase
- Rapid production of multiple other substances
  leukotrienes
  prostaglandins
  cytokines

CAUSES

- Insect venom (bee, wasp)
- Drugs (Table 12.1)
- Food (Table 12.2)
- Exercise
- Idiopathic

MANAGEMENT

- Identify cause and avoid if possible
- Specific immunotherapy for insect venom allergy
- Prophylactic antihistamines, e.g. cetirizine, for exercise-induced anaphylaxis
- Adrenaline self-injection

ALLERGIC RHINITIS AND NASAL POLYPS

CLINICAL FEATURES

- Rhinorrhoea, nasal blockage, postnasal drip, excessive sneezing, nasal itch
- Loss of smell and taste
- Nasal polyps complicate rhinitis in 2% of cases

- Allergic conjunctivitis frequently associated
- Nasal polyps are more common in young males with asthma, aspirin intolerance and sinusitis

PATHOPHYSIOLOGY

- IgE antibodies bound to mast cells are cross-linked by allergen, leading to the degranulation of mast cells
- Mast cell mediators are chemotactic, especially for eosinophils, which release further vasoactive and toxic mediators
- The response is regulated by T cells of the TH2 (T helper type 2) subtype

CAUSES

- Seasonal allergens: grass, tree, weed pollens
- Perennial allergens: animal danders including house dust mite, cat, moulds (may be seasonal in temperate climates)

MANAGEMENT

- Identify offending allergens by skin prick testing or RAST
- Avoid offending allergens where possible
- Intranasal corticosteroid sprays
- Oral antihistamines
- Specific immunotherapy in selected cases

DRUG ALLERGY

Table 12.1 Types of abnormal immune responses to drugs

Reaction	Drugs commonly responsible
Type I anaphylaxis	Beta-lactam antibiotics
Anaphylactoid	Aspirin, NSAIDs, radio-contrast media
Type II (rare) (antibody-dependent)	Penicillin-induced haemolytic anaemia
Type III (immune complex-mediated, serum sickness reaction)	Antibiotics, propylthiouracil
Type IV (delayed-type)	Topical preparations

MANAGEMENT

- Avoidance is desirable in all cases of known drug allergy
- Rapid desensitisation is possible in a hospital setting when a drug is urgently needed and there is no viable alternative

FOOD ALLERGY AND INTOLERANCE

Table 12.2 Food allergy and food intolerance

Food allergy	Food intolerance
IgE-mediated	Non-immunological mechanisms, e.g. enzymatic deficiency pharmacological effect of food toxic effect of food
Skin prick or RAST positive	Skin prick or RAST negative
Common foods implicated	Common foods implicated
Children cow's milk, egg, peanut, fish	artificial flavourings artificial colourings
Adults fish other seafood peanut nuts	dairy products preservatives wheat amines (e.g. in cheese, chocolate) salicylates (e.g. in tea, coffee, fruit)

MANAGEMENT

A diet which eliminates the majority of food chemicals and additives (elimination diet) followed by carefully controlled food challenges may be needed to identify food intolerance.

The *only* treatment for true food allergy is strict avoidance.

URTICARIA AND ANGIO-OEDEMA

CLINICAL FEATURES

- Urticarial lesions are raised, pruritic, erythematous wheals, ranging in size from several millimetres to centimetres in diameter.
- Angio-oedema is a subcutaneous or submucosal oedema, generally manifesting as non-pruritic swelling. Common sites include the lips, palms, soles, oral cavity, larynx, genitals and periorbital tissues.
- Acute urticaria is defined as being of less than six weeks' duration. Longer than this is arbitrarily defined as chronic.
- Angio-oedema and urticaria frequently occur concurrently.

PATHOPHYSIOLOGY

- Mast cell degranulation is the final common pathway, with release of preformed vasoactive mediators causing increased vascular permeability.
- Tissue fluid thus accumulates, causing local irritation and resultant itch.
- Mast cell mediators are also chemotactic for eosinophils, which release further inflammatory mediators.
- In the chronic form, an increasing infiltration of T lymphocytes is observed in affected tissues.

Table 12.3 *Causes of urticaria and angio-oedema*

Immunological	Non-immunological
Type I (IgE-mediated)	**Physical**
Foods, e.g. peanuts	Heat
Drugs, e.g. penicillin	Cold
Insect venom, e.g. bees	Pressure
Contact allergens, e.g. grass	Vibration
	Sunlight
	Exercise
Type III (Immune-complex-mediated)	**Pharmacological**
Autoimmune disease, e.g. SLE	Aspirin/NSAIDS
Neoplasm, e.g. lymphoma	Radio-contrast media
Viral disease common in children	Foods, e.g. preservatives

- In pure angio-oedema without urticaria, consider deficiency of C1-esterase inhibitor.
- The hereditary form (autosomal dominant) presents in infancy or early childhood, often with a positive family history.
- The acquired form is associated with malignancy, especially plasma cell dyscrasias and lymphoma, and autoimmune disease, e.g. SLE.
- C4 complement levels are reduced, indicating the need for the specific assay.

MANAGEMENT

- Where possible, identify the cause of the problem and avoid. An elimination diet and food challenging may be required.
- Oral antihistamines are the mainstay of therapy, e.g. loratadine, cetirizine.
- H2 receptor antagonists, e.g. famotidine, in combination with antihistamines, may improve success rates.
- Oral beta2-agonists, e.g. terbutaline, can be added in resistant cases.
- Corticosteroids should only be used for severe cases, and only in short courses.
- For C1-esterase inhibitor deficiency, concentrates of donor C1-esterase inhibitor can be administered for acute severe angio-oedema.

EOSINOPHILIC SYNDROMES

Eosinophilia is defined as an absolute count of >500 eosinophils per microlitre of peripheral blood.

CAUSES

- Hypereosinophilic syndrome. This is characterised by endomyocardial fibrosis, mitral and aortic valve regurgitation, thrombosis, and infiltration of multiple organs by eosinophils. Eosinophil count is >1500 for at least 6 months in the absence of other causes. Treatment is with prednisolone or hydroxyurea.

- Parasitic infections, e.g. hookworm, schistosomiasis, filariasis.
- Atopic disorders—asthma, allergic rhinitis, atopic dermatitis.
- Eosinophilic pneumonias.
- Episodic angio-oedema and eosinophilia.
- Drugs, e.g. antibiotics (penicillin, ampicillin, sulfonamides), naproxen, bleomycin, chlorpromazine, aspirin.
- Churg-Strauss syndrome.
- Dermatitis herpetiformis.
- Asthma.
- Allergic bronchopulmonary aspergillosis.
- Tropical pulmonary eosinophilia.
- Hodgkin's disease.
- Rheumatoid arthritis.
- Job's syndrome (Table 12.8).
- Mycosis fungoides.
- Eosinophilic fasciitis. This is characterised by inflammation of the dermis, subcutaneous tissues and deep fascia. It frequently follows exercise. Along with peripheral eosinophilia there will be a raised ESR and hyper-gammaglobulinaemia. Diagnosis is with deep fascial biopsy.
- Chronic granulomatous disease
- Eosinophilic gastroenteritis.

IMMUNODEFICIENCY

HIV INFECTION AND THE ACQUIRED IMMUNODEFICIENCY SYNDROME (AIDS)

HIV INFECTION

CLINICAL FEATURES

A. Primary infection
Results in an acute seroconversion illness in more than 50% of cases, up to 6 weeks after exposure.

Seroconversion illness
Fever
Maculopapular rash
Arthralgia/myalgia
Pharyngitis
Generalised lymphadenopathy
Headache
Meningoencephalitis
Oral candidiasis
Diarrhoea

B. Asymptomatic infection
May last from months to many years.

Progressive immunological decline may cause no symptoms until immunodeficiency is severe.

Generalised lymphadenopathy may persist throughout this time.

C. Complications suggestive of moderate immunodeficiency or immune dysregulation

Infective	*Autoimmune*
Herpes zoster	Immune thrombocytopenic purpura
Oropharyngeal candidiasis	Bell's palsy
Oral hairy leucoplakia	Polymyositis
Recurrent/persistent herpes	Sjögren's syndrome
simplex	Guillain-Barré syndrome
	Lymphocytic interstitial pneumonitis

D. Complications suggestive of severe immunodeficiency
AIDS-defining illnesses

Infections	*Malignancy*
Oesophageal candidiasis	Kaposi's sarcoma
Pneumocystis carinii pneumonia	Cerebral lymphoma
Cerebral toxoplasmosis	Burkitt's lymphoma
Cytomegalovirus retinitis	Immunoblastic lymphoma
Cytomegalovirus disease elsewhere	Cervical cancer
Cryptosporidiosis	
Mycobacterium avium complex infection	*Other*
Mycobacterium tuberculosis	HIV wasting syndrome
Cryptococcal meningitis	Progressive multifocal
Coccidioidomycosis	leucoencephalopathy
Histoplasmosis	HIV dementia

PATHOPHYSIOLOGY

- Human immunodeficiency virus is a retrovirus. There are two types which cause a similar clinical illness, HIV-1 and HIV-2.
- The principal cell ligand is the CD4+ molecule, found on CD4+ T lymphocytes, monocytes, macrophages, dendritic cells, Langerhans cells and thymocytes.
- To gain entry into these cells, a co-receptor is required. For CD4+ lymphocytes, this is a surface protein called fusin. For macrophages, a receptor called cc CKr5 is needed.
- Some CD4- cells can also be infected by HIV, e.g. neuronal and endothelial cells.
- Primary infection is associated with a high plasma viral load. Host defence mechanisms involving both the humoral and cellular arms of the immune system then cause a dramatic reduction in the plasma viral load in the majority of cases and for a prolonged period.

- While the plasma viral load may remain low for many years, HIV gradually accumulates in tissue, especially lymphoid tissue.
- Failure of the immune system to control viral replication may be the result of progressive emergence of mutant viral epitopes which prove increasingly more difficult to control.
- The immune deficiency which results in the clinical consequences of HIV infection is complex, involving both a reduction in number and a loss of normal function of CD4+ T cells, a loss of CD8+ T lymphocytes in the advanced stage of disease (after having been an important component in control of viral replication up to that point), reduction in functional ability of monocyte-macrophages, and ineffective B cell responses to foreign antigens.

Transmission of HIV
- Sexual—especially receptive anal or vaginal intercourse, and in association with other sexually transmitted infections.
- Transfusion of blood or blood products.
- Maternal-fetal transmission, either *in utero* or through breast milk; artificial insemination.
- Injecting drug use through use of shared needles.
- Organ transplantation.
- Occupational exposure, e.g. needle stick injury.

DIAGNOSIS
- Depends on demonstration of antibody to HIV-1 or HIV-2. IgG is the most reliable, as IgM is only detectable for a short time after the primary infection.
- IgG can be detected by ELISA (enzyme-linked immunosorbent assay) or immunoblotting techniques.
- Detection of HIV RNA by polymerase chain reaction is sensitive, and becomes positive before the antibody tests.

Surrogate markers
- CD4+ cell count gradually declines in the majority of cases over time. Counts of <500 cells per microlitre correlate with moderate immunodeficiency. Counts of <200 indicate severe immunodeficiency and a high risk of development of AIDS.
- p24 antigen is a protein which makes up the bulk of the core of the virus. It is frequently detectable in the serum at the time of primary infection, and later in the disease in the presence of a high viral load.
- Skin testing for delayed-type hypersensitivity tends to remain normal until the development of moderate to severe immunodeficiency.
- Increasing levels of beta2-microglobulin and neopterin reflect increasing cell turnover, therefore disease progression.
- Quantitation of HIV RNA levels in plasma is now the most sensitive indicator of disease activity, and the most reliable prognostic indicator.

- High or increasing plasma viral load.
- Low or falling CD4+ lymphocyte count.
- Increasing serum beta2-microglobulin, neopterin, p24 antigen.
- Persistent weight loss.

Table 12.4 *Infective complications of HIV infection*

Condition	Clinical features	Treatment
P. carinii pneumonia	Dry cough Dyspnoea Fever Inspiratory crackles	High-dose oral or IV co-trimoxazole IV pentamidine Prednisolone 1 mg/kg/day for 3 weeks if hypoxaemic (PaO_2 <70 mmHg)
Cryptococcal meningitis	Headache Fever Meningism Clouding of consciousness	IV amphotericin-B in the acute phase Fluconazole indefinitely
Cerebral toxoplasmosis	Seizures Focal neurological deficits Fever Clouding of consciousness	Pyrimethamine plus sulfadiazine or clindamycin
Cytomegalovirus retinitis	Asymptomatic or loss of vision	IV ganciclovir or foscarnet
Mycobacterium avium complex infection	Weight loss Fever Malaise Symptoms related to pancytopenia Diarrhoea	Combination anti-tuberculous chemotherapy. Drugs include azithromycin, clarithromycin, clofazimine, rifabutin, ciprofloxacin
Cryptosporidiosis	Intractable diarrhoea Abdominal pain Weight loss	Problematic: anti-diarrhoeals, paromomycin, azithromycin
Oral and oesophageal candidiasis	Asymptomatic or sore throat, odynophagia, dysphagia	Fluconazole Itraconazole Amphotericin-B in very severe cases

Table 12.5 *Non-infective complications of HIV infection*

Condition	Clinical features	Treatment
Kaposi's sarcoma (due to co-infection with Kaposi's sarcoma associated herpes virus)	Cutaneous, mucosal, or organ-based darkly pigmented, non-tender nodules	Radiotherapy Chemotherapy with vinblastine, adriamycin, bleomycin Interferon-alpha
Non-Hodgkin's lymphoma	May be enlarged lymph nodes, or organ-based	Radiotherapy Combination chemotherapy (CHOP)
HIV dementia	Cognitive disturbance Motor dysfunction (e.g. unsteady gait) Behavioural change (apathy, withdrawal)	Anti-retroviral drugs, especially high-dose zidovudine
Progressive multifocal leucoencephalopathy (due to co-infection with Creutzfeldt-Jakob virus)	Progressive focal neurological deficit(s)	Nil proven
Peripheral neuropathy	Predominantly sensory symptoms	Symptomatic, e.g. tricyclic antidepressants
Immune thrombocytopenic purpura	Bruising, bleeding	Anti-retroviral drugs, especially zidovudine Corticosteroids IV immunoglobulin Splenectomy

CHOP = cyclophosphamide, adriamycin, vincristine and prednisone.

TREATMENT

INDICATIONS FOR COMMENCING ANTI-RETROVIRAL DRUGS IN HIV INFECTION

- Clinical disease progression
- Symptomatic disease
- Increasing HIV viral load
- Stable viral load of moderate to high level
- Pregnancy
- Post-occupational exposure

Anti-retroviral drugs should be used in combination, to prevent or retard the emergence of resistant viral strains.

Table 12.6 Drugs used for HIV infection (anti-retroviral agents)

Class	Examples	Side effects
Nucleoside reverse transcriptase inhibitors	Zidovudine (AZT)	Headache, nausea, myositis, macrocytosis, bone marrow suppression
	Didanosine (DDi)	Nausea, vomiting, pancreatitis, painful peripheral neuropathy
	Zalcitabine (DDc)	Mucositis, painful peripheral neuropathy, pancreatitis
	Stavudine (d4T)	Painful peripheral neuropathy, liver function test abnormalities
	Lamivudine (3TC)	Rare: headache, nausea, diarrhoea
Non-nucleoside reverse transcriptase inhibitors	Nevirapine	Rash, Stevens-Johnson syndrome
Protease inhibitors	Nelfinavir	Diarrhoea, lipodystrophy, glucose intolerance
	Saquinavir	As for nelfinavir; poor absorption
	Indinavir	As for nelfinavir; renal calculi

CONGENITAL IMMUNODEFICIENCIES

Table 12.7 Clinical clues to congenital immunodeficiencies

Type of infection	Likely immune defect	Examples
Recurrent bacterial respiratory tract infections (otitis media, sinusitis, bronchitis)	Antibody deficiency	Selective IgA deficiency Agammaglobulinaemic syndromes Common variable immunodeficiency
Bronchiectasis	As above	As above
Infection due to encapsulated organisms, e.g. pneumococcus, meningococcus	Complement deficiencies Asplenia IgG2 deficiency	C5,6,7,8,9 deficiency Post-splenectomy IgG sub-class deficiency
Recurrent fungal or viral infection, e.g. persistent oropharyngeal candidiasis, invasive aspergillosis	A. T cell dysfunction or reduction B. Phagocyte deficiency	Severe combined immunodeficiency (SCID) Di-George syndrome Chronic granulomatous disease
P. carinii pneumonia	Antibody deficiencies T cell dysfunction or reduction	Hyper IgM syndrome SCID
Chronic diarrhoea, e.g. due to Giardia lamblia	Antibody deficiencies, or T cell dysfunction or reduction	

Table 12.8 Pathophysiology of congenital immunodeficiencies

Condition	Defect	Comment
Congenital antibody deficiency syndromes		
Selective IgA deficiency	No single defect	Most common congenital immunodeficiency: approx. 1 : 700
		May be asymptomatic
		Prone to anaphylaxis with transfusion—avoid unwashed erythrocytes and immune serum globulin (form IgE or IgG anti-IgA antibodies)
Common variable immunodeficiency	Not known	Recurrent respiratory tract infections
	Levels of IgG and IgA low	Presents in childhood or teenage years
	T cells usually normal	Increased incidence of lymphoma and autoimmune disease
X-linked agammaglobulinaemia	Defect in *Btk* gene	Recurrent respiratory infection
	Pre-B cells fail to mature	Absent lymphoid tissue
	Very low IgG, IgA, IgM	
Hyper IgM syndrome	Defect in gene encoding for CD40 ligand	Rare
	Activated T cells fail to provide B cell help	Recurrent bacterial *and* opportunistic infection
	Very low IgG and IgA; IgM elevated	
Primary T cell deficiencies		
Severe combined immunodeficiencies (SCID):		
a) X-linked	Gene defect in IL-2 receptor gamma chain	All SCID patients present in infancy with infection and growth failure
	Low T cells	Infection may be bacterial, viral, or fungal
	Elevated B cells	
	Low immunoglobulins	
b) Adenosine deaminase (ADA) deficiency	Defect in ADA gene	
	Absent T and B cells, and immunoglobulins	
c) MHC class II deficiency	Gene defect in proteins which regulate the expression of class II genes	

Table 12.8 Continued

Condition	Defect	Comment
d) Other	ZAP 70 defects Recombination activating gene defects	
Di-George syndrome	Abnormality of chromosome 22q11 Low B and T cells and immunoglobulins	Recurrent infection Congenital heart defects Hypoparathyroidism Unusual facies
Ataxia telangiectasia	Mutation in ATM gene, causing DNA fragility Reduced IgA, IgE, IgG2	Cerebellar ataxia Oculocutaneous telangiectasia Malignancies
X-linked lymphoproliferative syndrome	Infection with Epstein-Barr virus results in progressive disease	Abnormalities include hepatic failure and hypogammaglobulinaemia
Wiskott-Aldrich syndrome	Abnormal WASP gene, causing CD43 abnormalities Elevated IgE, reduced IgG, IgM, T cell abnormalities	Thrombocytopenia, eczema and recurrent infection
Phagocyte deficiencies		
Chronic granulomatous disease (usually X-linked)	Phagocytes unable to produce superoxide normally	Abnormal nitro blue tetrazolium dye reduction test Recurrent bacterial and fungal infection
Leucocyte adhesion deficiency	Defects in adhesion molecules	Rare. Autosomal recessive
Myeloperoxidase deficiency	Phagocytes have giant lysosomal granules, and impaired microbicidal activity	Recurrent pyogenic infections; nystagmus, peripheral neuropathy; partial oculocutaneous albinism
Job's syndrome	Abnormal neutrophil and monocyte chemotaxis	'Cold' cutaneous abscesses Raised serum IgE
Complement deficiencies		
C1, C2, C4		Associated with autoimmune diseases, especially SLE
C5-8		*Neisseria* infection

MULTISYSTEM AUTOIMMUNE DISEASE

Table 12.9 Antibodies associated with multisystem autoimmune disease

Disease	Associated antibodies
Systemic lupus erythematosus (SLE)	Anti-single-stranded DNA (not specific) Anti-double-stranded DNA (50–60%) Anti-Smith (sm: 30%) Anti-ribonucleoprotein (RNP: 30% in low titre) Anti-SS-A (30%) Anti-SS-B (15%) Anti-histone (drug-induced SLE: 95%)
Scleroderma and CREST	Anti-centromere (CREST: 70%; scleroderma 10%) Anti-nucleolar, Anti Scl-70 (scleroderma 40%) Anti-RNP, Anti-SS-A (scleroderma occasionally in low titre)
Sjögren's syndrome	Anti-SS-A (70%), Anti-SS-B (60%)
Mixed connective tissue disease (MCTD)	Anti-RNP (100%), Anti-SS-A (occasionally in low titre)
Polymyositis	Anti-PM1 (polymyositis: 50%; dermatomyositis: 10%)

Table 12.10 Antinuclear antibodies

Fluorescent pattern	Antigen	Important associated diseases
Rim	Double-stranded DNA	SLE
Homogeneous	Histone	SLE
Speckled	Extractable nuclear antigen	Sjögren's syndrome, MCTD, SLE, scleroderma
Nucleolar	RNA	Scleroderma

SYSTEMIC LUPUS ERYTHEMATOSUS (SLE)

CLINICAL FEATURES

- Incidence approximately 1:1000
- Female to male ratio 9 to 1
- Peak incidence 20 to 40 year age group
- More prevalent in African-American and Asian people

Table 12.11 Clinical features of SLE

Symptom or sign	Comment
Fatigue	Almost universal, non-specific
Skin and mucous membranes	Common
	Multiple types of rash:
	Butterfly rash
	Photosensitive eruption
	Generalised maculopapular
	Cutaneous vasculitis
	Livedo reticularis
	Mouth ulceration, sicca complex
Arthralgia	Very common
	Usually fingers, wrists, knees
Arthritis	Usually a non-deforming polyarthritis, but many possible variants
Myalgia	Frequent
Renal disease:	Multiple forms of glomerulonephritis
Proteinuria	may occur, with a wide range of
Haematuria	clinical manifestations
Nephrotic syndrome	
Hypertension	
Neurological disease:	Often non-specific
Headache	May be fulminant in severe form
Anxiety	Screen for concurrent
Depression	anti-phospholipid syndrome
Seizures	
Strokes	
Mononeuritis multiplex	
Cardiovascular:	
Pericarditis	
Non-infective endocarditis	
Raynaud's phenomenon	
Respiratory	
Pleuritis	
Interstitial pneumonitis	
Secondary anti-phospholipid syndrome	May occur in up to 50% of cases
Recurrent miscarriage	
Venous and arterial thrombosis	
Haematological:	
Thrombocytopenia	
Haemolytic anaemia	
Recurrent infection	Especially urinary tract
	Due to multiple immunological abnormalities

PATHOPHYSIOLOGY

- Genetic factors important: more common in HLA-B8 DR3/DR4 haplotypes.
- High concordance (approximately 50%) in monozygotic twins.
- Abnormalities in T cell number and function, with reduced suppressor cell activity, and consequent reduction in B cell control.
- Increase in number and activity of B cells, including autoreactive B cells.
- Reduced number and function of natural killer cells.
- High levels of circulating immune complexes, and decreased clearance by reticuloendothelial system.
- Abnormal cytokine profiles.

Table 12.12 *Autoantibodies in SLE*

Autoantibody	Significance
Antinuclear antibody:	Present in ~95% of cases, but not specific.
	Titre important, with high titres (>1:640) more specific
Homogeneous pattern	More specific pattern for SLE
Speckled pattern	Check for extractable nuclear antigens
Anti double-stranded DNA antibodies	More than 95% specific for SLE
	Associated with renal and neurological disease especially
	Useful guide to disease activity
Extractable nuclear antigens (ENA):	
Anti-Smith (sm)	Insensitive, highly specific
Anti-SSA (Ro)	Also found in Sjögren's syndrome, neonatal lupus, and pathogenic in congenital heart block
Anti-SSB (La)	Never found without SSA
	Non-specific
Anti-RNP	~50% sensitive, but found in mixed connective tissue disease and overlap syndromes

RENAL DISEASE IN SLE

- A wide range of renal abnormalities occur in SLE, predominantly glomerular.
- Approximately 30% of all lupus patients have significant renal disease.
- Glomerular pathology: class 1 (normal except for occasional mesangial deposits); class 2 (mesangial lupus nephritis); class 3 (focal segmental proliferative lupus nephritis—<50% glomeruli affected); class 4 (diffuse

proliferative lupus nephritis); class 5 (membranous lupus nephritis); class 6 (end stage).

- Diffuse proliferative disease carries an inevitable risk of chronic renal failure without heavy immunosuppressive therapy, and chronic dialysis is often required despite treatment.
- High titres of anti-ds DNA are associated with the more severe forms of renal disease.
- Pregnancy is a risk factor for an exacerbation of renal lupus, and should be delayed until the disease has been quiescent for approximately 6 months.

DRUG-INDUCED LUPUS

- Most commonly implicated drugs are hydralazine, alpha-methyldopa, procainamide and chlorpromazine. Others include isoniazid, penicillamine and phenytoin.
- Disease is usually limited to skin, joints, and serosal surfaces (pleuro-pericarditis).
- Homogeneous pattern ANA and anti-histone antibodies are present in 95% of cases.
- Disease resolves with withdrawal of offending drug.

NEONATAL LUPUS

- Results from the passage of IgG anti-SSA (Ro) antibodies from mothers with SLE or Sjögren's syndrome to the fetus via the placenta.
- Clinical features in the newborn include complete heart block, which is frequently irreversible and may be associated with congestive heart failure if the heart block develops early enough before delivery, skin rash, and haematological abnormalities including haemolytic anaemia and thrombocytopenia.
- Severity of maternal illness does not correlate with risk of development of neonatal lupus, but the risk is significant if previous pregnancies were affected.
- All but the cardiac lesion resolve by 3 months of age (commensurate with the half-life of maternal IgG).

LABORATORY INDICATORS OF ACTIVE DISEASE IN LUPUS

- Low serum complement levels: C3, C4 and total haemolytic complement.
- Raised acute phase reactants (often with the exception of C-reactive protein).
- Increasing levels of anti-ds DNA antibodies.

ANTI-PHOSPHOLIPID SYNDROME (APS)

CLINICAL FEATURES

- May be primary (PAPS) or secondary. These occur in roughly equal proportions.

- The secondary form is found in association with other autoimmune diseases, especially SLE, and has been described in HIV-infected patients.

Table 12.13 *Clinical features of APS*

Sign or symptom	Comment
Thrombosis	May be venous or arterial
	Venous thromboses may be recurrent and unusual, e.g. subclavian, cavernous sinus
	Arterial thromboses may cause myocardial or cerebral infarction
Recurrent spontaneous abortion	Usually first trimester
Intrauterine growth retardation and sudden fetal death	Related to placental insufficiency
Thrombocytopenia	
Livedo reticularis	
Neurological abnormalities including chorea	Due to cerebral vascular occlusion with thrombosis or vasculitis
HELLP syndrome	Haemolysis, elevated liver enzymes (often with hepatic infarction) and low platelets

PATHOPHYSIOLOGY

- Antibodies against membrane phospholipids are responsible for this syndrome.
- May be either IgG or IgM, with IgG more likely to be pathogenic.
- The presence of the antibodies in serum is not necessarily associated with disease.
- May take the form of anti-cardiolipin antibodies or lupus inhibitor.
- Lupus inhibitor causes elongation of the activated partial thromboplastin time, but *increases* the tendency to thrombosis *in vivo*.
- Anti-phospholipid antibodies stimulate platelet aggregation, and interfere with thrombolysis, perhaps through interaction with alpha-2 glycoprotein.

SJÖGREN'S SYNDROME (SS)

CLINICAL FEATURES

Sjögren's syndrome may be primary or secondary to other autoimmune disease such as rheumatoid arthritis or SLE.

It is more common in women, with a female to male ratio of 9:1.

Table 12.14 Clinical features of Sjögren's syndrome

Symptom or sign	Comment
Keratoconjunctivitis sicca	Manifests as dry, irritable eyes with markedly reduced tear production
	Confirm with Schirmer's test and slit lamp examination after using Rose-Bengal stain
Xerostomia	Markedly reduced saliva production may result in chronic dental caries and periodontitis, and difficulty with mastication and swallowing
Intermittent parotid gland swelling	
Dry skin and dry hair	Due to sebaceous gland damage
Arthralgia, arthritis	Non-deforming polyarthritis
Respiratory	Pleuritis, interstitial pneumonitis are rare
Neurological	Cerebral vasculitis is rare but may lead to multiple CNS abnormalities
Renal	Renal tubular acidosis due to interstitial nephritis
	Glomerulonephritis may cause renal failure very uncommonly
Gastrointestinal	Pancreatitis
Lymphadenopathy	May be due to non-Hodgkin's lymphoma in long-term disease

PATHOPHYSIOLOGY

- Infiltration of exocrine glands by mature lymphocytes and occasional plasma cells is the characteristic pathological abnormality.
- CD4+ T cells appear to be the major mediators of inflammation, but the triggers for this are unknown.
- Anti-SSA and SSB antibodies are likely to be pathogenic, and circulating immune complexes may also mediate some of the immune damage.
- Chronic inflammation in glandular structures may eventually lead to non-Hodgkin's lymphoma in a small percentage of cases.
- Sjögren's syndrome may occur in HIV infection, but in this instance the predominant cellular infiltrate is CD8+ T cells.
- In primary Sjögren's syndrome, SSA and SSB antibodies, positive ANA in a speckled pattern, high-titre rheumatoid factor, polyclonal hypergammaglobulinaemia, and an elevated ESR are usual. A hypokalaemic metabolic acidosis may result from renal tubular acidosis.

SCLERODERMA

CLINICAL FEATURES

Table 12.15 Clinical features of scleroderma

Sign or symptom	Comment

Skin changes:
  Thickening
  Calcinosis
  Raynaud's phenomenon
  Telangiectasia
  Ischaemia, infarction
	Scleroderma is defined as limited if the skin changes affect only the upper limbs below the elbows, and the face

Renal disease: hypertension	May be malignant, with associated renal failure

Gastrointestinal:
  Reflux oesophagitis
  Malabsorption
  Altered bowel habit
  Primary biliary cirrhosis
	Fibrosis of gut wall leading to motility disturbance
	Bacterial overgrowth secondary to motility disturbance

Respiratory:
  Interstitial pneumonitis
  Pulmonary hypertension
	Carries a poor prognosis
	May be isolated or secondary to interstitial fibrosis

Joint disease	Polyarthritis

Heart disease:
  Myocardial fibrosis
  Pericarditis
  Conduction disturbances
	Less common manifestations

Neurological: Acute myositis	
Thyroid: Hypothyroidism	Rare

Reproductive system:
  Impotence in men
  Reduced fertility in women	

Malignancy	Possible associations with breast and alveolar cell lung cancer

PATHOPHYSIOLOGY

- Tissue fibrosis is the hallmark of scleroderma.
- Excessive fibroblastic activity may be driven by overproduction of certain cytokines, e.g. platelet-derived growth factor.
- Macrophages and endothelial cells are likely producers of these pro-inflammatory mediators.

- The trigger for these abnormal events is not known.
- Most patients will have autoantibodies, either anti-Scl-70 or anti-poly-merase 3 in the diffuse variant, or anti-centromere in the limited form.
- The disease causes extreme morbidity as well as excess mortality, the latter especially due to pulmonary disease.

Table 12.16 *Comparison of diffuse and limited (CREST syndrome) scleroderma*

Manifestation	Scleroderma	CREST
Involved skin	Limbs and trunk	Limited to distal extremities
Disease progress	Rapid	Slow
Systemic disease	Early	Delayed although pulmonary hypertension may develop early
Lung involvement	Fibrosis common	Low DLCO common
Anti-centromere antibody	10%	70%
Anti-Scl-70 antibody	40%	Rare
Anti-nuclear antibody	90%; nucleolar or speckled	Invariable: speckled

CREST = calcinosis, Raynaud's, oesphageal dysfunction, sclerodactyly, telangiectasia. DCLO = diffusing capacity for carbon monoxide.

DIFFERENTIAL DIAGNOSIS OF THICKENED AND TETHERED SKIN

- CREST syndrome, scleroderma, or mixed connective tissue disease
- Eosinophilic fasciitis
- Localised morphea—small areas of sclerosis
- Chemicals—vinyl chloride, pentazocine, bleomycin, toxic oil syndrome
- Pseudoscleroderma—secondary to porphyria cutanea tarda, acromegaly, carcinoid syndrome
- Scleroedema—diabetics develop thick skin over the shoulders and upper back
- Graft-versus-host disease
- Silicosis

MIXED CONNECTIVE TISSUE DISEASE (MCTD)

CLINICAL FEATURES

- Signs and symptoms are a mixture of SLE, scleroderma, rheumatoid arthritis, and polymyositis.
- ANA is positive and anti-RNP antibodies need to be present to make the diagnosis.
- Renal disease is uncommon.
- Raynaud's syndrome is frequent.

RAYNAUD'S PHENOMENON

CLINICAL FEATURES

- White-blue-red colour changes in the distal extremities, usually precipitated by cold.
- Digital ulceration and gangrene can result.

PATHOPHYSIOLOGY

- Raynaud's phenomenon is the result of an inappropriate vasoconstriction of the arterial supply to a limb.
- Raynaud's disease applies to Raynaud's phenomenon with no other demonstrable underlying disease process.
- It is important to differentiate primary Raynaud's disease from Raynaud's phenomenon secondary to underlying connective tissue disease.
- Up to 10% of patients with Raynaud's phenomenon will develop a connective tissue disease.

Table 12.17 *Comparison of Raynaud's disease and connective tissue disease*

Manifestation	Raynaud's disease	Connective tissue disease
Sex ratio	Female predominant	Females and males
Age at onset	Typically menarche	Typically young adults
Digits involved	Usually all	Often a single digit
Digital ulcers	Rare	Common
Digital oedema	Rare	Common
Livedo reticularis	Common	Rare

CAUSES OF RAYNAUD'S PHENOMENON

- Primary Raynaud's disease
- Connective tissue disease
- Cryoglobulinaemia
- Cold agglutinins
- Hyperviscosity syndromes
- Jackhammer operators
- Drugs, e.g. vinblastine, bleomycin
- Thoracic outlet obstruction (unilateral)

VASCULITIDES

Table 12.18 *Classification of vasculitis by size of vessel involved*

Large artery	Medium artery	Small artery	Veins
Giant cell arteritis	Polyarteritis nodosa	Microscopic polyarteritis	Behçet's syndrome
Takayasu's arteritis	Churg-Strauss syndrome	Wegener's granulomatosis Henoch-Schönlein purpura	Hypersensitivity vasculitis

GIANT CELL ARTERITIS

CLINICAL FEATURES

- Majority of patients are elderly (>60 years)
- Majority of patients have symptoms of polymyalgia rheumatica; myalgias in limbs, especially the shoulder girdle, fatigue, low-grade fevers, weight loss
- Symptoms and signs will depend further on which large arteries are involved:
  - Temporal—headaches, scalp tenderness
  - Ophthalmic—blindness due to retinal infarction
  - Other branches of the external carotid—jaw claudication, throat pain

PATHOPHYSIOLOGY

- Cause unknown
- Vessel walls are infiltrated with CD4+ T cells, macrophages, and giant cells
- Laboratory abnormalities are non-specific; raised acute phase proteins, normochromic anaemia

TAKAYASU'S ARTERITIS

CLINICAL FEATURES

- Female predominance
- Fever, weight loss, fatigue
- Consequences of ischaemia to brain, heart, kidneys, and limbs, e.g. dizziness, visual blurring, stroke, ischaemic chest pain, hypertension, claudication
- Loss of upper limb pulses may occur
- Bruits may be audible over carotid arteries

PATHOPHYSIOLOGY

- Vasculitis affects the aorta and its primary branches
- Histopathology is identical to that of giant cell arteritis

POLYARTERITIS NODOSA

CLINICAL FEATURES

- Male to female ratio 2 : 1
- Constitutional symptoms—fever, weight loss, arthralgia, myalgia, fatigue
- Vasculitic organ damage:
  - Renal—hypertension, glomerulonephritis
  - Gastrointestinal—abdominal pain, visceral infarction due to mesenteric arterial vasculitis
  - Neurological—mononeuritis multiplex
  - Cutaneous—palpable purpura

PATHOPHYSIOLOGY

- Associated with viral infections such as hepatitis B
- Antigens may be present in walls of small and medium sized arteries, either by deposition or as part of the vessel wall, and incite a predominantly neutrophilic infiltration
- The triggers for the disorder are not known
- Laboratory abnormalities include normochromic anaemia, raised acute phase proteins
- Biopsy (e.g. sural nerve, skin) or angiography (e.g. mesenteric, coronary) may be needed to establish the diagnosis

CHURG-STRAUSS VASCULITIS

CLINICAL FEATURES

- Patients have a history of asthma and allergic rhinitis in the majority of cases
- Constitutional symptoms: fatigue, weight loss, fevers, night sweats, arthralgias
- Respiratory involvement: dyspnoea, cough
- Mononeuritis multiplex or symmetrical peripheral neuropathy
- Worsening of asthma usually accompanies the onset of the disease

PATHOPHYSIOLOGY

- Necrotising granulomatous arteritis of medium-sized vessels with a predominantly eosinophilic infiltrate
- The mechanism triggering the uncontrolled activity of eosinophils is unknown
- A peripheral eosinophilia, raised serum IgE, and acute phase response are usual

MICROSCOPIC POLYARTERITIS

CLINICAL FEATURES

- Constitutional symptoms; weight loss, fatigue, malaise, fever, night sweats
- Hypertension, active urinary sediment secondary to glomerulonephritis

- Haemoptysis and dyspnoea due to lung involvement
- Palpable purpura
- Mononeuritis

PATHOPHYSIOLOGY

- Initiating factors for this disease are not known
- Small vessel vasculitis with a segmental vascular necrosis which can affect almost any organ
- Anti-neutrophil cytoplasmic antibodies with specificity for the myeloperoxidase antigen are usually present (but these may also be found in a variety of other conditions, especially inflammatory bowel disease, and primary sclerosing cholangitis)
- Elevated acute phase proteins and a normochromic, normocytic anaemia are usual

HENOCH-SCHÖNLEIN PURPURA

CLINICAL FEATURES

- More common in young children than adults
- Palpable purpura, especially lower limbs and buttocks
- Arthritis and arthralgia
- Fever
- Abdominal pain, with occasional bloody diarrhoea
- Haematuria

PATHOPHYSIOLOGY

- Necrotising vasculitis of small vessels
- IgA is deposited in dermal capillary walls and glomerular mesangium
- Serum IgA may be elevated
- Diagnosis may be possible on clinical grounds or skin biopsy may be required

HYPERSENSITIVITY VASCULITIS

CLINICAL FEATURES

- Skin changes:
  Urticaria
  Palpable purpura
  Livedo reticularis
  Digital infarcts
- Other features of an underlying disease

PATHOPHYSIOLOGY

- The necrotising vasculitis is known as leucocytoclastic and affects venules and capillaries

CAUSES

- Connective tissue disease
- Viral infection, e.g. hepatitis B
- Drugs, e.g. penicillin, phenothiazines, phenylbutazone, propylthiouracil
- Essential mixed cryoglobulinaemia
- Paraproteinaemia
- Idiopathic

BEHÇET'S SYNDROME

CLINICAL FEATURES

- Female predominance
- Oral and genital ulcers
- Uveitis
- Asymmetrical large joint polyarthritis
- Thrombophlebitis
- Meningoencephalitis
- Aneurysms and thromboses of major vessels can occur
- Cerebral vasculitis may produce a variety of neurological abnormalities
- Pulmonary vasculitis may cause severe haemoptysis

PATHOPHYSIOLOGY

- Unknown aetiology
- Vasculitis affects medium to small arteries and veins

13

Rheumatology

IMPORTANT CLINICAL CLUES

CAUSES OF A MONOARTHRITIS

A. ACUTE MONOARTHRITIS

1. Septic arthritis
2. Gout
3. Pseudogout
4. Haemarthrosis, e.g. haemophilia
5. Seronegative spondyloarthritis (occasionally)

B. CHRONIC MONOARTHRITIS

1. Chronic infection, e.g. tuberculosis
2. Osteoarthritis
3. Seronegative spondyloarthritis
4. Vasculitis (rarely, e.g. polyarteritis nodosa, Wegener's granulomatosis—usually a large joint early in the disease course)

C. SWOLLEN TOE (1ST METATARSOPHALANGEAL JOINT)

1. Gout
2. Pseudogout
3. Reiter's syndrome

CAUSES OF A POLYARTHRITIS

A. ACUTE POLYARTHRITIS

1. Onset of chronic polyarthritis
2. Manifestation of a systemic disease, e.g. bacterial endocarditis, serum sickness

B. CHRONIC POLYARTHRITIS

1. Rheumatoid arthritis
2. Seronegative spondyloarthritis
3. Primary osteoarthritis

4. Gout
5. Pseudogout
6. Systemic lupus erythematosus (SLE)
7. Other connective tissue disease

CAUSES OF A SYMMETRICAL POLYARTHRITIS

1. Rheumatoid arthritis
2. Primary osteoarthritis
3. SLE
4. Other connective tissue disease

DIFFERENTIAL DIAGNOSIS OF A DEFORMING POLYARTHROPATHY

1. Rheumatoid arthritis
2. Seronegative spondyloarthropathy
3. Chronic tophaceous gout
4. Primary generalised osteoarthritis

DIFFERENTIAL DIAGNOSIS OF AN ARTHRITIS AND NODULES

1. Rheumatoid arthritis (seropositive)
2. SLE (rare)
3. Rheumatic fever (Jaccoud's arthritis—very rare)

Gouty tophi and xanthoma from hyperlipidaemia may cause confusion.

Table 13.1 *Synovial fluid analysis*

Disease	Appearance	White cells/mm³	Glucose	Viscosity	Crystals
Normal	Clear-straw Does not clot	75–200 (15% PMN)	Normal	Normal	None
RA	Cloudy-light yellow	10 000–75 000 (75% PMN)	Low	Poor	None
SLE	Clear-cloudy	1000–1500 (15% PMN)	Normal	Fair to poor	None
OA	Clear-straw	1000 (15% PMN)	Normal	Normal	None
Gout	Cloudy-yellow or white	10 000–20 000 (70% PMN)	Normal	Poor	Strongly negatively birefringent
Pseudogout	Cloudy-white	10 000–40 000 (70% PMN)	Normal	Fair to poor	Weakly positively birefringent
Bacterial infection	Cloudy-grey or yellow	50 000–100 000 (90% PMN)	Very low	Poor	None
TB	Cloudy-grey or yellow	25 000 (<50% PMN)	Low	Poor	None

PMN = polymorphonuclear leucocyte. RA = rheumatoid arthritis. SLE = systemic lupus erythematosus. OA = osteoarthritis. TB = tuberculosis.

Table 13.2 *Immune complexes (IC) and complement (C') in rheumatic diseases*

Disease	Serum IC	Serum C'	Synovial fluid IC	Synovial fluid C'
RA	Normal to increased	Normal	Increased	Low
SLE	Normal to increased	Normal to decreased	Increased	Low
Reiter's syndrome	Normal	Normal	Normal	Increased
Bacterial infection	Normal	Normal to increased	Normal	Increased
Crystal arthropathy	Normal	Normal	Normal	Normal to increased

RA = rheumatoid arthritis. SLE = systemic lupus erythematosus.

CAUSES OF RECURRENT ACHILLES TENDONITIS

1. Reiter's syndrome, ankylosing spondylitis, other seronegative spondyloarthropathies
2. Trauma

Table 13.3 *Comparison of important diseases causing mucocutaneous ulceration*

Manifestations	Reiter's syndrome	Enteropathic arthritis	Behçet's syndrome	Stevens-Johnson syndrome
Oral ulcers	+ (painless)	+	+ (painful)	+
Genital ulcers	+	–	+	–
Conjunctivitis	+ (common)	+	+	–
Uveitis	+ (10%)	+	+	–
Arthritis	+	+	+	–
Sacroiliitis	+	+	+ (rare)	–
Thrombophlebitis	+ (rare)	+	+ (common)	–
CNS disease	+ (rare)	–	+ (common)	–
Colitis	–	+	+ (discrete ulcers)	–

CNS = central nervous system. + = feature present.

DISEASES ASSOCIATED WITH ASEPTIC NECROSIS OF BONE

1. Steroid excess
2. SLE

3. Alcoholism
4. Fat embolism
5. Haemoglobinopathy
6. Diabetes mellitus
7. Hyperlipidaemia
8. Hyperuricaemia
9. Pancreatitis

CAUSES OF A CHARCOT (NEUROPATHIC) JOINT

1. Shoulder or knee affected—suspect syringomyelia
3. Knee affected—suspect tabes dorsalis
3. Foot or ankle affected—suspect diabetic neuropathy

CAUSES OF JOINT HYPERMOBILITY

1. Ehlers-Danlos syndrome, types I-VII; skin is hyperextensible in types I, II, V, VI
2. Marfan's syndrome: tall, with long and thin extremities; arm span is greater than height, and the ratio of upper to lower segments is low; high arched palate; bilateral lens dislocation; aortic dissection can occur
3. Osteogenesis imperfecta: pathological fractures; blue sclera; deafness due to otosclerosis
4. Congenital
5. Noonan's syndrome

DISEASE STATES

RHEUMATOID ARTHRITIS (RA)

CLINICAL FEATURES

1. Peak incidence between 35 and 45 years of age
2. HLA-DR4 or HLA-DR1 or both are frequently present
3. Female preponderance
4. In descending order, the joints most frequently involved are the metacarpophalangeals, proximal interphalangeals, wrists, knees, ankles, shoulders, elbows, hips, acromioclavicular joints, cervical spine and temporomandibular joints
5. Onset is abrupt in approximately 30% of patients
6. 70% of patients have exacerbations followed by remissions
7. Rheumatoid arthritis is associated with reduced life expectancy

AMERICAN RHEUMATISM ASSOCIATION REVISED CRITERIA FOR DIAGNOSIS OF RHEUMATOID ARTHRITIS (1987)

1. Morning stiffness (>1 hour).
2. Arthritis of 3 or more joint areas.

3. Arthritis of hand joints.
4. Symmetrical arthritis.
5. Subcutaneous (rheumatoid) nodules.
6. Serum rheumatoid factor.
7. Typical X-ray changes in hands
   a) Soft tissue swelling
   b) Joint space narrowing
   c) Joint erosions
   d) Juxta-articular osteoporosis.

Diagnosis of RA requires 4 or more criteria (N.B. 1–4 must have been present for >6 weeks).

EVIDENCE OF ACTIVE DISEASE

1. Erosions on serial X-rays
2. Raised ESR
3. Anaemia
4. High rheumatoid factor titre

POOR PROGNOSTIC INDICATORS

1. Chronic onset and duration >1 year
2. Continuous disease activity
3. Bone erosions
4. Rheumatoid nodules, and rheumatoid factor (positive in 70% of cases)
5. Extra-articular manifestations (rheumatoid nodules, vasculitis etc)

EXTRA-ARTICULAR MANIFESTATIONS

1. Eyes—scleritis, episcleritis, scleromalacia perforans, cataracts (from steroids, chloroquine). N.B. iritis rarely occurs.
2. Skin—Raynaud's phenomenon, leg ulcers (vasculitis), palpable purpura, calf swelling (ruptured Baker's cyst).
3. Lungs—interstitial pneumonitis progressing to fibrosis, pleuritis and pleural effusion, nodules, Caplan's syndrome.
4. Heart—pericarditis, conduction defects, aortic and mitral regurgitation.
5. Blood—anaemia (chronic disease, dietary folate deficiency, iron deficiency from gastrointestinal blood loss secondary to NSAIDs, Felty's syndrome).
6. Renal (rare)—vasculitis, amyloid, analgesic kidneys from prolonged analgesic use.
7. Nervous system—entrapment neuropathy (e.g. carpal tunnel), peripheral neuropathy, mononeuritis multiplex, cervical cord compression from subluxation.
8. Felty's syndrome—splenomegaly and neutropenia with rheumatoid arthritis.
9. Rheumatoid nodules—occur in approximately 25% of people with RA. They are limited to people with detectable rheumatoid factor.
10. Hepatic—nodular hyperplasia.

LABORATORY ABNORMALITIES IN RHEUMATOID ARTHRITIS

1. Normocytic anaemia
2. Raised acute phase reactants; leucocytosis, thrombocytosis, hypergamma-globulinaemia
3. Raised ESR and C-reactive protein
4. Rheumatoid factor (positive in up to 90% of patients at some stage)
5. Cryoglobulins may be present
6. Antinuclear antibodies may be present
7. Eosinophilia in approximately one-third

DIFFERENTIAL DIAGNOSIS OF A POSITIVE RHEUMATOID FACTOR

1. Rheumatoid arthritis
2. Sjögren's syndrome
3. Mixed cryoglobulinaemia
4. Subacute bacterial endocarditis
5. SLE
6. Scleroderma
7. Sarcoidosis
8. Idiopathic pulmonary fibrosis
9. Hypergammaglobulinaemic purpura
10. Asbestosis
11. Malignancies, e.g. lymphoproliferative disorders
12. Infectious mononucleosis
13. Influenza
14. Chronic hepatitis
15. Vaccinations
16. Tuberculosis
17. Syphilis
18. Brucellosis
19. Leprosy
20. Salmonellosis
21. Malaria
22. Kala-azar syndrome
23. Schistosomiasis
24. Filariasis
25. Trypanosomiasis

TREATMENT

Principles
1. Physiotherapy
2. Joint protection
3. Medications: (see also Therapeutics)
   - Non-steroidal anti-inflammatory drugs (NSAIDs)
   - Corticosteroids (low dose)

- Disease-modifying agents: methotrexate, gold salts, D-penicillamine, anti-malarials, sulfasalazine
- Immunosuppressants: azathioprine, cyclophosphamide
4. Surgery

ADULT-ONSET STILL'S DISEASE

CLINICAL FEATURES

- Onset in young adults
1. High spiking quotidian fever
2. Macular salmon-coloured rash on trunk and limbs
3. Arthritis of wrists, shoulders, hips and knees
4. 30% have progressive erosive arthritis
5. Weight loss, sore throat, lymphadenopathy and hepatosplenomegaly are common

TREATMENT

1. Similar to rheumatoid arthritis
2. Approximately 50% require immunosuppressive agents

OSTEOARTHRITIS

CLINICAL FEATURES

1. Joint pain worse on movement
2. Joints may be tender and display crepitus on movement
3. Mild inflammatory changes may be evident
4. Deformity occurs late in the course

PRIMARY OSTEOARTHRITIS

Types

1. Generalised
   - involves DIPs, PIPs, first carpometacarpal joints, hips, knees, and spine
   - mainly in post-menopausal women
   - mucous cysts may exist on the dorsolateral or dorsomedial aspect of the DIPs
2. Nodal—affects only the DIPs
3. Hip—more common in men
4. Erosive
   - affects DIPs and PIPs
   - recurrent painful flare-ups occur with eventual joint ankylosis
5. Diffuse idiopathic skeletal hyperostosis
   - occurs mainly in males >50 years
   - osteophytosis connects 4 or more vertebrae
   - associated with obesity and diabetes mellitus

SECONDARY OSTEOARTHRITIS

CAUSES

1. Trauma
2. Primary inflammatory arthritis
3. Congenital joint malformations
4. Haemochromatosis (affects MCPs and shoulders)
5. Ochronosis (homogentisic acid collects in connective tissues due to abnormality of tyrosine metabolism—mainly affects large joints)
6. Wilson's disease
7. Apatite microcrystals—associated with hypothyroidism, hyperparathyroidism and acromegaly
8. Neuroarthropathy (Charcot's joints)
9. Aseptic necrosis of bone
10. Haemophilia (repeated haemarthroses)

DIP = distal interphalangeal joint
PIP = proximal interphalangeal joint
MCP = metacarpophalangeal joint

SERONEGATIVE SPONDYLOARTHROPATHIES

CLASSIFICATION OF SACROILIITIS

1. Ankylosing spondylitis (HLA-B27 in >90%)—bilateral sacroiliitis.
2. Psoriatic arthritis (HLA-B27 in 50%)—unilateral or bilateral.
3. Reiter's syndrome (HLA-B27 in >80%)—unilateral or bilateral.
4. Enteropathic arthritis (HLA-B27 in 75%)—unilateral or bilateral.
5. Uveitis (idiopathic)—probably part of this spectrum (HLA-B27 in 50%).

ANKYLOSING SPONDYLITIS

CLINICAL FEATURES

1. Onset is usually in young adulthood with gradual development of low back pain and morning stiffness
2. Bilateral sacroiliitis
   X-ray changes
   a) Cortical outline lost early
   b) Juxta-articular osteosclerosis*
   c) Erosions
   d) Joint obliteration

---

*This also occurs in osteitis condensa ilii, a benign entity in females; the sacroiliac joints are normal.

3. Lumbar spine disease
   X-ray changes
   a) Loss of lumbar lordosis
   b) Squaring of vertebrae
   c) Syndesmophytes (thoracolumbar region)
   d) Bamboo spine (bony bridging of vertebrae)—late sign
   e) Osteoporosis
   f) Apophyseal joint fusion
4. Cauda equina syndrome (rare), pseudofractures after trauma
5. Peripheral joint disease—hip (50%), knee, shoulder
6. Achilles tendonitis, plantar fasciitis
7. Eyes—uveitis
8. Lungs—decreased chest expansion, apical fibrosis (aspergillomas can occur)
9. Heart—aortic regurgitation, conduction defects, aortitis (late)
10. Amyloidosis

PSORIATIC ARTHRITIS

CLINICAL FEATURES

1. Onset is usually in young adulthood, with a slight female preponderance.
2. The arthritis occurs in between 5 to 10% of people with a psoriatic rash, and is more likely if the rash is severe.
3. In most cases, the rash precedes the onset of arthritis.
4. There are 5 patterns of arthritis; in order of frequency they are:
   a) Asymmetrical oligoarthritis—usually of the hands and feet.
   b) Symmetrical polyarthritis—like rheumatoid arthritis, but rheumatoid factor is absent.
   c) Sacroiliitis with or without peripheral arthritis.
   d) Predominant distal interphalangeal (DIP) joint involvement with psoriatic nail changes. The nail changes include pitting, onycholysis, hyperkeratosis, ridging and discoloration.
   e) Arthritis mutilans.

REITER'S SYNDROME AND REACTIVE ARTHRITIS

CLINICAL TRIAD

1. Non-specific urethritis (e.g. *Chlamydia*) or infectious diarrhoea (e.g. *Salmonella*, *Shigella*, *Yersinia*, *Campylobacter jejuni*)
2. Conjunctivitis
3. Arthritis—toes, asymmetrical lower limb large joints, DIP joints

OTHER MANIFESTATIONS

1. Keratoderma blennorrhagica—rash like psoriasis on palms and soles
2. Sacroiliitis (may be unilateral)
3. Iritis
4. Aortitis, cardiac conduction defects

ENTEROPATHIC ARTHRITIS (INFLAMMATORY BOWEL DISEASE ARTHRITIS)

CLINICAL FEATURES

There are two types:
1. Ankylosing spondylitis—bears little relation to activity of the bowel disease.
2. Peripheral arthropathy—oligoarthritis that tends to parallel the activity of the bowel disease; a non-destructive asymmetrical arthritis affects especially the knees and ankles.

CRYSTALLINE ARTHROPATHIES

GOUT

CLINICAL FEATURES

1. Acute gouty arthritis—acute painful joint swelling, typically 3 days after trauma or surgery, or due to excess alcohol intake, major medical illness, or fasting.
2. Chronic tophaceous gouty arthropathy—asymmetrical joint involvement; tophi are found on the helix or antihelix of the ear, the ulnar surface of the forearm, and over the olecranon bursa and Achilles tendon.
3. Renal disease—uric acid stone disease, interstitial renal disease.

CAUSES

Primary
1. Underexcretion of uric acid (90%), due to
   a) reduced filtration of uric acid
   b) enhanced tubular reabsorption, or
   c) decreased tubular secretion
2. Overproduction of uric acid (10%)
   a) Idiopathic (association with obesity)
   b) Enzyme defects
      i) HG PRTase* deficiency (X-linked recessive): Lesch-Nyhan syndrome results (chorea, retardation, self mutilation)
      ii) PRPP† synthetase overactivity (X-linked recessive)

Secondary
1. Overproduction, e.g. myeloproliferative disease, malignancy (especially following cytotoxic therapy), psoriasis
2. Underexcretion, e.g. drugs (diuretics, low-dose salicylates), lead poisoning

---

*Hypoxanthine-guanine phosphoribosyltransferase
†5-Phosphoribosyl-1q-pyrophosphate

TREATMENT

1. Acute gouty arthritis—colchicine or NSAIDs
2. Preventive treatment—allopurinol, probenecid

Indications for allopurinol
1. More than two attacks of gout in 1 year (do not start until an acute attack has completely subsided).
2. Tophi or renal stone disease.
3. Asymptomatic hyperuricaemia if there is a strong family history of gout or renal stone disease and there is high renal excretion of uric acid.

PSEUDOGOUT

CLINICAL FEATURES

1. Usually affects the knees
2. May affect wrists, elbows, ankles and intervertebral discs
3. Usually occurs in older individuals
4. May occur in setting of osteoarthritis or true gout.

Calcium pyrophosphate crystals are rhomboid-shaped, weakly positive birefringent crystals that are found in polymorphonuclear cells or extracellularly in pseudogout.

CAUSES

1. Idiopathic.
3. Hereditary.
3. Endocrine diseases, e.g. primary hyperparathyroidism, hypothyroidism, hypophosphatasia.
4. Metabolic disease, e.g. haemochromatosis, Wilson's disease, ochronosis.

HYDROXYAPATITE ARTHROPATHY

Is due to deposition of calcium hydroxyapatite crystals

CLINICAL FEATURES

1. Knee and shoulder arthritis in elderly patients.
2. Synovial fluid can be screened using alizarin red S staining, but electron microscopy or X-ray diffraction is required for definitive diagnosis.

N.B. Gout, pseudogout, calcium hydroxyapatite arthropathy or infection should all be considered in a dialysis patient who presents with a red, swollen joint.

INFECTIOUS ARTHRITIS

If synovial fluid has a low sugar and a high lactate, suspect infection.

Table 13.4 Infectious arthritis

Causative organism	Clinical features	Diagnosis
Neisseria gonorrhoea	Increased incidence in menstruating women. May be associated with tenosynovitis, fever, and a vesicopustular rash. Knee, wrist or ankle typically affected	Joint fluid culture (positive in 30%)
Staphylococcus aureus	Joints most commonly affected are knees, hips, shoulders, ankles, wrists, elbows, fingers, toes. Serious underlying systemic disease predisposes	Blood and joint fluid cultures
Streptococci	As for *S. aureus*	Blood and joint fluid cultures
Haemophilus influenzae	As for *S. aureus* (most common in children)	Blood and joint fluid cultures
Gram-negative infection, e.g. *Pseudomonas, Serratia*	As for *S. aureus* (injecting drug use a risk factor)	Blood and joint fluid cultures

LYME DISEASE

Spirochaetal disease (*Borrelia burgdorferi*) transmitted by a tick (*Ixodes dammini*).

CLINICAL FEATURES

1. Early (stage I)—Erythema chronicum migrans (red papule that grows into an expanding lesion with partial central clearing). Fever, neck stiffness, arthralgia, lymphadenopathy. Elevated ESR, AST can occur. Occurs several days to a month after tick bite.
2. Stage II—Nervous system disease, e.g. Bell's palsy, peripheral neuropathy, meningoencephalitis. AV nodal conduction abnormalities or myocarditis. 30–50% have arthritis. Occurs weeks to months after symptoms of stage I.
3. Late (stage III)—Recurrent or chronic arthritis (often associated with HLA-DR2 and HLA-DR4). Occurs several years later.

DIAGNOSIS
- Serology with ELISA technique.

Treatment

- Tetracycline. In late or severe disease, intravenous penicillin or ceftriaxone.

NON-ARTICULAR RHEUMATISM

FIBROMYALGIA

Clinical features

1. Chronic diffuse musculoskeletal pain (>3 months)
2. High tender point count at muscle attachment sites
3. More common in women
4. Aggravated by physical activity or weather change
5. May occur after viral illness

POLYMYALGIA RHEUMATICA

Clinical features

1. Aching and stiffness in the proximal musculature
2. Older people
3. Slight female preponderance
4. May have mild constitutional symptoms
5. Oligoarticular synovitis can occur in knees, wrists and shoulders
6. Granulomatous hepatitis and myocarditis are rare
7. Elevated ESR
8. Predisposes to giant cell arteritis

TREATMENT

1. Rapid response to moderate dose prednisolone is universal
2. Maintenance doses of prednisolone are typically <10mg per day

THERAPEUTICS

Table 13.5 *Mechanism of action of drugs used to treat rheumatic disorders*

Drug	Mechanism of action
NSAIDs	Inhibit arachidonic acid metabolism via blockade of cyclo-oxygenase(cox)II, thereby reducing production of inflammatory mediators, e.g. prostaglandins and thromboxanes
Glucocorticoids	Decrease production of pro-inflammatory cytokines, decrease action of T helper cells, macrophages, B cells

Table 13.5 Continued

Drug	Mechanism of action
Penicillamine	Possible action via reduction of macrophage function (through inhibition of IL-1 release)
Gold salts	Possible action via reduction of IL-1 production, inhibition of neutrophil chemotaxis, decreased production of toxic oxygen metabolites from phagocytes
Hydroxychloroquine	Possible action via reduction of IL-1 production, inhibition of neutrophil chemotaxis, decreased production of toxic oxygen metabolites from phagocytes
Methotrexate	Inhibits enzyme dihydrofolate reductase, which leads to impairment of thymidylate synthesis and impairment of DNA synthesis. The anti-inflammatory effect results from the impairment of leucocyte function
Cyclophosphamide	An alkylating agent which cross-links DNA and has a pronounced effect on reducing the function of lymphocytes
Cyclosporin A	Inhibits production of IL-2 by T lymphocytes, thus reducing induction of cytotoxic T cells and T-cell-dependent B cell responses
Azathioprine	Has a cytotoxic action on dividing cells and therefore inhibits clonal proliferation during the induction phase of the immune response

Table 13.6 Side effects of drugs used in rheumatoid arthritis

Drug	Side effects
Aspirin and NSAIDs	Gastric erosions, peptic ulcer, gastrointestinal bleeding (not cox II-specific NSAIDs)
	Asthma in aspirin-sensitive individuals
	Platelet dysfunction
	Renal impairment (including glomerulonephritis, interstitial nephritis)
	Salicylate hepatitis
Gold	Rash
(Intramuscular gold: give a test dose first. Check blood count and urinalysis prior to each dose)	Diarrhoea
	Glomerulonephritis
	Thrombocytopenia
(Oral gold: check blood count and urinalysis monthly)	Granulocytopenia

Table 13.6 *Continued*

Drug	Side effects
D-penicillamine (Check blood count and urinalysis every 2 weeks for 6 months, then monthly)	Diarrhoea, nausea Rash Glomerulonephritis Thrombocytopenia Granulocytopenia Dysgeusia
Chloroquine (Ophthalmic examination every 6 months)	Retinopathy—'bull's eye' lesion, which is irreversible Corneal opacities Skin tanning Nausea and vomiting
Glucocorticoids	Myopathy Weight gain Lipodystrophy Glucose intolerance Hypertension Skin atrophy Mood changes Easy bruising
Methotrexate (Follow liver function tests)	Bone marrow suppression Liver fibrosis, cirrhosis Interstitial pneumonitis Nausea, vomiting, diarrhoea
Sulfasalazine	Diarrhoea Nausea Vomiting Male infertility Neutropenia, aplastic anaemia Cholestasis, hepatitis, pancreatitis

14

Infectious Diseases

IMPORTANT CLINICAL CLUES

NIGHT SWEATS

CAUSES (MNEMONIC MEDIAN)

1. **M**alignancy e.g. lymphoma, carcinoma
2. **E**ndocrine e.g. menopause, thyrotoxicosis, nocturnal hypoglycaemia
3. **D**rugs e.g. cholinergics, withdrawal of anticholinergics
4. **I**nfections e.g. abscess, tuberculosis, endocarditis
5. **A**lcohol withdrawal
6. **N**eurological disease e.g. hypothalamus, sympathetic nervous system

SOME IMPORTANT SKIN SIGNS IN INFECTIOUS DISEASES

Sign	Diagnosis
Koplick's spots (tiny white spots)	Measles
Rose spots (red macules or papules)	Typhoid
Horder's spots (red macules)	Psittacosis
Target lesions (erythema multiforme)	Mycoplasma pneumonia, herpes simplex
Erythema nodosum	Beta-haemolytic streptococcal infection
Erythema migrans (annular red lesion with partial central clearing; can be multiple)	Lyme disease

IMPORTANT ORGANISMS

Table 14.1 Bacteria

Organism	Clinical syndromes	Treatment
Group A, beta-haemolytic streptococci	Impetigo Pharyngitis Otitis media Sinusitis Erysipelas Cellulitis Scarlet fever (due to toxin release) Acute rheumatic fever Post-infectious glomerulonephritis	Penicillin Erythromycin
Group D, mainly *Strep. bovis*	Endocarditis (may be associated with carcinoma of the colon or prostatism) Bacteraemia	Penicillin
Enterococcus, mainly *E. faecalis*	Endocarditis Bacteraemia Urinary tract infection	Penicillin plus gentamicin or streptomycin
Streptococcus pneumoniae	Pneumonia Empyema Pericarditis Otitis media Sinusitis Meningitis Spontaneous peritonitis	Penicillin Cephalosporins Erythromycin
Staphylococcus aureus	Boils Folliculitis Osteomyelitis Bacteraemia Pneumonia Endocarditis Food poisoning Toxic shock syndrome Scalded skin syndrome	Flucloxacillin Vancomycin Imipenem
Staph. epidermidis	Endocarditis IV line infection Blood culture contaminant	Flucloxacillin Vancomycin
Escherichia coli	Urinary tract infection/ stone formation	Cephalosporins

Table 14.1 Continued

Organism	Clinical syndromes	Treatment
	Intra-abdominal sepsis Spontaneous peritonitis Cholangitis	Aminoglycosides Ampicillin
Proteus mirabilis	Urinary tract infection	Ampicillin
Klebsiella pneumoniae	Pneumonia Lung abscess Empyema	Cephalosporins Aminoglycosides Ciprofloxacin
Enterobacter	Nosocomial pneumonia Nosocomial bacteraemia	Aminoglycosides 3rd generation cephalosporins
Serratia	Nosocomial pneumonia Nosocomial bacteraemia	Aminoglycosides 3rd generation cephalosporins
Pseudomonas aeruginosa	Neutropenic sepsis Nosocomial pneumonia Urinary tract infection Infective exacerbations of cystic fibrosis	Ceftazidime Aminoglycosides Imipenem Aztreonam Ciprofloxacin
Salmonella typhi	Gastroenteritis Bacteraemia Typhoid fever	Ampicillin Chloramphenicol 3rd generation cephalosporins
Haemophilus influenzae	Pneumonia Bronchitis Sinusitis Meningitis Epiglottitis	Amoxycillin with clavulanic acid 3rd generation cephalosporins Imipenem
Bordatella pertussis	Whooping cough	Erythromycin
Legionella pneumoniae	Pneumonia	Erythromycin
Listeria monocytogenes	Meningitis Bacteraemia	Penicillin Ampicillin
Corynebacterium diphtheriae	Diphtheria	Antitoxin Penicillin or erythromycin may prevent transmission to others
Bacteroides	Intra-abdominal infection Pelvic inflammatory disease Pneumonia Lung abscess	Metronidazole Clindamycin Imipenem

Table 14.1 *Continued*

Organism	Clinical syndromes	Treatment
Clostridium tetani	Tetanus First muscles involved are often those in distributions of cranial nerves V, VII, IX, X and XII (see tetanus prophylaxis guidelines below)	Human tetanus immune globulin Penicillin
Clostridium botulinum	Botulism (neurotoxicity)	Equine antitoxin

Table 14.2 *Tetanus prophylaxis guidelines*

History of active immunisation	Tetanus toxoid	Tetanus immune globulin	
		Fresh clean minor wound	Other wounds
Uncertain	Yes	No	Yes
Never immunised	Yes	No	Yes
Incomplete (<3 doses)	Yes	No	Yes
Complete	No (unless >10 years since last dose)	No (unless >5 years since last toxoid)	No (unless >5 years since last toxoid)

Table 14.3 *Mycobacteria*

Organism	Clinical syndromes	Treatment
Mycobacterium tuberculosis	Pneumonia Vertebral infection (Pott's disease) Meningitis Kidney or urinary tract infection	Isoniazid Rifampicin Ethambutol Pyrazinamide Streptomycin
Mycobacterium avium-intracellulare	With HIV infection: —diarrhoea —bone marrow infection —fever —weight loss Without HIV infection: —chronic lung disease	Rifabutin Azithromycin Ciprofloxacin Clarithromycin

Table 14.4 Fungi

Organism/condition	Clinical syndromes	Diagnosis/treatment
A. Deep Mycoses		
Cryptococcus neoformans	Meningoencephalitis Pneumonia (in immunosuppressed) Punched-out bone lesions	CSF: India ink stain Serum antigen test Biopsy Amphotericin-B Flucytosine Fluconazole
Blastomyces dermatitidis Blastomycosis	Lung infection Skin, especially face: painless, non-pruritic crusty rash, ulcerations Punched-out bone lesions Prostatic and epididymal lesions	Culture (sputum, pus or urine) Amphotericin-B Fluconazole
Histoplasma capsulatum Histoplasmosis	Acute influenza-like illness Chronic cavitating lung disease Acute disseminated disease	CXR-calcified nodules Culture—sputum, bone marrow, blood, urine, biopsy specimens Amphotericin-B Fluconazole
Coccidioides immitis Coccidioidomycosis	Lung infection: pneumonitis, hilar adenopathy, pleural effusion, cavitatory lesions Skin infection: maculopapular rash, erythema nodosum Bone, meningeal lesions	Sputum culture Silver stain on biopsies Amphotericin-B Fluconazole Intrathecal amphotericin for neurological disease
B. Opportunistic deep mycoses		
Aspergillus species	Pneumonia Fungal abscess Invasive bronchopulmonary disease Allergic bronchopulmonary aspergillosis Otitis externa Endophthalmitis Disseminated disease	CXR—fungus ball Biopsy Amphotericin-B
Candida species	Skin infection Oral and vaginal thrush Fungaemia Endocarditis Endophthalmitis Oesophagitis	Wet smear for pseudohyphae Culture of skin scrapings Blood culture Ketoconazole Fluconazole

Table 14.4 *Continued*

Organism/condition	Clinical syndromes	Diagnosis/treatment
	Cystitis, nephritis	Amphotericin-B plus flucytosine for disseminated disease
Mucormycosis	Nasal and paranasal sinus infection—necrotic midline lesion Cavitating pneumonia	Biopsy, histology Culture Surgery Tight diabetic control Amphotericin-B
Sporotrichosis	Skin infection—lesions along ascending lymph vessels of the limb Cavitating pneumonitis (rare)	Biopsy, culture Oral potassium iodide for skin lesions Amphotericin

CSF = cerebrospinal fluid. CXR = chest X-ray.

Table 14.5 *Fungal-like bacterial infections*

Condition	Clinical syndromes	Diagnosis/treatment
Actinomycosis	Mandibular lump with chronic draining sinus Suppurative pneumonitis, emphysema, draining sinuses Periappendiceal abscess, fistulae Pelvic abscess associated with an intrauterine device	Anaerobic culture Penicillin Surgical drainage
Nocardiosis	Lung—chronic pneumonitis, abscess Brain abscess	Biopsy Microscopy Culture Trimethoprim-sulfamethoxazole Surgical drainage

Table 14.6 *Mycoplasma*

Organism	Clinical syndromes	Treatment
Mycoplasma pneumoniae	Pneumonia Pleural effusion Bronchitis	Erythromycin Roxithromycin Tetracycline

Internal Medicine

Table 14.7 Viruses

Organism	Clinical syndromes	Treatment
Herpes simplex virus (HSV)	Perioral infection Genital lesions Encephalitis Pneumonia Oesophagitis Cutaneous infection	Aciclovir Valaciclovir Foscarnet
Cytomegalovirus (CMV)	Immunocompetent individuals: mononucleosis-type syndrome Immunodeficient states: retinitis, hepatitis, encephalitis, pneumonia, oesophagitis, gastroenteritis	Ganciclovir Foscarnet
Varicella-zoster virus (VZV)	Chicken pox Shingles Pneumonia Encephalomyelitis	Aciclovir Valaciclovir Famciclovir
Epstein-Barr virus (EBV)	Fever Pharyngitis (infectious mononucleosis) Lymphadenopathy Hepatitis	Nil proven
Influenza	Upper respiratory tract infection Pneumonia	Amantadine Zanamivir
Creutzfeldt-Jakob virus	Progressive multifocal leucoencephalopathy	Nil

Table 14.8 Parasites

Organism	Clinical syndromes	Diagnosis/treatment
Entamoeba histolytica	Dysentery Hepatic abscess	Trophozoites in stool Serology (+ve in 90% with hepatic abscess) Metronidazole Paromomycin
Giardia lamblia	Diarrhoea	Stool examination, duodenal aspirate Metronidazole Tinidazole
Toxoplasma gondii	Mononucleosis-like syndrome Rash Fever Congenital infection In HIV patients: encephalitis, pneumonia	Serology Isolation from blood or biopsy Pyrimethamine Sulfadiazine Clindamycin

Table 14.8 Continued

Organism	Clinical syndromes	Diagnosis/treatment

Cryptosporidiosis	Diarrhoea
	Cholangitis (in
	  immunosuppressed)
		In AIDS patients;
		  paromomycin
		Azithromycin
		Clarithromycin

Malaria	1. *Plasmodium vivax* or
	   ovale—tertian malaria
	2. *P. malariae*—quartan
	   malaria
	3. *P. falciparum*—fever of
	   variable pattern.
	   Complications include
	   cerebral malaria,
	   blackwater fever (massive
	   intravascular haemolysis),
	   acute respiratory
	   distress, splenic rupture
		Thick and thin film
		  blood smear
		  examination
		Acute malaria:
		  chloroquine (except
		  resistant falciparum)
		Exoerythrocytic stages:
		  primaquine
		Falciparum: quinine
		  and pyrimethamine

Table 14.9 Helminths

Organism	Clinical syndromes	Diagnosis/treatment
Hookworm	Iron deficiency anaemia	Stool microscopy for ova and parasites Iron supplements Pyrantel pamoate Mebendazole
Dog hookworm	Eosinophilic ileocolitis	Mebendazole
Pork tapeworm	Larval stage: cysticercosis Expanding lesion in brain (nodule or cyst) Adult worm: GI tract	CT scan Serology Praziquantel, steroids

Pinworm	Anal pruritus	Stool microscopy for
		  ova and parasites
		Scotch tape examination
		  of anus
		Pyrantel pamoate
		Mebendazole

Roundworm
*(Ascaris
lumbricoides)*
	Intestinal obstruction
	Cholangitis
	Visceral larval migrans
		Ova in faeces
		Serology
		Pyrantel pamoate
		  or mebendazole—
		  piperazine is slightly
		  more toxic

Trichinosis	Muscle pain, eosinophilia, periorbital oedema	Muscle biopsy Serology Thiabendazole

Table 14.9 *Continued*

Organism	Clinical syndromes	Diagnosis/treatment
Schistosomiasis	1. Acute disease— *S. mansoni* (spur on side), *S. japonicum*: prolonged febrile illness, eosinophilia, seizures	Serology Eggs in faeces
	2. Liver fibrosis— *S. mansoni, S. japonicum*: periportal fibrosis and portal hypertension; may be associated glomerulonephritis and hypertension	Liver biopsy Eggs in faeces
	3. Haematuria and bladder carcinoma—*S. hematobium* (spur on tail)	Eggs in urine or tissue Praziquantel

DISEASE STATES

PYREXIA OF UNKNOWN ORIGIN

DEFINITION

This is a term applied when an individual has fevers of more than 38.3°C without a diagnosis for more than 2 weeks despite intensive investigation.

IMPORTANT CAUSES

1. Neoplasms
   a) Lymphoma, leukaemia, malignant histiocytosis
   b) Hepatic, renal, lung tumours
   c) Disseminated carcinoma
   d) Atrial myxoma
2. Infections
   a) Bacterial—tuberculosis, brucellosis, abscess formation (e.g. pelvic, abdominal), endocarditis, pericarditis, osteomyelitis, cholangitis, pyelonephritis
   b) Viral—hepatitis, HIV infection, Ross River virus
   c) Parasitic and fungal—malaria, Q fever, toxoplasmosis
3. Connective tissue diseases
   a) Rheumatoid arthritis, SLE
   b) Vasculitis—polyarteritis nodosa, temporal arteritis
4. Miscellaneous
   a) Drug fever—e.g. antibiotics (sulfonamides, penicillin, cephalosporins, isoniazid, ethambutol, nitrofurantoin), antiepileptics (phenytoin, bar-

biturates), antithyroids (iodides, thiouracil), antiarrhythmics, (quinidine, procainamide), antihypertensives (methyldopa)
b) Inflammatory bowel disease
c) Granulomatous disease—sarcoidosis, granulomatous hepatitis, lethal midline granuloma
d) Multiple pulmonary emboli
e) Familial Mediterranean fever
f) Factitious fever

N.B. extreme pyrexia (>41.1°C [106°F]) can occur with CNS or drug fevers, heat stroke, malignant hyperthermia or HIV infection.

Table 14.10 Sexually transmitted diseases

Disease state/ organism	Clinical manifestations	Diagnosis and treatment
Gonorrhoea	Urethritis	Gram stain and culture
	Cervicitis	
	Pharyngitis	Ceftriaxone
	Arthritis	Doxycycline
	Tenosynovitis	Erythromycin
	Proctitis	Ciprofloxacin
	Endocarditis	
	Meningitis	
Chlamydia trachomatis	Urethritis	Culture
	Cervicitis	
	Pelvic inflammatory disease	Doxycycline
Syphilis	1. Primary syphilis—chancre (clean, indurated ulcer)	Dark field examination Serology (see Table 14.11)
	2. Secondary syphilis—occurs 2–8 weeks later: rash, alopecia, condylomata lata	For early infection use penicillin, doxycycline or erythromycin
	3. Tertiary syphilis—neurosyphilis (tabes dorsalis, general paresis, meningovascular syphilis)	For late infection use same drugs for longer period
Pelvic inflammatory disease (*N. gonorrhoea*, *C. trachomatis*, *Mycoplasma hominis*, Gram-negative bacteria)	Endometritis Salpingitis Tubo-ovarian abscess Pelvic peritonitis	Culture Cefoxitin Clindamycin Gentamicin Doxycycline

SEROLOGICAL TESTS FOR SYPHILIS

- Syphilitic infection results in production of antilipid and specific anti-treponemal antibodies.
- Non-treponemal tests measure antibodies to lipid and are sensitive.
- Treponemal tests measure specific anti-treponemal antibody.

Table 14.11 *Serological tests for syphilis*

Non-treponemal tests (VDRL, RPR)	Treponemal tests (FTA-ABS, MHA-TP)	Interpretation
–	–	Does *not* exclude early (or rarely late) syphilis
–	+	Treated syphilis *or* treponemal disease; rarely secondary *or* late syphilis
+	–	Biological false positive: leprosy, TB, leptospirosis, hepatitis, varicella, infectious mononucleosis, connective tissue disease
+	Borderline FTA-ABS	Repeat test
+	Beaded FTA-ABS	Connective tissue disease
+	+	Syphilis or other treponemal disease

VDRL = Venereal Disease Research Laboratory test.
RPR = Rapid plasma reagin test.
FTA-ABS = Fluorescent treponemal antibody-absorbed test.
MHA-TP = *T. pallidum* haemagglutination assay.

TOXIC SHOCK SYNDROME *(Staphylococcus aureus* toxin*)*

CLINICAL FEATURES

- Usually associated with tampon use
- May occur with non-purulent wounds
- Fever
- Hypotension
- Diffuse macular erythroderma, followed by generalised desquamation
- Conjunctival injection
- Diarrhoea, vomiting
- Myalgia, rhabdomyolysis
- Abnormal liver function tests
- Thrombocytopenia
- Hypocalcaemia

DIFFERENTIAL DIAGNOSIS

- Toxic epidermal necrolysis
- Scarlet fever
- Kawasaki's syndrome
- Rocky Mountain spotted fever

SEPTIC SHOCK

CLINICAL FEATURES

- Impaired tissue perfusion
- Hypotension
- Multi-organ failure
- Blood cultures are positive in approximately 50% of cases
- Mortality rate is about 25%

CAUSES

- Gram-negative organisms in 70% (especially *E. coli, Klebsiella, Proteus, Pseudomonas*)
- Gram-positive cocci in 20–30% (especially *S. aureus* and *Strep. pneumoniae*)

TOXIC STREPTOCOCCAL SYNDROME

CLINICAL FEATURES

- Hypotension, plus 2 of the following:
1. Renal failure
2. Coagulopathy
3. Liver impairment
4. Adult respiratory distress syndrome
5. Rash
6. Soft tissue necrosis
7. Positive blood cultures in most cases
8. Mortality approximately 30%

CAUSE

- Infection with Group A streptococci, usually skin or soft tissue infection
- Caused by production of streptococcal pyrogenic exotoxin A

INFECTION RISK IN SOLID ORGAN TRANSPLANT RECIPIENTS

IN FIRST MONTH

1. Infection residing in allograft itself
2. Reactivation of latent infection—CMV, varicella-zoster, *Toxoplasma gondii*, Epstein-Barr virus, *Strongyloides stercoralis*
3. Wound, chest or catheter-related infection after operation

FROM 2 TO 6 MONTHS

- Life-threatening opportunistic infection (e.g. aspergillosis, *P. carinii*, *Listeria*, *Nocardia*, CMV, mycobacteria)

FROM 6 MONTHS ONWARD

As for general population, unless on increased doses of immunosuppression

THERAPEUTICS

Table 14.12 Antibiotics

Antibiotic	Antimicrobial activity	Major clinical indications
1. Benzylpenicillin	Streptococci, pneumococci, *Neisseria* spp., susceptible anaerobes, *Clostridium perfringens*, *Listeria*, *Borrelia*	Lobar pneumonia, endocarditis, meningitis, pharyngitis, syphilis, gonorrhoea, diphtheria, Lyme disease
2. Ampicillin	As 1., plus *E. coli*, *Proteus* spp., *Shigella*, *Salmonella*, some *H. influenzae*	Otitis media, lower respiratory tract infection, urinary tract infection
3. Amoxycillin/ clavulanic acid	As 2., plus *Klebsiella*, *Bacteroides fragilis*	Respiratory, urinary tract infection, soft tissue infection, surgical prophylaxis
4. Antipseudomonal penicillins (ticarcillin, piperacillin)	As 2., plus *P. aeruginosa*, *Bacteroides fragilis*	Febrile neutropenia, pseudomonal infection
5. Ticarcillin/ clavulanic acid	As 4., plus resistant streptococci, staphylococci, *B. fragilis*	As 4., plus anaerobic, mixed infections
6. Penicillinase-resistant penicillins (flucloxacillin, methicillin)	Staphylococci	Staphylococcal infection
7. Imipenem	Staphylococci, *Strep. faecalis*, *P. aeruginosa*, *Bacteroides*	Serious infections, nosocomial infection resistant to less costly agents

Infectious Diseases

Table 14.12 Continued

Antibiotic	Antimicrobial activity	Major clinical indications
8. First-generation cephalosporins (e.g. cephalexin, cefaclor)	Streptococci, *E. coli*, *Proteus* spp., *Shigella*, *Salmonella*, *Klebsiella*	Urinary tract, skin and soft tissue infection
9. Second-generation cephalosporins		
a) cefuroxime	*H. influenzae*, *Staph. aureus*, streptococci, gonococci	Meningitis
b) cefoxitin	*B. fragilis*, gonococci (less activity against Gram-positives)	Anaerobic infections
10. Third-generation cephalosporins (ceftriaxone, cefotaxime, ceftazidime)	Gram-negative organisms, *P. aeruginosa* (especially ceftazidime)	Serious sepsis, febrile neutropenia, meningitis
11. Fluoroquinalones (norfloxacin, ciprofloxacin)	Broad spectrum; ciprofloxacin has some activity against methicillin-resistant *Staph. aureus* (MRSA)	Urinary, respiratory tract infection, osteomyelitis
12. Aminoglycosides	Aerobic Gram-negative bacilli (in combination treatment)	Sepsis, febrile neutropenia, *P. aeruginosa* in combination treatment
13. Monobactams (aztreonam)	Enterobacteriaceae, *Pseudomonas*	As 12. above
14. Trimethoprim-sulfamethoxazole	Enterobacteriaceae, *Pneumocystis carinii*, *Brucella*, *Nocardia*	
15. Metronidazole	*B. fragilis*, *Clostridia*, *C. difficile*, *Entamoeba*, *Giardia*	Serious anaerobic infections, amoebic liver disease, giardiasis, trichomoniasis
16. Macrolides		
a) Erythromycin*	*S. pyogenes*, pneumococcus, *Neisseria*, *Mycoplasma*, *Legionella*, *Campylobacter*	Legionnaire's disease, *Mycoplasma* pneumonia
b) Roxithromycin	As for erythromycin	As for erythromycin
c) Clarithromycin	As for erythromycin, plus	Main use is with atypical

355

Table 14.12 *Continued*

Antibiotic	Antimicrobial activity	Major clinical indications
	M. avium-intracellulare, M. chelonei, B. burgdorferi, H. pylori	mycobacterial infection at this time, combination therapy for *H. pylori*
d) Azithromycin	As for clarithromycin	As for clarithromycin
17. Tetracycline*	*Actinomyces*, rickettsiae, chlamydiae, *Mycoplasma*, Lyme disease, brucellosis	Chlamydial infection, brucellosis, Whipple's disease, acne
18. Vancomycin	Staphylococcus, streptococcus, *C. difficile*	MRSA, pseudomembranous colitis, penicillin-allergic patients
19. Chloramphenicol	*S. pneumoniae, N. meningitides, H. influenzae, Salmonella*	Penicillin-allergic patients with serious infection
20. Clindamycin	Anaerobes, staphylococcus, streptococcus	Anaerobic infection

*Bacteriostatic.

Table 14.13 *Anti-fungal therapy*

Anti-fungal agent	Spectrum of activity	Clinical uses
Amphotericin-B	All fungal infections except *Pseudoallescheria boydii* and chromoblastomycosis	Serious or life-threatening fungal infections
Flucytosine	Cryptococci, *Candida*, chromoblastomycosis	Cryptococcal or *Candida* meningitis, *Candida* cystitis, chromoblastomycosis
Azoles		
a) Ketoconazole	*Histoplasma, Blastomycosis, Candida, P. boydii*	Non-life-threatening *Histoplasmosis, Blastomycosis*, chronic mucocutaneous candidiasis, paracoccidioidomycosis
b) Fluconazole	Cryptococci, *Candida, Histoplasma, Blastomycosis*, paracoccidioidomycosis	Candidal infection, cryptococcal meningitis
c) Itraconazole	As for fluconazole, but with enhanced activity against *Aspergillus, Sporothrix schenckii, Histoplasma* and *Blastomycosis*	*Histoplasmosis, Blastomycosis*, coccidioidomycosis, sporotrichosis

Table 14.14 *Antiviral therapy (excluding antiretroviral drugs)*

Antiviral drug	Spectrum of activity	Clinical uses
Aciclovir	Herpes simplex types I and II Varicella-zoster virus Epstein-Barr virus	Primary and recurrent herpes simplex, either genital, perianal, oral, or encephalitis Shingles Disseminated zoster
Ganciclovir	CMV	Herpes zoster ophthalmicus CMV infection in immunosuppressed hosts
Famciclovir	Herpes simplex Varicella-zoster	As for aciclovir
Foscarnet	All human herpes viruses Hepatitis B	As for ganciclovir

15

Medical Dermatology

PRURITUS

Any generalised persistent pruritus with scratch marks that is unrelieved by emollients and wakens the patient from sleep needs evaluation to exclude systemic disease.

SYSTEMIC CAUSES

1. Cholestasis, e.g. primary biliary cirrhosis
2. Chronic renal failure
3. Pregnancy
4. Lymphoma, myeloma
5. Polycythaemia rubra vera, mycosis fungoides
6. Carcinoma, e.g. breast, stomach, lung
7. Endocrine disease, e.g. diabetes mellitus, hypothyroidism and hyperthyroidism, carcinoid
8. Iron deficiency

PIGMENTATION

CAUSES

1. Liver disease, e.g. haemochromatosis, Wilson's disease, primary biliary cirrhosis, porphyria
2. Malignancy (related to cachexia or ectopic ACTH production)
3. Endocrine disease, e.g. Addison's disease, the oral contraceptive pill or pregnancy, Cushing's syndrome, acromegaly, phaeochromocytoma, hyperthyroidism
4. Chronic renal failure
5. Connective tissue disease, e.g. SLE, scleroderma, dermatomyositis
6. Drugs, e.g. neuroleptics, chloroquine, busulfan, gold, lead
7. Radiation
8. Malabsorption
9. Chronic infection, e.g. infective endocarditis

PHOTOSENSITIVITY

CAUSES

1. Drugs, e.g. neuroleptics, antibiotics (sulfonamides, tetracycline), sulfonylureas
2. Porphyria cutanea tarda
3. SLE
4. Pellagra

RASH ON THE PALMS AND SOLES: DIFFERENTIAL DIAGNOSIS

1. Syphilis
2. Acute infections, e.g. infectious mononucleosis (non-specific macular erythema), gonococcaemia (purpuric tender pustules), toxic shock syndrome (page 352), hand, foot and mouth disease (linear or oval vesicles)
3. Erythema multiforme
4. Reiter's syndrome (erythematous pustular eruptions)
5. Pustular psoriasis
6. Drug reaction, or mercury or arsenic poisoning

RED MAN SYNDROME (ERYTHRODERMA OR EXFOLIATIVE DERMATITIS)

CAUSES

1. Malignancy
   a) Mycosis fungoides (infiltration of the skin by T cells)
   b) Lymphoma, leukaemia
   c) Carcinoma (rare)
2. Drugs, e.g. phenytoin, allopurinol
3. Generalisation of a pre-existing dermatitis, e.g. psoriasis, atopic dermatitis

Patients present with oedema (hypoalbuminaemia from skin loss), loss of muscle mass and extrarenal water loss: 60% recover in 8 months.

ALLERGIC SKIN DISEASE

ATOPIC DERMATITIS

CLINICAL FEATURES

1. Dry skin
2. Pruritic scaling of the flexures
3. May affect any part of the body, or become generalised or secondarily infected
4. Occurs in atopic individuals

TREATMENT

TREATMENT

1. Moisturisers
2. Topical steroids
3. Antihistamines to control itch
4. Identification and modification of exacerbating factors, e.g. diet, allergens

ALLERGIC CONTACT DERMATITIS

COMMON CAUSES

1. Nickel sulphate (jewellery)
2. Potassium dichromate (cement, leathers, paint)
3. Paraphenylenediamine (hair dyes, cosmetics)
4. Para-aminobenzoic acid (sunscreen)
5. Formaldehyde (cosmetics, shampoos)

IMMUNOLOGICAL SKIN DISEASE

PSORIASIS

CLINICAL FEATURES

1. Psoriasis is common, affecting up to 3% of the population
2. The rash has a predilection for the elbows, buttocks, knees and scalp
3. Usual rash is plaque-like with a silvery scale and an erythematous base
4. Erythrodermic psoriasis, generalised pustular psoriasis and psoriasis associated with arthropathy can be classified as severe forms of the disease
5. Nail abnormalities are very common, especially onycholysis and pitting
6. Guttate psoriasis is an acute form of disease with small psoriatic lesions, often following streptococcal sore throat
7. Steroids, gold and antimalarial drugs can exacerbate psoriasis

TREATMENT

1. Topical corticosteroids
2. Topical tar preparations
3. Topical synthetic vitamin D analogue (calcipotriol)
4. Ultraviolet-B (UVB)
5. Psoralen with ultraviolet-A (PUVA)
6. Etretinate is a derivative of vitamin A that is used in the treatment of psoriasis and psoriatic arthropathy. Adverse effects include teratogenicity (the drug has a half-life of up to 160 days), hepatitis, hypertriglyceridaemia, cheilitis, xerosis, alopecia and bony hyperostosis
7. Methotrexate for treatment of severe skin disease and psoriatic arthropathy

ERYTHEMA NODOSUM

<small>CLINICAL FEATURES</small>

• Presents with tender, red palpable lesions on the pretibial area

<small>CAUSES</small>

1. Sarcoidosis
2. Steptococcal infections (beta-haemolytic)
3. Inflammatory bowel disease
4. Drugs, e.g. sulfonamides, penicillin, bromides, iodides, sulfonylureas, oestrogen
5. Tuberculosis
6. Other infections (less common), e.g. lepromatous leprosy, histoplasmosis, blastomycosis, coccidioidomycosis, toxoplasmosis, *Yersinia, Chlamydia,* lymphogranuloma venereum
7. SLE
8. Behçet's syndrome
9. Anti-phospholipid syndrome

ERYTHEMA MULTIFORME

<small>CLINICAL FEATURES</small>

1. Presents with multiple target (bulls-eye) lesions, bullae on an urticarial base, and mouth ulcers
2. Stevens-Johnson syndrome is a severe form with widespread blistering and mouth ulcers

<small>CAUSES</small>

1. Idiopathic
2. Drugs, e.g. sulfonamides, phenytoin
3. Infection, e.g. herpes simplex virus, enterovirus, *Mycoplasma pneumoniae,* histoplasmosis, *Yersinia enterocolitica*
4. Malignancy
5. Sarcoidosis

<small>PATHOLOGY</small>

• Subepidermal vesicles

<small>TREATMENT</small>

1. Disease is usually self-limiting
2. Corticosteroids are unproven but may be helpful in some cases

361

BULLOUS LESIONS

PEMPHIGUS VULGARIS

CLINICAL FEATURES
1. Usually presents in the fifth to seventh decade
2. Oral ulcers, and blisters on the limbs and trunk (especially at sites of trauma or pressure) that are painful and easily broken
3. Nikolski's sign is positive (affected superficial skin can be moved over the deeper layer)

PATHOLOGY
1. Skin biopsy reveals acantholysis (rounded keratinocytes resulting from detachment of intercellular adhesion) and intraepithelial vesicles
2. Immunofluorescence shows IgG (intercellular substance antibody) and C3 deposits in the interepithelial spaces
3. Titre of IgG anti-intercellular substance is useful to monitor disease activity

TREATMENT
• Requires aggressive immunosuppression

BULLOUS PEMPHIGOID

CLINICAL FEATURES
1. Presents predominantly in the elderly
2. Large, tense, not easily broken bullae on an erythematous base
3. Predilection for flexures
4. Oral ulcers rare
5. Infrequently associated with malignancy

PATHOLOGY
1. Skin biopsy—subepidermal vesicles with IgG or IgM and complement in a linear pattern along the basement membrane zone
2. Immunofluorescence reveals IgG anti-basement-membrane zone antibodies in 70%
3. Circulating anti-basement-membrane zone antibodies do not correlate with disease activity

TREATMENT
• Immunosuppression

DERMATITIS HERPETIFORMIS

CLINICAL FEATURES
1. Presents with pruritic vesicles on knees, elbows, buttocks (no mouth lesions)

2. Usually 3rd or 4th decade
3. Coeliac disease (often asymptomatic) is almost always present
4. HLA-B8 and DR3 associated in 90%

PATHOLOGY

1. Skin biopsy shows subepidermal vesicles beneath which are found neutrophils in dermal papillae
2. Immunofluorescence reveals IgA in a granular pattern and complement in the dermal papillae and along the basement membrane zone of involved and uninvolved skin
3. Serum IgA anti-reticulin and anti-endomysial antibodies are present in the majority of cases

TREATMENT

• Dapsone (skin disease) and a gluten-free diet (coeliac disease)

SKIN DISEASE ASSOCIATED WITH UNDERLYING SYSTEMIC DISEASE

ACANTHOSIS NIGRICANS

CLINICAL FEATURES

• Is characterised by hyperpigmentation of the intertriginous areas

CAUSES

1. Malignancy: adenocarcinoma, lymphoma
2. Endocrine disease, e.g. acromegaly, Cushing's syndrome, hypothyroidism, diabetes mellitus and insulin resistance states, lipodystrophies (especially leprechaunism), Stein-Leventhal syndrome
3. Obesity
4. Congenital

PYODERMA GANGRENOSUM

This is an ulcerating disease of the skin and soft tissue, often affecting the lower legs.

CAUSES

1. Inflammatory bowel disease
2. Rheumatoid arthritis
3. Paraproteinaemia, e.g. IgA myeloma
4. Myeloproliferative disorders

LUPUS AND THE SKIN

CLINICAL FEATURES

There are 3 types: systemic lupus erythematosus (SLE)
 discoid lupus (DLE), and
 subacute cutaneous lupus erythematosus (SCLE)

- DLE causes erythematous papules and plaques with follicular hyperkeratosis and scaling. It most commonly affects face, scalp and ears.
- SCLE causes 2 types of lesions: psoriatic-like plaques (like DLE, but they do not atrophy or scar and involve the trunk), and a violaceous annular rash with fine scales in sun-exposed areas.

DIAGNOSIS

- In SCLE, antinuclear antibody (ANA) is positive in 60%, dsDNA antibody is positive in 30%, and SS-A/SS-B antibodies are positive in 60% of patients.
- In DLE, ANA and dsDNA antibodies are positive in only 5%, while SS-A/SS-B antibodies are absent.

Table 15.1 Diagnostic features in lupus

Disease	Positive immunofluorescence (lupus band test)	
	Involved skin	Uninvolved (normal appearing) skin
SLE	95%	50%
DLE	95%	0%
SCLE	50%	30%

THE PHAKOMATOSES

NEUROFIBROMATOSIS

TYPE I (VON RECKLINGHAUSEN'S DISEASE: CHROMOSOME 17)

1. Neurofibromas of peripheral nerves
2. More than six 1.5 cm café-au-lait spots
3. Hamartomas of the iris (Lisch nodules)
4. Axillary freckling (Crowe's sign)
5. Pseudo-arthrosis of the tibia
6. Predisposed to nervous system neoplasms including plexiform neurofibromas, optic gliomas, phaeochromocytomas, ependymomas, meningiomas, astrocytomas, and change to sarcoma

TYPE II (CHROMOSOME 22q)

1. Bilateral acoustic Schwannomas
2. Predisposed to meningiomas, gliomas, Schwannomas of peripheral and cranial nerves

Most common presentation is unilateral deafness. If detected early, surgery can preserve the auditory nerve.

TUBEROUS SCLEROSIS

CLINICAL FEATURES

1. Autosomal dominant, or sporadic
2. Triad of convulsions, mental retardation (with calcification in the temporal lobes) and adenoma sebaceum (fibromas on the cheeks and forehead)
3. Other features may include the shagreen patch (thick yellow skin on the lower back), cardiac rhabdomyoma, renal angioleiomyoma and pulmonary fibrosis

VON HIPPEL-LANDAU DISEASE (autosomal dominant)

CLINICAL FEATURES

1. Haemangioblastomas of the retina, cerebellum and spinal cord
2. Cysts in the kidney, epididymis, pancreas
3. Haemangiomas elsewhere (e.g. liver, pancreas, kidney)
4. Phaeochromocytoma
5. Renal and pancreatic cancer

STURGE-WEBER SYNDROME (congenital, non-hereditary disorder)

CLINICAL FEATURES

1. Capillary or cavernous haemangiomas (port wine stains) in the V cranial nerve distribution, upper or middle branch, with an intracranial venous haemangioma of the leptomeninges
2. Associated with seizures and mental retardation

ATAXIA-TELANGIECTASIA

CLINICAL FEATURES

- Triad of cerebellar ataxia, oculocutaneous telangiectasia on the bulbar conjunctiva and skin, and immunodeficiency (decreased IgA and IgE, and thymic atrophy)

CUTANEOUS MALIGNANCY

MELANOMA

RISK FACTORS

1. Commoner in fair-skinned people
2. Associated with blistering sunburn in early life

3. The dysplastic naevus syndrome comprises tan-coloured irregular lesions typically <6 mm in diameter on sun-exposed and unexposed skin—the incidence of malignant transformation may be up to 1% per year. Inheritance is autosomal dominant.
4. Family history of melanoma or other skin cancers
5. Large numbers of benign pigmented naevi
6. Immunosuppression, including HIV infection

DIAGNOSIS

1. Early diagnosis improves survival
2. Tumour depth of invasion is most important prognostic feature

TREATMENT

1. Melanoma is curable in 95% of people when it is contained within the epidermis or upper dermis
2. Surgery is the only proven treatment modality

CUTANEOUS T-CELL LYMPHOMA

1. MYCOSIS FUNGOIDES

Clinical features
1. Initially, discrete plaques or nodules on the skin
2. May progress to coalescent lesions
3. Lymph nodes and viscera may become involved in time

Diagnosis
- Biopsy reveals T lymphocytes which are monoclonal expressing CD3 and CD4 in the epidermis and dermis (Sézary cells)

Treatment
1. Topical chemotherapy with nitrogen mustard
2. Radiotherapy
3. Psoralen with ultraviolet-A (PUVA)
4. Systemic chemotherapy

2. SÉZARY SYNDROME

Clinical features
1. Generalised erythroderma
2. Keratoderma of palms and soles
3. Pruritus
4. Sézary cell count of >1000/mm^3 in the peripheral blood

Diagnosis
- Biopsy reveals T lymphocytes which are monoclonal expressing CD3 and CD4 in the epidermis and dermis (Sézary cells)

Treatment
1. Topical chemotherapy with nitrogen mustard
2. Radiotherapy

3. Psoralen with ultraviolet-A
4. Systemic chemotherapy

SKIN DISEASE ASSOCIATED WITH UNDERLYING MALIGNANCY

MALIGNANCIES WHICH METASTASISE TO THE SKIN

1. Carcinomas of:
   a) Breast
   b) Gastrointestinal tract
   c) Lung
   d) Kidney
   e) Ovary
2. Melanoma
3. Leukaemias (especially acute myeloid)

CAUSES OF EXCESSIVE SWEATING (HYPERHYDROSIS)

1. Thyrotoxicosis
2. Phaeochromocytoma
3. Acromegaly
4. Hypoglycaemia
5. Autonomic dysfunction, e.g. Riley-Day syndrome
6. Physiological, e.g. emotional stress, fever, menopause

CAUSES OF SADDLE NOSE DEFORMITY AND ULCERATION

1. Wegener's granulomatosis
2. Midline granuloma (non-caseating granuloma without vasculitis)
3. Tumour—carcinoma, lymphoma
4. Infection, e.g. tuberculosis, leprosy, syphilis, histoplasmosis
5. Cocaine sniffing

Table 15.2 *Cutaneous clues to underlying malignancy*

Skin change	Possible underlying malignancy
Extramammary Paget's disease	Genitourinary or gastrointestinal
Acanthosis nigricans	Gastrointestinal, especially stomach
Pyoderma gangrenosum	Leukaemia
Necrolytic migratory erythema	Glucagonoma
Torre's syndrome (multiple sebaceous tumours of the skin)	Carcinoma of the colon, breast
Cowden's syndrome (trichilemmomas, verrucous papules, oral fibromas)	Carcinoma of breast, thyroid

Table 15.2 Continued

Skin change	Possible underlying malignancy
Gardener's syndrome (soft tissue tumours, sebaceous cysts)	Carcinoma of the colon
Acquired ichthyosis	Hodgkin's disease
Hirsutism	Adrenal or ovarian tumour
Hypertrichosis	Carcinoid; carcinoma of breast, gastrointestinal, lymphoma
Erythema gyratum repens (concentric erythematous bands)	Carcinoma of breast
Sweet's syndrome (acute febrile neutrophilic dermatosis)	Leukaemia
Dermatomyositis	Especially gastrointestinal
Multiple mucosal neuromas	Medullary carcinoma of the thyroid
Cutaneous amyloidosis	Myeloma
Tylosis (palmar-plantar keratoderma)	Carcinoma of the oesophagus
Pemphigus	Thymoma
Paraneoplastic pemphigus (associated with erythema multiforme)	Lymphoma, leukaemia
Epidermolysis bullosa acquisita	Myeloma

16

Psychiatry

DISEASE STATES

MOOD DISORDERS

1. Adjustment disorder with depressed mood
2. Dysthymia
3. Major depression
4. Cyclothymia
5. Mania and bipolar disorder

ADJUSTMENT DISORDER WITH DEPRESSED MOOD

CLINICAL FEATURES

1. Depressed mood occurs in response to psychosocial stressors
2. The mood disturbance may seem disproportionate to the apparent severity of the psychosocial stressors

TREATMENT

1. Supportive counselling
2. Antidepressant drugs on occasions

DYSTHYMIA (CHRONIC DEPRESSION)

CLINICAL FEATURES

1. A depressed mood is present most of the time during a 2-year period
2. Mild vegetative symptoms such as disturbance of sleep and appetite may be present
3. Patients will often have difficulties with low self-esteem and interpersonal relationships

TREATMENT

1. Supportive therapy
2. Cognitive therapy
3. Problem solving therapy
4. Antidepressants

MAJOR DEPRESSION

CLINICAL FEATURES

1. Depressed mood
2. Significant weight gain or loss
3. Diminished interest in almost all activities
4. Change in appetite
5. Insomnia or hypersomnia
6. Psychomotor agitation or retardation
7. Loss of energy
8. Feelings of worthlessness or guilt
9. Poor concentration
10. Suicidal ideation or attempts
11. Delusions or hallucinations (known as major depression with psychotic features)

Melancholic sub-type is characterised by diurnal mood variation (feels worse in the morning), psychomotor changes (retardation, agitation), early morning wakening (2 or more hours before usual time of wakening) and an inability to enjoy activities that are usually pleasurable.

TREATMENT

1. Cognitive-behavioural therapy
2. Interpersonal therapy
3. Antidepressants combined with psychosocial counselling
4. Electroconvulsive therapy:
   a) delusional depression (psychotic features)
   b) melancholia
   c) severe treatment-resistant depression
5. Circadian rhythm manipulation: sleep deprivation or phototherapy, used mainly in the context of seasonal affective disorder

CYCLOTHYMIA

CLINICAL FEATURES

Multiple episodes of hypomania or depression occur which are mild enough not to interfere with occupational or social functioning.

TREATMENT

1. Psychotherapy
2. Lithium may be of benefit in some instances

MANIA AND BIPOLAR DISORDER

CLINICAL FEATURES

Mood is euphoric during manic episodes, and often associated with

a) Inflated self-esteem
b) Impulsive behaviour

c) Insomnia
d) Pressured speech
e) Flight of ideas
f) Easy distractibility
g) Psychomotor agitation
h) Sexual indiscretions

TREATMENT

1. Lithium carbonate
2. Carbamazepine
3. Sodium valproate
4. Antipsychotic agents, e.g. haloperidol, during the acute phase

PSYCHOTIC DISORDERS

SCHIZOPHRENIA

DIAGNOSTIC CRITERIA

A. Inclusion criteria
1. Disorder of thought form and content, including delusions and hallucinations
2. Disturbance in behaviour
3. Marked decline in everyday functioning
4. Disturbance in volition
5. Problem persistent for at least 6 months

B. Exclusion criteria
1. No concomitant mood disorder
2. No obvious organic cause, e.g. drug use

SUB-TYPES OF SCHIZOPHRENIA

1. Catatonic
2. Disorganised
3. Paranoid
4. Undifferentiated
5. Residual

GENETICS

1. General population—risk approximately 1-2%
2. Monozygotic twins—approximately 78% concordance rate
3. Dizygotic twins—approximately 18% concordance rate
4. One parent schizophrenic—offspring risk approximately 10%
5. Both parents schizophrenic—offspring risk approximately 50%
6. Second-degree relative schizophrenic—patient risk approximately 2%

TREATMENT

• Involves the use of antipsychotic medication and psychosocial treatment

DRUGS WHICH MAY PRODUCE PSYCHOTIC SYMPTOMS

1. Amphetamines
2. Phencyclidine
3. Anticholinergics
4. Glucocorticoids
5. Heavy metals
6. Marijuana (may exacerbate symptoms)

ANXIETY DISORDERS

1. Adjustment disorder with anxious mood
2. Panic disorder
3. Post-traumatic stress disorder
4. Generalised anxiety disorder
5. Obsessive-compulsive disorder

ADJUSTMENT DISORDER WITH ANXIOUS MOOD

CLINICAL FEATURES

Is an excessive response to a psychosocial stress with anxiety symptoms that interfere with the ability to function normally.

TREATMENT

1. Supportive counselling
2. Short course of anxiolytic agents (<2 weeks)

PANIC DISORDER

CLINICAL FEATURES

1. Recurrent, discrete episodes of extreme anxiety
2. Symptoms include dyspnoea, dizziness, sweating, palpitations, tremulousness, chest or abdominal pain
3. Often associated with agoraphobia
4. More common in females
5. Depressive features may also be present

DIFFERENTIAL DIAGNOSIS

1. Hyperthyroidism
2. Phaeochromocytoma
3. Hypoglycaemia
4. Alcohol withdrawal

TREATMENT

1. Cognitive-behavioural therapy
2. Short-term use of anxiolytic medication
3. Selective serotonin reuptake inhibitors or tricyclic antidepressants

POST-TRAUMATIC STRESS DISORDER

CLINICAL FEATURES

1. Follows an extremely traumatic event outside the range of normal human experience
2. May be short-lived or cause chronic symptomatology
3. Symptoms include nightmares, flashbacks, avoidance of reminders of the event

TREATMENT

1. Behavioural therapy
2. Psychotherapy
3. Antidepressants, particularly the selective serotonin reuptake inhibitors

GENERALISED ANXIETY DISORDER

CLINICAL FEATURES

1. Chronic excessive anxiety and worry about trivial issues
2. Chronic apprehension about life circumstances
3. Recurrent somatic symptoms, e.g. restlessness, autonomic hyperactivity

TREATMENT

1. Behavioural therapy
2. Psychotherapy
3. Selective serotonin reuptake inhibitors or tricyclic antidepressants

OBSESSIVE-COMPULSIVE DISORDER

CLINICAL FEATURES

1. Compulsions are repetitive, intentional behaviours that are irrational and resisted
2. Obsessions are distressing, unwanted thoughts, ideas or impulses that are irrational and resisted
3. Anxiety symptoms are prominent
4. Sex distribution is equal

TREATMENT

1. Behavioural therapy
2. Antidepressants with serotoninergic effects, e.g. fluoxetine, sertraline, clomipramine and tricyclic antidepressants
3. Surgery for severe resistant disease

SOMATOFORM DISORDERS

1. Somatisation disorder
2. Conversion disorder
3. Hypochondriasis
4. Chronic pain disorder
5. Body dysmorphic disorder

SOMATISATION DISORDER

CLINICAL FEATURES

1. Recurrent multiple somatic complaints in absence of evidence of underlying physical disease
2. Female preponderance

TREATMENT

- Supportive

CONVERSION DISORDER

CLINICAL FEATURES

1. Loss of an aspect of physical functioning in the absence of any physiological disturbance
2. Differs from malingering in that it is unintentional

TREATMENT

- Focuses on management of the symptom

EATING DISORDERS

ANOREXIA NERVOSA

CLINICAL FEATURES

1. Female preponderance
2. Weight loss of 15% or more of body weight
3. Body mass index of <16
4. Preoccupation with weight and desire to be thinner (disturbed body image)

ADVERSE CONSEQUENCES

1. Protein-calorie malnutrition
2. Bradycardia, cardiac muscle wasting, ventricular arrhythmias, sudden death
3. Constipation
4. Abdominal pain
5. Endocrine disturbances including amenorrhoea and lanugo hair
6. Osteoporosis
7. Death

BULIMIA

CLINICAL FEATURES

1. Eating binges are followed by purging
2. Concomitant depression and anxiety are common

ADVERSE CONSEQUENCES

1. Fluid and electrolyte abnormalities
2. Upper gastrointestinal bleeding (Mallory Weiss tears)
3. Tooth decay
4. Parotid and salivary gland hypertrophy
5. Hyperamylasaemia

Table 16.1 Drugs used in the treatment of psychiatric disease

Class of drug	Examples	Indications	Side effects
Benzodiazepines	Clonazepam Diazepam Oxazepam Lorazepam Alprazolam	Anxiety disorders (for short-term use) Anticipatory anxiety of panic disorder Epilepsy	Sedation Tolerance Dependence Withdrawal syndrome—muscle aches, agitation, insomnia Potentiate effects of alcohol
Tricyclic antidepressants*	Amitriptyline Imipramine Dothiepin Clomipramine Nortriptyline Desipramine Doxepin Trimipramine	Major depression Obsessive-compulsive disorder Panic disorder (in some instances) Neuropathic pain	Anticholinergic—dry mouth, blurred vision, urinary retention, constipation Gastrointestinal—nausea, vomiting, reversible cholestasis Cardiovascular—postural hypotension, tachycardias, arrhythmias (increased QRS complex an early sign) CNS—sedation, lower seizure threshold, tremor, ataxia Leucopenia
Reversible inhibitors of monoamine oxidase	Moclobemide Phenelzine Tranylcypromine	Severe depression Phobias	Postural hypotension, dry mouth, blurred vision, constipation CNS stimulation—restlessness, insomnia

375

Table 16.1 Continued

Class of drug	Examples	Indications	Side effects
			Interaction with tyramine-containing food causing acute hypertensive crisis
Lithium carbonate**		Acute mania and hypomania Prevention of recurrent mania	Gastrointestinal—nausea, vomiting, diarrhoea Renal—nephrogenic diabetes insipidus, interstitial fibrosis Thyroid—goitre, hypothyroidism Cardiovascular—sinus node dysfunction CNS—ataxia, seizures, coma, tremor
Selective serotonin reuptake inhibitors	Fluoxetine Sertraline Paroxetine Fluvoxamine Citalopram	Depression Anxiety disorders	Nausea, anorexia, insomnia Dangerous interaction with MAO inhibitors, causing tremor, hyperthermia and hypotension
Neuroleptic drugs Phenothiazines	Chlorpromazine Fluphenazine Thioridazine Trifluoperazine	Schizophrenia Other psychotic disorders Huntington's disease Tourette's syndrome	Anticholinergic side effects—dry mouth, blurred vision, urinary retention; Hyperprolactinaemia; Obstructive jaundice; Acute dystonia;[†] Tardive dyskinesia;[‡] Neuroleptic malignant syndrome;[§] Hypotension; Impotence; Retinal pigmentation, lenticular opacities; Pigmentation, photosensitivity Sedation; weight gain

Table 16.1 *Continued*

Class of drug	Examples	Indications	Side effects
Butyrophenones	Haloperidol	As for phenothiazines	As for phenothiazines
Atypical neuroleptics	Clozapine Risperidone Olanzapine	Schizophrenia	Fewer anticholinergic side effects than phenothiazines; High incidence of agranulocytosis (clozapine only)

CNS = central nervous system.

*Tricyclics: Plasma levels correlate poorly with clinical response, which can take up to 4 weeks. Contraindications include glaucoma, prostatic hypertrophy and cardiac arrhythmias. The most sedating are amitriptyline, dothiepin, doxepin and trimipramine; the least sedating are nortriptyline and desipramine.

**Lithium: $t^1/_2$ is 24 hours—monitor serum samples (take sample 10 hours after the last dose): takes 7–19 days to achieve a full therapeutic effect.

Contraindicated in renal disease (as lithium is renally excreted): diuretics can *increase* toxicity.

†Dystonia: Usually in first week of therapy and characterised by limb extension, neck stiffness and jaw opening; responds to anti-parkinsonian drugs e.g. benztropine.

‡Tardive dyskinesia: Delayed reaction following chronic use, characterised by involuntary repetitive movements of the lips, tongue and other extremities, and more common in those >60 years or with pre-existing brain pathology; irreversible in 50% on stopping the drug.

§Neuroleptic malignant syndrome: Rare, characterised by hyperthermia, muscle rigidity, altered consciousness and autonomic dysfunction, typically in young adult males. Lasts 5–10 days after stopping potent neuroleptics.

Index

Index

Index